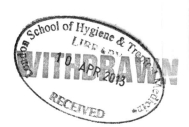

D1326640

# International perspectives on mental health

Edited by Hamid Ghodse

RCPsych Publications

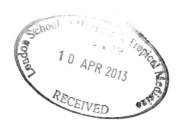

RCPsych Publications is an imprint of the Royal College of Psychiatrists,
17 Belgrave Square, London SW1X 8PG
http://www.rcpsych.ac.uk

British Library Cataloguing-in-Publication Data.
A catalogue record for this book is available from the British Library.
ISBN 978-1-908020-00-0

Distributed in North America by Publishers Storage and Shipping Company.

Printed in the UK by Bell & Bain Limited, Glasgow.

# Contents

# Contributors

**Samir Al-Adawi**  Lecturer, Department of Behavioural Medicine, College of Medicine and Health Sciences, Sultan Qaboos University, Muscat, Oman, email adawi@squ.edu.om

**Tsuyoshi Akiyama**  Director of the Department of Psychiatry, Kanto Medical Center, Clinical Professor of Psychiatry, Tokyo University, Japan, email akiyama@sa2.so-net.ne.jp; and member of the International Committee, Japanese Society of Psychiatry and Neurology

**Atalay Alem**  Assistant Professor of Psychiatry, Addis Ababa University, Ethiopia, email atalayalem@yahoo.com

**Akleema Ali**  PhD Student, Faculty of Social Sciences, Department of Behavioural Sciences, University of the West Indies, St Augustine, Trinidad, West Indies

**Mazen Alkhalil** MD  General Adult Psychiatrist, Al-Basheer Hospital, Harasta, Damascus, Syria, email mazenalkhalil@yahoo.com

**Dimitris Anagnostopoulos** MD  Assistant Professor of Child and Adolescent Psychiatry, First Psychiatric Department of Athens University, Athens, Greece

**Daniel Okitundu Luwa E. Andjafono**  Psychiatry Department, School of Medicine, University of Kinshasa, Democratic Republic of Congo

**F. Antun** MD PhD FRCP FRCPsych DPM  Professor of Psychiatry, Adviser and WHO National Focal Point for Mental Health, Ministry of Health, Beirut, Lebanon, email antun@cyberia.net.lb

**J. B. Asare** MD FRCPsych FWACP FGCP&S  Retired Chief Psychiatrist, Ghana, email jbasarek@yahoo.co.uk

**Iyas Assalman** MD  FTSTA3 in Psychiatry, West Midlands Deanery, UK, email iyasassalman@hotmail.com

**Sherif Atallah**  Consultant Psychiatrist and Medical Director, Behman Hospital, Cairo, Egypt

**Esmina Avdibegovic**  Department of Psychiatry, University of Tuzla, Bosnia and Herzegovina

**Sayed Azimi**  Mental Health Adviser, World Health Organization, Kabul, Afghanistan

**Charles Baddoura**  Professor of Psychiatry, Saint Joseph University, Beirut, Hospital of the Cross, Lebanon

**Benjamin J. Baig**  Clinical Lecturer in Psychiatry, Division of Psychiatry, University of Edinburgh, Royal Edinburgh Hospital, Edinburgh EH10 5HF, UK,email bbaig@staffmail.ed.ac.uk

**Vicky Banks** MB BS MRCGP FRCPsych  Consultant in Older Persons' Mental Health and Deputy Medical Director, Hampshire Partnership Foundation Trust, and Associate Dean, Royal College of Psychiatrists, email Vicky.Banks@hantspt-sw.nhs.uk

**Mariano Bassi**  Direttore Dipartimento Salute Mentale, Azienda USL Città di Bologna, Italy; Vice President of the Italian Society of Psychiatry (Società Italiana di Psichiatria – SIP)

**Julian Beezhold**  Consultant Psychiatrist, Norfolk and Waveney Mental Health Foundation Trust, UK

**Edgard Belfort**  Professor of Psychiatry, Venezuela Central University; Chairman, Child and Adolescent Psychiatric Service, Caracas Psychiatric Hospital; Administrative Secretary, Latin American Psychiatric Association (APAL), Av. Libertador. Edif. Majestic No. 148, Caracas 1050, Venezuela, email secretariaapal@cantv.net, belfort.ed@excite.com; Zonal Representative (Northern South America), World Psychiatric Association

**Shoshana Berenzon**  Researcher, National Institute of Psychiatry 'Ramon de la Fuente Muñíz', Mexico City, Mexico

**Carol A. Bernstein** MD  President, American Psychiatric Association, Associate Professor of Psychiatry, New York University School of Medicine, USA, email carol.bernstein@nyumc.org

**Alexey Bobrov**  Deputy Director for Education, Moscow Research Institute of Psychiatry, Moscow, Russia

**Jacek Bomba**  Chair of Psychiatry, Jagiellonian University Collegium Medicum, Kopernika 21 A, 31 501 Kraków, Poland, email jacek.bomba@uj.edu.pl

**Michel Botbol** MD  Psychiatrist, World Psychiatric Association Zonal Representative for Western Europe (Zone 6); Chair of the Therapeutic Section of the Child and Adolescent College of the French Federation of Psychiatry, 116 Rue du Moulin des Pres, 75013 Paris, France, email mbotbol@wanadoo.fr

**Pauv Bunthoeun**  Deputy Director of the National Programme for Mental Health, Ministry of Health, Cambodia

**S. Byambasuren** MD PhD  Policy and Coordination Department, Ministry of Health, Government Building 8, Olympic Street 2, Ulaanbaatar, Mongolia, email tsetsegdary@yahoo.co.uk

**Elisaldo A. Carlini**  Professor Titular do Departamento de Psicobiologia da Universidade Federal de São Paulo – UNIFESP, São Paulo, Brazil

**Ismet Ceric**  Department of Psychiatry, Clinical Hospital Centre Sarajevo, Medical Faculty, University of Sarajevo, 71000 Sarajevo, Bosnia and Herzegovina

**Eric F. C. Cheung** Consultant Psychiatrist, Castle Peak Hospital, Hong Kong Special Administrative Region, China

**Dixon Chibanda** MMed Psychiatry MPH Consultant Psychiatrist, Harare Hospital, Zimbabwe

**Siow-Ann Chong** Senior Consultant Psychiatrist, Vice Chairman, Medical Board (Research) of the Institute of Mental Health, Buangkok Green Medical Park, 10 Buangkok View, Singapore 539747, email siow_ann_chong@imh.com.sg

**Chantharavady Choulamany** Psychiatrist, Mental Health Unit, Mahosot Hospital, Vientiane, Lao PDR, email chantharavady_c@hotmail.com

**George Christodoulou** MD FRCPsych Emeritus Professor of Psychiatry, Honorary President, Hellenic Psychiatric Association, Greece, email gchristodoulou@ath.forthnet.gr

**Nikos Christodoulou** MBBS MSc MRCPsych University College London Hospital, London, UK

**Deborah C. Cohen** MBA Senior Writer, American Psychiatric Association, USA

**Bulent Coskun** Professor of Psychiatry, Kocaeli University Medical School; Director of Community Mental Health, Research and Training Centre, Kocaeli University, Kocaeli, Turkey, email bcoskun@isbank.net.tr

**Ken Courtenay** Consultant Psychiatrist, Barnet, Enfield and Haringey Mental Health NHS Trust, Unit 5, St George's Estate, London N22 5QL, UK, email Ken.Courtenay@beh-mht.nhs.uk

**Marcelo E. Cruz** MD Global Network for Research in Mental and Neurological Health, USA; Panandean Corporation for Research and Development, Ecuador, and Ecuadorean Academy of Neurosciences

**Martin Curtice** MB ChB MRCPsych LLM Consultant in Old Age Psychiatry, Queen Elizabeth Psychiatric Hospital, Edgbaston, Birmingham B15 2QZ, UK, email Martin.Curtice@bsmht.nhs.uk

**Ramy Daoud** Resident in Psychiatry, Behman Hospital, Cairo, Egypt

**Harutyun Davtyan** Head of the Men's Department, Avan Mental Hospital, Yerevan, Armenia

**Veronique Delvenne** Vice-Présidente, Société Belge Francophone de Psychiatrie et des Disciplines Associées de l'Enfance et de l'Adolescence, Professor of Child and Adolescent Psychiatry, Free University of Brussels, Espace Thérapeutique Enfants-Adolescents-Parents, 24 Rue Ketels, 1020 Brussels, Belgium, email v.delvenne@skynet.be

**M. Parameshvara Deva** FRCPsych Honorary Professor of Psychiatry, UPNG; Head of Department of Psychiatry, SSB Hospital, Kuala Belait, Brunei, email devaparameshvara@yahoo.com

**R. J. A. ten Doesschate** Psychiatrist, Adhesie, Deventer, The Netherlands, email r.tendoesschate@adhesie.nl

**Jozef Dragašek** MD PhD 1st Department of Psychiatry, Faculty of Medicine, University of P. J. Safarik, Košice, Slovak Republic, email jozef.dragasek@upjs.sk

**Valsamma Eapen** PhD FRCPsych   Chair of Child Psychiatry, University of New South Wales, Sydney, Australia, email valsa_eapen@hotmail.com

**Julian Eaton**   Mental Health Adviser, CBM International, PO Box 8451, Wuse, Abuja, Nigeria, email julian_eaton@cbm-westafrica.org

**Roman Evsegneev**   Head, Department of Psychiatry, Belarusian Medical Academy for Postgraduate Training, Minsk, Belarus

**Hafizullah Faiz**   Project Coordinator Mental Health, HealthNet TPO, Jalalabad, Afghanistan

**Marcos Pacheco de Toledo Ferraz**   Professor Titular do Departamento de Psiquiatria da Universidade Federal de São Paulo – UNIFESP, São Paulo, Brazil

**Angelo Fioritti**   Direttore Programma Salute Mentale e Dipendenze Patologiche, Azienda USL Rimini, via Coriano 38, 47900 Rimini, Italy, email afioritti@auslrn.net; Elected President of the Italian Society for Addiction Psychiatry (Società Italiana Psichiatria delle Dipendenze – SIPD)

**W. Wolfgang Fleischhacker**   Department of Biological Psychiatry, Medical University Innsbruck, Austria, email wolfgang.fleischhacker@uibk.ac.at

**Elisabete Fradique** MD   Psychiatrist, Portugal, email elisabete.fradique@gmail.com

**Wolfgang Gaebel**   Department of Psychiatry and Psychotherapy, Heinrich-Heine-Universität, Rhineland State Clinics, Bergische Landstrasse 2, D-40629, Düsseldorf, Germany, email wolfgang.gaebel@uni-duesseldorf.de

**Saveta Draganic Gajic**   School of Medicine, University of Belgrade, Institute of Mental Health, Belgrade, Serbia

**Susanna Galea**   Clinical Lecturer and Specialist Registrar in Addictive Behaviour, Department of Mental Health, St George's Hospital Medical School, London, UK, email sgalea@sghms.ac.uk; Member of the Royal College of Psychiatrists; Member of the Association of Maltese Specialists in Psychiatry

**Khachatur Gasparyan**   Yerevan State Medical University, Yerevan, Armenia

**Dan Georgescu**   Department of Old Age Psychiatry, Königsfelden Hospital, Brugg, Switzerland, email dan.georgescu@pdag.ch

**Suhaila Ghuloum**   Consultant Psychiatrist, Psychiatry Department, Hamad Medical Corporation, PO Box 3050, Doha, Qatar, email sghuloum@hmc.org.qa

**Ayana Gibbs**   Wellcome Clinical Research Fellow, Section of Cognitive Neuropsychiatry, Division of Psychological Medicine, Institute of Psychiatry, King's College London, UK

**Giovanni de Girolamo**   Dipartimento Salute Mentale, Azienda USL Città di Bologna; formerly responsible for the National Mental Health Project, National Institute of Health (Progetto Nazionale Salute Mentale, Istituto Superiore di Sanità), Rome, Italy

**Semyon Gluzman**   Executive Secretary, Ukrainian Psychiatric Association, Kiev, Ukraine, email upa2@i.com.ua

**Natallia Golubeva** Forensic Psychiatrist, Department of Forensic Psychiatry, State Medical Forensic Service, Minsk, Belarus, email doctor_golubeva@mail.ru

**Javier González** Coordinator, Latin American Fellows' Programme; Latin American Psychiatric Association (APAL), Venezuela

**Alexander Grinshpoon** Director, Mental Health Services, Ministry of Health, Jerusalem, Israel

**Nady el-Guebaly** Professor, Department of Psychiatry, University of Calgary, Canada, email nady.el-guebaly@calgaryhealthregion.ca; Past President, Canadian Psychiatric Association; President, International Society of Addiction Medicine

**Oye Gureje** Professor of Psychiatry, University of Ibadan, Nigeria, email gureje.o@skannet.com.ng

**Isaak Gurovich** Deputy Director, and Head of Department of Organisation of Mental Healthcare, Moscow Research Institute of Psychiatry, Moscow, Russia

**M. K. Al-Haddad** Professor of Psychiatry, Arabian Gulf University, Bahrain

**Arega Hakobyan** Head of the Outpatient Department, Avan Mental Hospital, Yerevan, Armenia

**Mevludin Hasanovic** Department of Psychiatry, University of Tuzla, Bosnia and Herzegovina

**Zoe Hawkins** BM BCh MA Advisor to the Ministry of Health for Mental Health, Epilepsy and Health Research, Democratic Republic of Timor-Leste, email zoe.hawkins@doctors.org.uk

**Bruce Hershfield** MD Assistant Professor, Johns Hopkins University School of Medicine, Baltimore, MA, USA

**Frederick W. Hickling** DM MRCPsych(UK) DFAPA, Professor of Psychiatry, Department of Community Health and Psychiatry, University of the West Indies, Mona, Kingston 7, Jamaica email frederick.hickling@uwimona.edu.jm

**P. P. G. Hodiamont** Psychiatrist, Tilburg University, The Netherlands, email p.p.g.hodiamont@uvt.nl

**Siarhei Holubeu** Forensic Psychiatrist, Department of Forensic Psychiatry, State Medical Forensic Service, Minsk, Belarus

**Se-fong Hung** Hospital Chief Executive, Kwai Chung Hospital, Hong Kong Special Administrative Region, China, email hungsf@ha.org.hk

**Mohammed A. Ibrahim** Chairman, Psychiatry Department, Hamad Medical Corporation, Doha, Qatar, email psychiatry@hmc.org.qa

**Fuad Ismayilov** Head of the 4th Department, Baku City Psychiatric Hospital No. 2, Baku, Azerbaijan, email fouad@azerin.com

**Sladjana Strkalj Ivezic** Day Hospital and Community Rehabilitation Centre, Psychiatric Hospital Vrapce, Bolnicka cesta 32, 10090 Zagreb, Croatia, email sladjana.ivezic@bolnica-vrapce

**Abdul-Monaf Al-Jadiry** Professor of Psychiatry, Baghdad Medical School, Baghdad, Iraq; currently Professor of Psychiatry, Faculty of Medicine,

The Jordanian University; c/o Kent and Medway NHS and Social Care Partnership Trust, Rochester Health Centre, Delce Road, Rochester, Kent ME1 2EL, UK

**Rachel Jenkins** MB BChir MD (Cantab) FRCPsych FFOHM FRSPH   Director and Professor of Psychiatry, WHO Collaborating Center and Section for Mental Health Policy, Institute of Psychiatry, London, UK

**Arun Jha** MPhil MRCPsych   Consultant Psychiatrist and Chairman, Psychiatry Section, Nepalese Doctors' Association; Logandene, Ashley Close, Hemel Hempstead, Hertfordshire HP3 8BL, UK, email arun.jha@ HPT.nhs.uk

**Jan Olav Johannessen**   Chief Psychiatrist, Division of Psychiatry, University Hospital of Stavanger, Post Box 1163 Hillevaag, 4095 Stavanger, Norway, email jojo@sir.no

**M. Rezaul Karim** FCPS   Professor of Psychiatry and Principal, Sylhet MAG Osmani Medical College, Sylhet, Bangladesh, email psyrkarim@yahoo.com

**Felix Kauye**   Chief Government Psychiatrist, Ministry of Health, Zomba Mental Hospital, Zomba, Malawi, email felixkauye@yahoo.com

**Mounir Khani** MD   American Board of Psychiatry and Neurology, Clinical Associate Professor of Psychiatry, American University of Beirut Medical Center, Beirut, Lebanon

**Marietta Khurshudyan**   Expert, National Assembly, Standing Committee on Health Issues, Yerevan, Armenia

**Pius A. Kigamwa**   Department of Psychiatry, University of Nairobi, Kenya

**Fred Kigozi**   Medical Director/Senior Consultant Psychiatrist, Butabika National Referral Teaching Hospital, Uganda, email buthosp@infocom. co.ug

**Anne Kleinberg**   Secretary General, Estonian Psychiatric Association, Tallinn, Estonia, email anne.kleinberg@lastehaigla.ee

**Stanislav Kostyuchenko**   Lecturer, Psychiatry Department, Kiev Medical Academy of Postgraduate Training, Ukraine

**Valery Krasnov**   Director, and Head of Department of Affective Spectrum Disorders, Moscow Research Institute of Psychiatry, Russia, email krasnov@mtu-net.ru

**Ajmal-Khan Kudlebbai**   Staff Grade Forensic Psychiatrist, Three Bridges Regional Secure Unit, West London Mental Health NHS Trust, London, UK

**Tamás Kurimay** MD PhD   President, Hungarian Psychiatric Association, Director of Psychiatry, Department Chair, Saint John Hospital and North-Buda Integrated Hospitals, Budapest, Hungary, email tamas.kurimay@ janoskorhaz.hu

**Martina Rojnic Kuzman**   Department of Psychiatry, Zagreb University Hospital Centre and Zagreb School of Medicine, Croatia

**Eero Lahtinen** MD PhD   Senior Medical Officer, Health Department, Health Promotion Group, Sjötullsgatan 8, Helsingfors, Finland, email eero.lahtinen@stm.fi

**Linda C. W. Lam**  Professor, Department of Psychiatry, The Chinese University of Hong Kong, Hong Kong Special Administrative Region, China

**Zahid Latif**  Department of Community Rehabilitation Psychiatry Services, Cavan/Monaghan Mental Health Services, St Davnet's Hospital, Monaghan, Ireland

**Alisher Latypov** MA MHS  Country Manager in Tajikistan, Global Initiative on Psychiatry; Sub-regional Drug Epidemiology Expert, United Nations Development Programme, email alisher_latypov@fulbrightweb.org

**Ledia Lazëri**  National Professional Officer at the WHO Country Office, Albania, and Coordinator of the Albanian Development Centre for Mental Health, email ledial@who-albania.org

**Itzhak Levav**  Adviser, Mental Health Services, Ministry of Health, Jerusalem, Israel, email Itzhak.Levav@moh.health.gov.il

**Slobodan Loga**  Department of Psychiatry, University of Sarajevo, Bosnia and Herzegovina

**Juan J. López-Ibor**  Professor and Chairman, Director, Institute of Psychiatry and Mental Health, San Carlos Complutense University, Madrid, Spain, email jli@lopez-ibor.com

**Nasser Loza**  Consultant Psychiatrist and Director, Behman Hospital, 32 Marsad Street, Cairo 11421, Egypt, email nloza@behman.com

**Chitsanzo Mafuta**  Registrar Psychiatric Clinical Officer, Ministry of Health, Zomba Mental Hospital, Zomba, Malawi, email chitsanzomafuta@yahoo.co.uk

**Vladimir Magkoev** MD  Narcology Specialist, Drug Demand Reduction Programme, Tajikistan

**Hari D. Maharajh**  Senior Lecturer, Faculty of Medical Sciences, Department of Psychiatry, University of the West Indies, Mt Hope, Trinidad, West Indies, email drharim@carib-link.net

**Djibo Douma Maiga**  Head of National Mental Health Programme, Ministry of Health, Niamey, Republic of Niger

**Ahmed Mohamed Makki** MD  Reporter, Health Committee, Shura Council, Past Deputy Minister of Health, Yemen

**Walter Mangezi** MMed Psychiatry  Lecturer, Department of Psychiatry, Faculty of Health Sciences, University of Zimbabwe, email wmangezi@yahoo.co.uk

**João Marques-Teixeira** MD PhD  Psychiatrist and Psychotherapist, Portugal, email marquesteixeira@netcabo.pt

**James MacCabe**  MRC Training Fellow in Health of the Public Research, Department of Psychiatry, PO 63, Institute of Psychiatry, London SE5 8AF, UK, email james.maccabe@iop.kcl.ac.uk

**A. P. McGeorge** QSO FRANZCP  Oceania Vice-President, World Federation for Mental Health, New Zealand, email peter.mcgeorge@gmail.com

**Elena Medina-Mora**  General Director, National Institute of Psychiatry 'Ramon de la Fuente Muñiz', Mexico City, Mexico, email medinam@imp.edu.mx

**Nalaka Mendis**   Professor of Psychiatry, University of Colombo, Sri Lanka, email nalaka@sri.lanka.net

**Samuel Mampunza Ma Miezi**   Psychiatry Department, School of Medicine, University of Kinshasa, Democratic Republic of Congo

**John Mifsud**   Consultant Psychiatrist, Our Lady of Mount Carmel Psychiatric Hospital, Malta; Honorary Senior Lecturer, Department of Psychiatry, University of Malta, email psy@shadow.net.mt; Member of the Association of Maltese Specialists in Psychiatry

**Milica Pejovic Milovancevic**   School of Medicine, University of Belgrade, Institute of Mental Health, Belgrade, Serbia

**Gholamreza Mirsepassi** MD FRCPsych DPM   Vice President, Iranian Psychiatric Association, Tehran, Iran

**Malik Hussain Mubbashar**   Sheikh Sayed Hospital, Lahore, Pakistan

**Florence Muga**   Consultant Psychiatrist, National Department of Health, Papua New Guinea, email florencemugawebster@yahoo.co.uk

**Ulrich Müller**   Department of Psychiatry and Psychotherapy, Heinrich-Heine-Universität, Düsseldorf, Germany

**Ildephonse Muteba Mushidi**   Psychiatry Department, School of Medicine, University of Kinshasa, Democratic Republic of Congo

**Mridula S. Naga**   Consultant Psychiatrist, Brown Sequard Mental Health Care Centre, BeauBassin, Mauritius, email manish@intnet.mu

**Livia Nano**   Psychologist at the Albanian Development Centre for Mental Health, Tirana, Albania

**Ruhullah Nassery**   National Coordinator for Mental Health in Primary Health Care, Ministry of Public Health, Kabul, Afghanistan

**Kris Naudts**   Deputy Director, Forensic Psychiatry Teaching Unit, Department of Forensic Mental Health Science, Institute of Psychiatry, King's College London, UK

**Alexander Nawka** MD   Department of Psychiatry, 1st Faculty of Medicine, Charles University, Prague, Czech Republic

**Jedrin Ngungu**   Specialist Registrar, Norfolk and Waveney Mental Health Foundation Trust, email ngunguj@yahoo.com (former Acting Medical Director for a year at Chainama Hills Hospital, Zambia)

**Zulfia Nisanbaeva** MD   Lecturer, Department of Psychiatry, Tajik State Medical University (Avicena); Chair, In-patient Forensic Psychiatry Commission, Tajikistans

**Frank G. Njenga**   Chiromo Lane Medical Centre, University of Nairobi, Kenya, email fnjenga@africaonline.co.ke

**Adel Al-Offi**   Consultant Psychiatrist, Ministry of Health, Bahrain

**Michel Okitapoy On'okoko**   Social and Transcultural Psychiatry, McGill University, Montreal, Canada, email michel.okitapoy@mail.mcgill.ca; Psychiatry Department, School of Medicine, University of Kinshasa, Democratic Republic of Congo

**Izet Pajevic**   Department of Psychiatry, University of Tuzla, Bosnia and Herzegovina

**Soumana Pate**   Director of PRAHN, Niamey, Niger

**Vikram Patel**   Senior Lecturer, London School of Hygiene and Tropical Medicine, and the Sangath Society, Goa, India

**Siddhartha Paul** MPhil (Psychiatry)   Student, Sylhet MAG Osmani Medical College, Sylhet, Bangladesh

**Alfredo Pemjean**   Ministerio de Salud, Unidad de Salud Mental, MacIver 541, Santiago, Chile, email apemjean@rdc.cl

**Blanka Kores Plesnicar**   Associate Professor, Department of Psychiatry, University Clinical Centre Maribor, Slovenia, email blanka.kores@sb-mb.si

**Dimitris Ploumpidis** MD   Associate Professor of Psychiatry, First Psychiatric Department of Athens University, Athens, Greece

**David Price**   Consultant Adult Psychiatrist at St Brendan's Hospital, Bermuda, email David.Price@bermudahospitals.bm

**Dainius Puras**   Department of Psychiatry, Vilnius University, Vilnius, Lithuania, email dainius.puras@mf.vu.lt

**Jirí Raboch** MD   Director, Psychiatric Department, 1st Medical School, Charles University, 120 00 Prague 2, Ke Karlovu 11, Czech Republic, email raboch@mbox.cesnet.cz

**Maja Silobrcic Radic**   Croatian National Institute of Public Health, Croatia

**Blanca Reneses**   Deputy Director, Institute of Psychiatry and Mental Health, San Carlos Complutense University, Madrid, Spain

**Marta B. Rondon**   Assistant Professor, Department of Psychiatry and Mental Health, Universidad Peruana Cayetano Heredia and Attending Psychiatrist, Hospital E Rebagliati, Essalud, Lima, Peru

**Alan Rosen**   Director of Clinical Services and Senior Psychiatrist, Royal North Shore Hospital and Community Mental Health Services, Sydney; Associate Professor, School of Public Health, University of Wollongong; Clinical Associate Professor, Department of Psychological Medicine, University of Sydney, New South Wales, Australia, email arosen@nsccahs.health.nsw.gov.au

**Omer El-Rufaie** FRCPsych   Professor of Psychiatry, Faculty of Medicine and Health Sciences, United Arab Emirates University, Al Ain, UAE

**Reehan Sabri**   Consultant Psychiatrist, Mental Health Unit, RIPAS Hospital, Bandar Seri Begawan, Brunei Darussalam BA 1710, email reehansabri@hotmail.com

**Majid Sadeghi** MD   Associate Professor of Psychiatry, Tehran University of Medical Sciences, School of Medicine, Department of Psychiatry, Roozbeh Hospital, Tehran, Iran, email sadeghmj@sina.tums.ac.ir

**Sabah Sadik**   National Advisor for Mental Health, Iraq

**Maan A. Bari Qasem Saleh** PhD   Associate Professor, Faculty of Medicine, Aden University, Yemen, email maanymha@yahoo.com

**Shekhar Saxena**   Coordinator, Mental Health: Evidence and Research, Department of Mental Health and Substance Abuse, WHO, Geneva, Switzerland

**Geoff Searle** MB BS BSc FRCPsych Crisis Team Consultant, Dorset Healthcare Foundation Trust, Core and Quality Training Programme Director, Wessex Deanery

**Héctor Sentíes** Education Director, National Institute of Psychiatry 'Ramon de la Fuente Muñiz', Mexico City, Mexico

**Fakhruzzaman Shaheed** MD Assistant Registrar, Psychiatry, Sylhet MAG Osmani Medical College and Hospital

**Pramod M. Shyangwa** MD Associate Professor, Department of Psychiatry, BPK Institute of Health Sciences, Dharan, Nepal, email pshyangwa@yahoo.com

**Donald Silberberg** MD Global Network for Research in Mental and Neurological Health, USA; University of Pennsylvania, Philadelphia, USA

**Helena Silfverhielm** National Board of Health and Welfare (Socialstyrelsen), S-106 30 Stockholm, Sweden, email Helena.Silfverhielm@socialstyrelsen.se

**Osman Sinanovic** Department of Neurology, University of Tuzla, Bosnia and Herzegovina

**Hamed Al-Sinawi** Senior Registrar, Department of Behavioural Medicine, Sultan Qaboos University Hospital, Muscat, Oman, email senawi@squ.edu.om

**Jan Skandsen** Medical Director, Department of Child and Adolescent Psychiatry, Division of Psychiatry, University Hospital of Stavanger; President of the Norwegian Association for Child and Adolescent Psychiatry, Stavanger, Norway

**Armen Soghoyan** Yerevan State Medical University, Yerevan, Armenia, email soghoyan@yahoo.com;

**Claes Göran Stefansson** National Board of Health and Welfare (Socialstyrelsen), Stockholm, Sweden

**Bjarte Stubhaug** Medical Director, Division of Psychiatry, University Hospital of Bergen, Norway; President of the Norwegian Psychiatric Association

**Guk-Hee Suh** Associate Professor of Psychiatry, Hallym University College of Medicine, Seoul, Republic of Korea; Visiting Lecturer, Imperial College School of Medicine, London, UK, email suhgh@chol.com

**Anastas Suli** Head of the Psychiatric Department of the University Hospital Centre, 'Mother Teresa', Tirana, and Chairman of the National Steering Committee for Mental Health, Albania

**Ka Sunbaunat** Director of the National Programme for Mental Health, Ministry of Health, No. 151-153, Kampuchea Krom Blvd, Phnom Penh, Cambodia

**Alija Sutovic** Department of Psychiatry, University Clinical Centre Tuzla, Medical Faculty, University of Tuzla, 75000 Tuzla, Bosnia and Herzegovina

**Adnan Takriti** Editor-in-Chief, Arab Journal of Psychiatry, Consultant Psychiatrist, PO Box 5370, Amman 11183, Jordan, email takriti@nets.com.jo

**Nicoleta Tataru**   Senior Consultant Psychiatrist, Oradea, Romania, email nicoleta_tataru@hotmail.com; President of the Romanian Association of Geriatric Psychiatry, Member of the Honorary Board of the Romanian Association of Psychiatry, and Member of the Board of the International Psychogeriatric Association and of the Association of European Psychiatrists

**Udgardo Juan L. Tolentino Jr**   Executive Assistant, National Program for Mental Health and Substance Abuse, Department of Health, Philippines, email edtol.md@pacific.net.ph

**Dusica Lecic Tosevski**   Professor of Psychiatry, School of Medicine, University of Belgrade, Serbia, email dusica.lecictosevski@eunet.rs

**Clare Townsend** MD   University of Queensland, Australia

**G. Tsetsegdary** MD PhD   Policy and Coordination Department, Ministry of Health, Ulaanbaatar, Mongolia

**Pichet Udomratn** MD   Department of Psychiatry, Faculty of Medicine, Prince of Songkla University, Hat Yai, Songkhla, 90110, Thailand, email upichet@medicine.psu.ac.th

**Peter Ventevogel**   Technical Adviser Mental Health, HealthNet TPO, Kabul, Afghanistan, email peterventevogel@yahoo.co.uk

**Mutabara Vohidova** MD   National Project Officer, United Nations Office on Drugs and Crime Sub-Office in Tajikistan

**Johannes Wancata**   Department of Social Psychiatry, Medical University Vienna, Austria

**M. A. Zahid**   Department of Psychiatry, Faculty of Medicine, Kuwait University, PO Box 24923 Safat 13110, Kuwait, email zahid@hsc.edu.kw

**Adel Al-Zayed**   Assistant Professor, Department of Psychiatry, Faculty of Medicine, Kuwait University, Kuwait

**Jürgen Zielasek**   Department of Psychiatry and Psychotherapy, Heinrich-Heine-Universität, Düsseldorf, Germany

**Slavko Ziherl**   Professor, University Psychiatric Hospital, Studenec 48, 1260 Ljubljana, Slovenia, email ziherls@siol.net

# Preface

The publication of specially commissioned country profiles has been one of the main features of *International Psychiatry*, a journal with a focus on mental health policy, administration, the audit and management of mental health services and training in psychiatry around the world. These profiles are original articles which have gone through the journal's normal peer-review process. The authors were asked to restrict their profile to about 1500 words, and not more than 12 references and 2 tables, graphs or figures. Each profile includes a section on the demography of the country so that information on service provision and training can be seen in context.

Country profiles are also expected to cover the following areas: mental health policy and legislation; mental health service delivery; psychiatric training (both undergraduate and postgraduate), including the number and type of residence programmes, examinations and the type of qualification bestowed; psychiatric subspecialties and allied professions (e.g. child psychiatry, psychotherapy, psychiatric nursing); main areas of research; workforce issues, including the number of psychiatrists in the country; psychiatric associations (if any) and frequency of meetings; human rights issues (if any); and any other issues likely to be of interest to international colleagues and in particular to Members and Fellows of the Royal College of Psychiatrists in the UK and abroad. Within this structure individual profiles differ in both style and content, reflecting varying levels of the general development of the country as well as sociocultural differences and different attitudes to the practice of psychiatry.

Each issue of *International Psychiatry* includes new country profiles, effectively building up a data bank about mental health and psychiatric practice in many parts of the world. The series has generated considerable interest and highlighted the fact that many people, for a variety of reasons, want to find out about the state of mental health services in other countries. However, such information has not previously been easily available and the College has received a number of enquiries relating to this, namely from psychiatrists planning to visit other countries, often for teaching purposes or to provide services, as well as other doctors, nurses and social workers interested in finding out about mental health services elsewhere, sometimes because a patient may be returning to their native land. Journalists are another source of enquiry, often because there has been a major incident that has brought mental health needs and psychiatry in a particular country into focus. Students wishing to do their electives in another country also seek information. It is worth noting that enquiries about mental health and psychiatry are not limited to individuals from the UK but have been received from all continents.

Given this level of interest it was decided to assemble all of the country profiles published in *International Psychiatry* in one volume. This will facilitate access to the published information and highlight the similarities and differences between countries. It is a unique collection of authoritative papers from 91 countries around the world, each one written by an experienced senior practitioner familiar with all aspects of psychiatry in their country.

In the globalised world of today, with significant movement of populations across the world and constant dialogue between professionals in different countries, it is important that we all have a better understanding of practice in different countries. The individual country profiles, as published in *International Psychiatry* and collected together in this volume, make a huge contribution to increasing that shared understanding. Until now there has been no worldwide view of psychiatry and mental health. This book fills that gap and, more importantly, encourages the reader to think about different approaches to mental health and psychiatric practice, education and training rather than blindly accepting that local practice is the only way. It will undoubtedly be recommended for supplementary reading on courses on global mental health and will be a 'must have' for university libraries in medicine, psychiatry and behavioural medicine.

*Hamid Ghodse*

# Africa

# Democratic Republic of Congo

Michel Okitapoy On'okoko, Rachel Jenkins, Samuel
Mampunza Ma Miezi, Daniel Okitundu Luwa E. Andjafono
and Ildephonse Muteba Mushidi

The delivery of mental healthcare in the Democratic Republic of Congo (DRC), formerly Zaire, is influenced by geography, politics, legislation and the structure of the health system, as well as traditional beliefs and culture.

The DRC is in Central Africa; the Central African Republic and Sudan border to the north, Uganda, Rwanda and Burundi to the east, Zambia and Angola to the south, and the Republic of Congo to the west; and it is separated from Tanzania by Lake Tanganyika to the east. The country occupies 2 345 408 km², which is slightly greater than Spain, France, Germany, Sweden and Norway combined. For administrative purposes the country is divided into 11 provinces, each with a provincial headquarters.

The population is over 66 million, with 47% aged under 15 years and 4% over 60. Average life expectancy at birth is 46 years for men and 49 years for women. There are around 350 ethnic groups; the largest groups are the Kongo, Luba and Mongo peoples. There are also around 600 000 Pygmies, the aboriginal people of the DRC. Although some 700 local languages and dialects are spoken, there is widespread use of French (the official language); the most common local languages are Kongo, Tshiluba, Swahili and Lingala. Eighty per cent of the population are Christian, 10% Muslim and 10% follow traditional beliefs or syncretic sects (Central Intelligence Agency, 2008).

Before independence in 1960, the DRC was under Belgian colonial rule. The economy, despite the country's vast natural resources, has greatly declined since the mid-1980s. Recent conflicts, which began in 1996, have dramatically reduced national output and government revenue and increased the external debt, as well as resulting in famine and disease and 5 million conflict-related deaths (US State Department, 2009).

Despite a current lull in overall violence, the plight of people across the eastern DRC remains dire. Thousands have been displaced following renewed violence or rumours of impending violence. Achieving mental health for the population of the DRC is a priority for its economic recovery, achievement of physical health goals and creating resilience among the local people.

# Mental health policy and legislation

The DRC's mental health policy was formulated in 1999. Its essential components are advocacy, promotion, prevention, treatment, rehabilitation and education; there is also a substance misuse policy. The national mental health programme was also formulated in 1999 (World Health Organization, 2005). The Ministry of Health is responsible for the organisation, management and planning of mental health sectors, and it is represented at provincial, district and community level.

The DRC has ratified the international legal instruments concerning the rights and protection of people who are mentally ill, but there is as yet no DRC law defining the rights and protection of people with mental illness or regulating the procedures for voluntary or involuntary admission to a psychiatric hospital.

# Mental disorders in the DRC

Popular beliefs persist about supernatural causes of disease in general and psychiatric problems in particular (Okitapoy, 1993; Okitapoy *et al*, 1996).

Mental disorders are probably at least as common in the DRC as they are elsewhere, but there are no national epidemiological data. Statistics from two psychiatric centres, the Soins de Sante Mentale (SOSAME) Psychiatric Centre in Bukavu (a post-crisis region) and the Katwambi Centre Neuropsychopathologique (CNPP) (in Kasai province), show the following:

- 80% of patients are under the age of 40, 36% aged 21–30
- there are 1.02 female patients for each male patient
- half the patients are without employment
- 6–15% of patients have schizophrenia
- 6–31% have other psychotic disorders
- 22% suffer from anxiety disorders (related to war trauma for 18%, to sexual abuse for 3.5% and to other factors for the remaining 0.5%)
- 13–23% of patients have mood disorders (manic episodes, depressive disorders and bipolar disorders).

# Psychiatric services

## *Historical background*

In 1926, a psychiatric institution situated along the Congo River called Mount Stanley Lazaret was created by order of the colonial authority, and from 1928 was open to patients with mental illness, tuberculosis and leprosy. In 1960, the centre became the Mount Stanley Psychiatric Institute but in 1969 it closed. It was replaced by the CNPP–Mount Amba in 1973, associated with the University of Kinshasa medical faculty. In 1957, the CNPP opened in Katwambi.

## Current mental health services

Mental healthcare is delivered by private institutions as well as general and company hospitals. According to the current national health sector plan (Ministère de la Santé, 1999), mental health should be integrated into primary care. The national mental health programme is responsible for carrying out this integration. Under the general health decentralisation policy, it is planned to establish a mental health programme in each province and district, with support for the health zones and basic health units.

However, the mental health infrastructure still remains very centralised in Kinshasa, the capital, and some provinces. There are two university institutions: the CNPP–Mont Amba in Kinshasa and the Department of Neuropsychiatry of Sendwe Hospital in Lubumbashi. There is one state hospital, operated by the Roman Catholic Brothers of Charity (the CNPP–Katwambi). In addition, there are mental health centres, 90% of which are run by Roman Catholic organisations. There are also some private clinics run by Congolese neuropsychiatrists in Kinshasa.

There are no budgetary allocations for mental health. Primary funding comes in the form of out-of-pocket expenditure by the patient or the patient's family. The cost of psychiatric treatment is considered high in relation to average earnings (World Health Organization, 2005).

## Mental health workforce

Specialist human resources in mental health are also very centralised. Currently, there are 34 neuropsychiatrists for a population of over 66 million, of whom only 2 are in the provinces – the other 32 are in Kinshasa. Thirteen Congolese neuropsychiatrists are abroad (Belgium, France, Canada, the USA, and South Africa). In addition, four general practitioners have had 6 months' training in neuropsychiatry. There are 0.01 psychologist clinicians and 0.03 psychiatric nurses per 100000 population, but again they are mainly in Kinshasa. There are no occupational therapists or social workers qualified in mental health (World Health Organization, 2005, 2006).

# Education and training

Medical training lasts 7 years and is available at a number of universities, including Kinshasa, Lubumbashi and Kisangani. Specialist training in neuropsychiatry for doctors and nurses is available only at the CNPP, University of Kinshasa, and lasts 5 years. That CNPP is mandated: to provide care to the community; to act as a training centre for mental health professionals at all levels, including academic and scientific personnel working in the field of neurology and psychiatry; and to serve as a biopsychosocial research centre for the University of Kinshasa.

As mental health is being integrated into primary care, regular training of primary care professionals is carried out in the field of mental health.

To facilitate access to mental healthcare despite the shortage of specialists outside Kinshasa, there is a training programme of 6 months in psychiatry (at the Kinshasa CNPP) for general practitioners.

There is no training available for occupational therapy or social work.

The government also partially supports some charitable organisations like SOSAME and some non-governmental organisations that provide mental health services and training (Réseau des ONG d'Action en Santé Mentale, 2007).

# Human rights

Human rights violations have been perpetrated by rebels, militiamen and other armed groups. According to Amnesty International (2007), the transitional power-sharing government since 2003 has made little progress in advancing the law and respect that are essential to securing human rights. Meanwhile, the eastern DRC partially remains under the control of some armed groups. Insecurity, unlawful killings, human rights abuses, ethnic tension, widespread rape and sexual exploitation of women and girls, torture and illegal detention, as well as the recruitment and use of child soldiers continue in many parts of the country, in some instances perpetrated by government forces. Guarantee of the safety and dignity of people returning to the country, including refugees, remains difficult (Human Rights Watch, 2007; Integrated Regional Information Networks, 2009).

# Conclusions

The DRC represents a chronic emergency, with endemic poverty, conflict, violence, forced dislocation of ethnic groups, torture and rape as weapons of war, which have all had devastating effects on the population. These serious violations of international humanitarian law must be addressed to create peace, respect for human rights and dignity, equity and accountability. These factors need also to be taken into account in mental health policy, legislation and implementation for the well-being of the Congolese population.

The national mental health programme needs to be allocated a government budget so that it can be implemented. It will then be possible to begin to work towards mental health promotion, training in mental health for staff at all levels, epidemiological research, improvement of infrastructure, effective integration of mental health in primary care, and liaison with family, traditional and religious healers in the management of people with mental problems.

# References

Amnesty International (2007) Democratic Republic of Congo. In *The State of the World's Human Rights. Amnesty International.* See http://archive.amnesty.org/report2007/eng/ Homepage (accessed February 2010).

Central Intelligence Agency (CIA) (2008) Democratic Republic of Congo. In *World Factbook* (2008). CIA.

Human Rights Watch (HRW) (2007) *Report on Human Rights, Democratic Republic of Congo*. HRW.

Integrated Regional Information Networks (IRIN) (2009) *Democratic Republic of Congo*. IRIN.

Ministère de la Santé (1999) *Politique et plan directeur de développement de la santé mentale en République Démocratique du Congo*. [Policy and Plan of Development for Mental Health in the Democratic Republic of Congo.] Ministère de la Santé.

Okitapoy, O. M. (1993) *Communauté thérapeutique: L'expérience du Service de psychiatrie (salle 7), Hôpital Gecamines Sendwe de Lubumbashi, Zaïre*. [The Therapeutic Community: The Experience at the Psychiatry Service (Room 7), Hôpital Gecamines Sendwe de Lubumbashi, Zaire.] Médecine d'Afrique Noire.

Okitapoy, O. M., Malanda, S., Penge, O., *et al* (1996) Ethno-psychiatric approach to adultery and mental health in Kinshasa. In *Psychotherapy in Africa* (eds S. N. Madu, P. K. Baguma & A. Pritz), pp. 178–182. World Council of Psychotherapy.

Réseau des ONG d'Action en Santé Mentale (ROASAM) (2007) *Programme d'appui a l'intégration de la santé mentale dans les soins de santé primaires et dans les services sociaux*. [Programme of Support for the Integration of Mental Health into Primary Healthcare and Social Services.] ROASAM.

US State Department (USSD) *(2009) Country Reports on Human Rights*. USSD.

World Health Organization (2005) Democratic Republic of Congo. In *Mental Health Atlas*. WHO.

World Health Organization (2006) *Country Statistics Concerning the Health System of the Democratic Republic of Congo*. WHO.

# Egypt

Ramy Daoud, Sherif Atallah and Nasser Loza

For over a thousand years, the Hippocratic system of medicine prevailed in Europe. It went into oblivion during the Dark Ages, when there was a reversion to the demoniacal theories of mental illness. Hippocrates' works survived, however, in the library at Alexandria, where they were translated into Arabic. These and other classical works were retranslated into Latin and Greek from the 12th century on, ushering in the Renaissance.

Around 1284 CE, the Sultan of Egypt, Al Mansour Kalawoon, bequeathed one of his palaces in Cairo for the construction of a general hospital with a department of psychiatry. It soon became one of the most famous hospitals throughout the Islamic world. It was, and still is, known as Dar Al Shefa, literally the House of Healing (Okasha *et al*, 1993). Two features were remarkable for that era: the care of mental patients in a general hospital, and the involvement of the community in the welfare of the patients, which foreshadowed modern trends by six centuries (Baasher, 1975).

The mentally disturbed usually received baths, fomentation, compresses, bandaging and massage with various oils. Blood letting, cupping and cautery were also widely used. A familiar term for an antidepressant in the medieval period was *mufarrih an nafs*, 'gladdening of the spirit'. Those suffering from insomnia would be placed in a separate hall to listen to harmonious music and to hear skilled story tellers recite their tales (Buergel, 1975; Dols, 1992).

## Mental health resources

Today, the population of Egypt is around 61 000 000 (National Information Centre, 1997). There is one psychiatric bed for every 6000 citizens; psychiatric hospital beds represent less than 10% of the total. These are largely concentrated in Cairo, bringing the ratio there to 1 bed per 2200 – the four public psychiatric hospitals in Cairo provide 5800 beds, and the remaining 1200 beds are distributed over the rest of Egypt (Ministry of Health, 1998). Psychiatric hospitals are currently experiencing difficulties in the provision of care, treatment and rehabilitation, as they have limited resources.

Egypt has one psychiatrist for every 130000 citizens, compared with one physician for every 500. Clinical psychologists total around 250 in the whole country, most of them also concentrated in the capital. The nurses working in the mental health field are general nurses – most have little or no training in psychiatric care. The more highly qualified nurses graduating in Egypt generally prefer to work abroad, often in the Gulf, where remuneration is much higher. There are many social workers practising in all psychiatric facilities, but they are mostly generic social workers, who have minimal graduate training in psychiatric social work. There is no training for occupational therapy in Egypt (Okasha & Karam, 1998).

## Training

There are 13 medical schools in Egypt, each with a department of psychiatry (mainly providing out-patient services). Undergraduate training in psychiatry is often limited to a few days in the curriculum. There is a 4-year postgraduate psychiatric training programme in several of these schools. In 1948, Cairo University started a diploma in psychological medicine and neurology.

## Health expenditure

According to United Nations Development Programme (UNDP), health expenditure, estimated as a percentage of gross domestic product (GDP), is 1% in Egypt. This is far below the minimum expenditure of 5% of GDP recommended by the World Health Organization, and may be compared with 13.7% in the USA (World Health Organization, 1996). The Ministry of Health budget constitutes 1.9% of the national budget (Ministry of Health, 1998). The allocation of resources is directed towards endemic problems such as malnutrition, parasitic infestations (e.g. bilharzia), tuberculosis and maternal and child morbidity.

In a postal survey conducted by Okasha & Karam (1998) looking at psychiatric services in several Arab countries, there was a consensus among Arab psychiatrists about the need for:

- public mental health education
- an increase in the number of psychiatrists
- upgrading of the training and education of mental health professionals
- the development of preventive and community mental healthcare services.

## Research in Egypt

Egypt is the most productive country in the Middle East in terms of the number of articles published per year over the past 30 years (176 articles).

However, using another method of measuring research productivity – the number of articles per million of the population – Egypt would rank average to low (1.5 articles per million).

The region seems to lack a strategic, policy-oriented position on the research agenda. Furthermore, funding for academic research is limited and depends on the interests of the different financing organisations. On the other hand, collaboration between different centres at the Arab, regional or international level will doubtless contribute to the development of research in the Arab world (Okasha & Karam, 1998).

## Policies and future directions

Egypt has a Mental Health Act dating back to 1944 and a documented health policy. Four years ago, the Ministry of Health adopted a new strategy, of centralisation of mental health services. In collaboration with several international agencies, this has facilitated the implementation of several projects to upgrade mental health services:

- a Finnish project on human resource development and the introduction of community-based services
- a UNDP project that concentrates on improving treatment services and rehabilitation for addiction
- a World Health Organization project on the inclusion of psychiatry in primary care services, as well as support for community-based services.

## Mental health and culture

As in the majority of developing countries, patients tend to present with somatic psychological symptoms. This presentation of mental ill health is reflected in the pattern of consultation. Patients tend to pass through different healthcare 'filters' before they reach psychiatric clinics and hospitals. According to Goldberg & Huxley (1992), almost two-thirds of patients with psychiatric symptoms attend only their general practitioner, and only 50% of those would be recognised as having a psychiatric disorder.

In this context, traditional and religious healers play a major role in primary psychiatric care in Egypt. They deal with minor neurotic, psychosomatic and transitory psychotic states using religious and group psychotherapies, suggestion and devices such as amulets and incantations (Okasha, 1966). It was estimated that 60% of out patients at the university clinic in Cairo, which generally serves people from low socio economic classes, have been to traditional healers before attending a psychiatrist (Okasha & Hassan, 1968). In rural areas, community care is implemented without the need for healthcare workers. Egyptians, especially those living in the countryside, have a special tolerance of mental disorders and an ability to assimilate those with a chronic mental illness. For example, these patients, and those with mild or moderate learning disabilities, may cultivate crops along with, and under the supervision of, family members.

Thus, the real challenge for mental health professionals is the first filter, that is, patients acknowledging their mental health problems. However, this challenge cannot be met without a reorganisation of both the health-providing structures and the approach to medical education and training. The latter cannot be systemically tackled without the guidance of action-oriented and policy-oriented research.

# References

Baasher, T. (1975) The Arab countries. In *World History of Psychiatry* (ed. J. G. Howells), pp. 547–578. New York: Bruner/Mazel.

Buergel (1975) Der Mufarrih an nafs des Ibn Cladi Ba'albakk, ein Lehrbuch der Psychohygiene aus dem 7. Jahrhundert der Hijra. In *Proceedings of the Sixth Congress of Arabic and Islamic Studies* (ed. F. Rundgren), p. 204. Leiden.

Dols, M. W. (1992) *In Majnun: The Madman in Medieval Islamic Society (ed.* D. E. Immisch), p. 133. Oxford: Clarendon Press.

Goldberg, D. P. & Huxley, P. (1992) *Common Mental Disorders: A Biosocial Model.* London: Routledge.

Ministry of Health (1998) *Statistics.* Cairo: Ministry of Health.

National Information Centre (1997) *Statistical Yearbook.* Cairo: National Information Centre.

Okasha, A. (1966) A cultural psychiatric study of EI-Zar cult in U.*A.R. British Journal of Psychiatry*, **112**, 1217–1221.

Okasha, A., Kamel, M. & Hassan, A. H. (1968) Preliminary psychiatric observations in Egypt. *British Journal of Psychiatry*, **114**, 949–955.

Okasha, A. & Karam, E. (1998) Mental health services and research in the Arab world. *Acta Psychiatrica Scandinavica*, **98**, 406–413.

Okasha, A., Seif EI-Dawla, A., Khalil, A. H., *et al* (1993) Presentation of acute psychosis in an Egyptian sample: a transcultural comparison. *Comprehensive Psychiatry*, **34**, 4–9.

World Health Organization (1996) *Recommendations for Mental Health Services.* Geneva: WHO.

# Ethiopia

## Atalay Alem

Ethiopia, in the Horn of Africa, is one of the ancient independent nations of the world and has a rich diversity of peoples and cultures. The country covers 1.1 million km$^2$ (Central Statistical Authority, 2000a). It has a population of about 70 million people (Central Statistical Authority, 2002), 80 different ethnic groups and some 200 dialects. Ethiopia is the second most populous nation in sub-Saharan Africa, after Nigeria (Hailemariam & Kloos, 1993). Forty-eight per cent of the population are under 15 years of age and over 80% live in rural areas (Central Statistical Authority, 1995). Islam and Christianity are the main religions.

Ethiopia maintained its independence during the colonial period. Over the past 30 years the country has undergone several manmade and natural disasters, such as war and political turmoil on the one hand, and famine and drought on the other. A federal system of government is now in place: there are nine regional states in the country and elections take place every 5 years.

Ethiopia is one of the least developed and most agrarian countries in the world; its estimated per capita gross national product in 1998 was $100 (Population Reference Bureau, 2000). About 65% of the country's people live below the absolute poverty line (World Bank, 1994). The literacy rate is estimated to be 38% for males and 23% for females (Central Statistical Authority, 2000b).

## Health status of the country

The main health problems in Ethiopia are malnutrition and infectious diseases, as has been the case for many years. Life expectancy at birth was recently estimated at 53 years (Ministry of Health, 2002). The crude birth rate is 39.9 per 1000 population per year and the crude death rate is 12.6 per 1000 per year. The infant mortality rate is 112.9 per 1000 live births and the mortality rate for the under-5s is 187.8 per 1000 live births. The maternal mortality rate is estimated at 871.0 per 100 000 live births. Only 28% of the population have access to potable water and 11% to a proper sewerage system. It is estimated that only 60% of the population are able to receive basic health services (Ministry of Health, 2002).

## Health policy

The Ministry of Health, which is the government body responsible for organising, running and monitoring health services in the country, was established in 1948.

In 1993, a national health policy and strategy were implemented (Transitional Government of Ethiopia, 1993). The main objective of the policy is to provide people with an acceptable standard of comprehensive primary healthcare in an integrated, decentralised and equitable fashion. The emphasis is on making health services available to the rural and neglected areas of the country. A four-tier healthcare system has been adopted. Health centres in the rural areas, each with five satellite health posts each serving 5000 people, form the broad base of the pyramidal system, which progresses up to district, regional and specialised hospitals.

In line with the policy, autonomy has been given to the regional governments to plan, implement and manage health services in the regions through their respective health bureaus. The health service has been under-funded, but in recent years its share of government expenditure has increased from below 5% of gross domestic product to 7% (Ministry of Health, 2002).

## Mental health services

Ethiopia still remains one of those African countries that do not have a mental health policy, national mental health programme or mental health act (World Health Organization, 2001). Most Ethiopians use traditional methods to treat mental illness and those who do seek to use modern treatments usually do so only after they have tried several traditional means (Alem, 2000).

Families and other concerned individuals are closely involved in the care of people who are mentally ill. However, many families keep relatives with an acute, severe illness at home under restraint (even in chains) until they are no longer aggressive or violent. Once their disruptive behaviour is over, many of these sufferers become vagrants. Not uncommonly such people may be seen walking naked or dishevelled in the streets of villages and towns. They typically receive any sort of care only after they have committed an offence and have been made the subject of a court order (Alem, 2000).

Modern psychiatric services are provided by Amanuel Mental Hospital (the only mental hospital in the country), the out-patient clinic at the University Department of Psychiatry and the psychiatric unit at a military hospital. All these institutions are located in the capital city, Addis Ababa. The military hospital has 30 beds for psychiatric patients. However, until late 1986 there were only two indigenous psychiatrists in the country, one working in the university and the other in the army. In 2003, there were 11 Ethiopian psychiatrists in the country (all of whom had trained abroad): nine working in the above-mentioned institutions and two in private practice. This gives a psychiatrist : population ratio of 1:6 000 000.

The Amanuel Mental Hospital was built by the Italians to serve as a general hospital during their occupation of the country in the 1940s. After the Italians left, it was converted to a mental asylum because it was far from the centre and deemed appropriate for the isolation of 'insane' people from the rest of the community. Now, as the city has increased its geographical size, the hospital is no longer on its outskirts but it is still located in an impoverished neighbourhood.

Initially the hospital had very few beds and its prime function was as a place of incarceration for mentally ill offenders. Gradually more buildings were added and the number of beds increased, to the current level of 360, although for many years the hospital accommodated over 500 in-patients. In those days the hospital was run by expatriate psychiatrists from Eastern Europe. From 1984 Ethiopian doctors gradually took over the responsibility for running the hospital and the situation started to change. The number of Ethiopian staff has increased and the patient:bed ratio has become 1:1.

The Amanuel Mental Hospital is the only mental health institution in the country to provide a forensic service. However, until hospital beds become available for the close observation and careful examination of alleged offenders by psychiatrists, they stay in the central prison in Addis Ababa. At any given time, one will find about 100 such persons in the central prison awaiting psychiatric assessment (Alem, 2000), sometimes for as long as a year, without any treatment. They are kept in crowded prison cells and are probably maltreated by prison guards and other inmates because of their disruptive behaviour.

The Ethiopian Psychiatric Association was established late in 2002, but formal meetings have not yet begun.

In 1985, the Ministry of Health and the University Department of Psychiatry, in collaboration with the World Health Organization, decided to train psychiatric nurses as the best alternative to provide a primary mental health service in the country. A training programme started in 1987. General nurses are recruited to it from the regional and district hospitals. The training takes one year and is designed to enable the nurses to identify and treat common psychiatric disorders. On completion of the training, the nurses go back to the institution from which they were recruited and set up psychiatric units.

Psychiatrists and general doctors working in psychiatry do most of the teaching of psychiatric nurses. A total of 232 nurses have been trained so far and currently there are 43 psychiatric units in the regional and district hospitals and two health centres outside Addis Ababa, each operated by two psychiatric nurses who graduated from the programme. The nurses receive periodic supervision at their place of work and refresher training by psychiatrists from Addis Ababa. Despite many difficulties, the services run by these nurses are very impressive.

In some regional hospitals the psychiatric nurses are able to admit patients to the medical wards and to provide an in-patient service for them. When they are faced with particularly difficult cases, the psychiatric nurses refer patients to Addis Ababa. After a treatment plan has been decided, the patients are referred back to the psychiatric nurses for follow-up and maintenance treatment. Periodic shortages of the necessary drugs are the greatest problem these nurses face in their practice (Alem, 2000).

# Education

For many years Addis Ababa University was the only one in Ethiopia. It had the country's only medical school until 25 years ago, when the Gondar School of Health Sciences started training doctors, followed by the Jima Institute of Health Sciences a few years later.

The teaching of psychiatry to medical students was started in Addis Ababa University in 1966 by Professor Robert Giel from the University of Groningen, The Netherlands, who established a psychiatric unit in the Department of Internal Medicine. Dr Fikre Workneh, the first Ethiopian psychiatrist, came from the USA (where he had trained) and joined the university in 1972. In 1973 the Department of Psychiatry was created and the teaching was done by one person for many years, although expatriate psychiatrists sometimes assisted him. Expatriate psychiatrists also taught psychiatry to medical students at the other two medical schools for some time, but for the past 15 years psychiatrists from Addis Ababa are the ones who have done most of the teaching in those institutions.

Since there was no postgraduate training programme for psychiatry in Ethiopia, doctors had to go abroad to do their training. Currently there are five trainees abroad – two in the UK, two in South Africa and one in Russia; they are expected to return to Ethiopia within 1–2 years to practise psychiatry.

In January 2003 the Department of Psychiatry, Faculty of Medicine, Addis Ababa University, started a 3-year postgraduate training programme with a first intake of seven doctors. The department has only three academic staff, all of whom are general adult psychiatrists: one Associate Professor and two Assistant Professors. The department has been able to solicit assistance for the teaching of its postgraduate students from universities and individuals abroad. The Department of Psychiatry at the University of Toronto, Canada, has committed itself to assisting the programme by sending two teachers for three 1-month blocks every year for 3 years. This is part of the University of Toronto's commitment to developing international partnerships for collaborative edu-cation and research. In addition to the Toronto-based faculty teaching in Ethiopia, psychiatrists from the University of Addis Ababa will visit Toronto to present research papers and to teach. The programme is also an opportunity to share expertise in mental health service delivery, research and education, and advocacy for mental health issues in both countries.

Volunteers from The Netherlands, England, Australia, Sweden and the USA also have contributed greatly in the postgraduate training programme, which is proving a success. More institutional collaborations are being sought to strengthen the programme until the department becomes self-sufficient.

# Research

Despite the facts that the number of psychiatrists in Ethiopia has always been minimal, the resources are limited and the infrastructure is poorly developed, quite a few research papers have been published in international and local journals since the 1960s. Particularly over the past 10 years, mental health research in the country has changed significantly. Epidemiological studies in different population groups such as children, adults, islanders, semi-nomads, displaced people and women have been conducted in towns and rural settings. Some of these studies are ongoing. For example, a cohort of patients with schizophrenia and bipolar dis-order is being followed in Butajira District, a rural setting, to describe the course and outcome of these disorders, which is one of the few such studies in the world in these settings (Kebede *et al*, 2003). A good number of publications have appeared in international and local journals from these studies. External funding sources and collaboration with universities abroad have contributed greatly to mental health research in Ethiopia.

# References

Alem, A. (2000) Human rights and psychiatric care in Africa with particular reference to the Ethiopian situation. *Acta Psychiatrica Scandinavica Supplementum*, **399**, 93–96.

Central Statistical Authority (1995) *Statistical Abstract of Ethiopia*. Addis Ababa: CSA.

Central Statistical Authority (2000a) *Statistical Abstract of Ethiopia*. Addis Ababa: CSA.

Central Statistical Authority (2000b) *Demographic and Health Survey of Ethiopia*. Addis Ababa: CSA.

Central Statistical Authority (2002) *Statistical Abstract of Ethiopia*. Addis Ababa: CSA.

Hailemariam, A. & Kloos, H. (1993) Population. In *The Ecology of Health and Disease in Ethiopia* (eds H. Kloos & Z. A. Zein), pp. 47–66. Boulder, CO: Westview Press.

Kebede, D., Alem, A., Shibre, T., *et al* (2003) Onset and clinical course of schizophrenia in Butajira, Ethiopia. *International Journal of Social Psychiatry and Psychiatric Epidemiology*, **38**, 625–631.

Ministry of Health (2002) *Health and Health Related Indicators*. Addis Ababa: Ministry of Health.

Population Reference Bureau (2000) *World Population Data Sheet*. Washington, DC: PRB.

Transitional Government of Ethiopia (1993) *Health Policy of the Transitional Government of Ethiopia*. Addis Ababa: TGE.

World Bank (1994) *Better Health in Africa: Experience and Lessons Learned*. Washington, DC: World Bank.

World Health Organization (2001) *Atlas: Country Profile of Mental Health Resources*. Geneva: WHO.

# Ghana

J. B. Asare

Ghana is a West African state that attained independence from Great Britain in 1957 and became a republican state in 1960. Its population is about 22 million (2004 estimate), distributed in ten regions. The World Health Organization (WHO) has estimated that 650000 of the population are suffering from severe mental disorder and 2 166 000 are suffering from moderate to mild mental disorder (see http://www.who.int/mental_health/policy/country/ghana/en).

Mental health activities started with the enactment of the Lunatic Asylum Ordinance in 1888 by the colonial government of the Gold Coast (as Ghana was then known). The ordinance allowed law-enforcement agencies to arrest people suspected of having a mental illness (at least those who were roaming about in towns, villages or the bush) to be confined in an abandoned prison in Accra. That facility soon became overcrowded, necessitating the provision of the Lunatic Asylum in 1906. The Asylum eventually became Accra Psychiatric Hospital (Ewusi-Mensah, 2001). Two other purpose-built psychiatric hospitals, the Ankaful Psychiatric Hospital and Pantang Hospital, were opened in 1965 and 1975, respectively. The first President of Ghana had a vision of making Pantang a pan-African mental health village for research into neuropsychiatric conditions but his vision was not realised before his overthrow in 1966.

## Mental health policy and legislation

Ghana's mental health policy was formulated in 1994, and revised in 2000 and 2004. The policy objective is to provide facilities at the tertiary, regional, district and sub-district levels for the management of psychiatric cases. In pursuit of this, each regional hospital is meant to have a psychiatric wing with 10–20 beds.

The policy of the Ministry of Health is to shift the focus of mental health treatment from institutionalised care to community care, integrated into general healthcare (according to the draft Mental Health Bill 2010). Decentralisation of mental health services has been pursued with the aim of increasing access, which has involved training more psychiatric nurses, medical officers in the district hospitals and non-mental health personnel. Ten general duty doctors were trained to head the regional wings, but only three of them could be engaged in the regions, while the others have augmented the staff at the specialist hospitals. The other policies set out in the Bill cover the formation of a technical coordinating committee, training, the rehabilitation of people who are mentally ill and periodic review of conditions of service for mental health personnel.

After the promulgation of the Lunatic Asylum Ordinance of 1888, the National Redemption Council Decree (NRCD 30) of 1972 followed. This was an institution-based law that did not address human rights adequately but was an improvement on the previous law. Unsuccessful attempts were made in 1992, 1996 and 2000 to revise the law. Since 2004, a more comprehensive Bill has been prepared with the technical assistance of the WHO and will soon be put before Parliament. The new Bill adopts an approach based on human rights, in accordance with international agreements (such as the United Nations Charter) on the health needs of people with mental disorders (WHO, 2005). The Bill applies to the private as well as the public sector. It addresses community care, which involves orthodox, traditional and spiritual practices, and the monitoring of activities in order to bring dignity to people suffering from mental illness. The Bill also ensures that standards of care and patients' rights are adhered to in order to prevent physical and sexual abuse.

## Mental health service delivery

Mental health services are provided by psychiatric hospitals, regional hospitals and some district hospitals. In-patient facilities are available at the three psychiatric hospitals, one teaching hospital, three regional hospitals and the military hospital; in addition, four of the five private facilities have in-patient psychiatric facilities. Three regional hospitals have 10–20 beds in psychiatric wings. Two substance misuse centres are available at Korlebu Teaching Hospital and Pantang Hospital, where the centre operates as a therapeutic community. The other regional hospitals admit psychiatric patients to medical wards supervised by general medical officers and assisted by community psychiatric nurses.

Community psychiatric nurses have been trained to provide aftercare to discharged patients in the community, to undertake mental health promotion, and to refer cases to regional hospitals or specialist facilities. Currently, there are 181 community psychiatric nurses, but in only 94 of the 170 districts.

There are three specialists (two on contract) working in Accra Psychiatric Hospital, which has 1200 patients, supported by three medical officers, a resident, seven medical assistants and 248 nurses. Pantang Hospital, which has 500 patients, has two specialists, supported by three medical assistants, one resident, 196 nurses and a clinical psychologist.

Ankaful Psychiatric Hospital has two specialists supported by two medical assistants, one clinical psychologist and 85 nurses, for a patient population of 300.

## Psychiatric training

Psychiatric undergraduate training takes place at the University of Ghana Medical School at Korlebu Teaching Hospital, in Accra, where there are two lecturers (supported by eminent Ghanaian specialists living overseas) as well as two lecturers in the Department of Psychology, and at the University of Medical Sciences at Komfo Anokye Teaching Hospital, in Kumasi. Both universities offer postgraduate training programmes for the Fellowship of the West African College of Physicians and the Ghana College of Physicians and Surgeons. The West African College was established by the Anglophone West African countries; senior specialists in the region provide training and conduct examinations at approved centres. The Ghana College has a local programme that trains its students and examines them using external assessors; it was established to increase the local demand for specialists and to tackle emigration by doctors.

Psychiatric nurses are trained in two centres. The 3-year training required to become a registered mental nurse (RMN) takes place at Pantang Hospital. The 18-month post-basic RMN training for the state-registered nurse qualification takes place at Ankaful Psychiatric Hospital.

## Psychiatric subspecialties and allied professions

Although some psychiatrists have expertise in the subspecialties, they end up practising as general psychiatrists as there are insufficient numbers of these. The Accra Psychiatric Hospital has a children's ward, female and male psychogeriatric wards and male and female forensic wards. The Ministry of Education, supported by the Department of Social Welfare, is responsible for special education, including institutions for people with intellectual disability. There is one such government facility and a private facility in Accra.

There are a number of non-governmental organisations (NGOs) working in the area of mental health. Prominent among them is BasicNeeds, which both promotes mental health and provides mental health services to deprived areas in the northern and southern parts of Ghana.

## Main areas of research

Ghana has been one of the four African countries involved in the Mental Health and Poverty Alleviation Project, which is sponsored by the UK Department for International Development (DfID). As a component of this project, the team has concerned itself with the development of mental health information systems; this involves development of software and the training of staff in the recording of data. There is also an ongoing project to set up a community-based mental health service at Kintampo (Akpalu *et al*, 2010).

## Workforce issues

The mental health service in Ghana is facing many challenges. The stigma attached to the psychiatric profession deters people from joining it. The few health personnel to have been fully trained, particularly the nurses, often emigrate, which counteracts the increase in the numbers trained (each school trains 200 students a year). Most of the wards are overcrowded with long-stay patients who are not accepted at home. Ghana has 13 psychiatrists for a population of 22 million, which represents a huge treatment gap for patients who need professional psychiatric attention. Since psychiatric services are free and the hospital facilities depend on government funding (which is insufficient) and do not generate any funds, they are always under-resourced. The budget for mental health was only 2.3% of the total health budget for 2009. A large proportion of this goes on staff costs, drugs and feeding of patients. The service operates an essential drug list. Many of the patients, however, cannot afford the new-generation drugs.

## Human rights

In some spiritual and traditional settings, aggressive psychiatric patients are chained or locked up. Some lose their jobs, particularly in the private sector, when employers get to know that their worker is a psychiatric patient. In the public sector, as well as in spiritual and traditional settings, patients may receive treatment against their will. Fortunately, the new Mental Health Bill seeks to address these concerns.

## References

Akpalu, B., Lund, C., Doku, V., *et al* (2010) Scaling up community based services and improving quality of care in the state psychiatric hospitals: the way forward for Ghana. *African Journal of Psychiatry*, in press.

Ewusi-Mensah, I. (2001) Post-colonial psychiatric care in Ghana. *Psychiatric Bulletin*, **25**, 228–229.

WHO (2005) *Resource Book on Mental Health. Human Rights and Legislation.* World Health Organization.

# Kenya

Frank G. Njenga and Pius A. Kigamwa

Following a 10-year war of liberation (fought by the Mau Mau against the British), Kenya attained full independence from colonial rule in 1963. For 10 years the country enjoyed rapid economic growth (6–7% per annum) but this slowed steadily to near stagnation in the 1990s. Poor governance, abuse of human rights, internal displacements of citizens, large numbers of refugees from neighbouring countries and the AIDS pandemic conspired to reduce Kenyans' life expectancy to 47 years (in the UK it is presently 77 years). Some 42% of the population now live below the poverty line, and 26% of Kenyans exist on less than US$1 per day. The annual per capita income in Kenya is US$360 (in the UK it is $24 000) (World Bank, 2002). AIDS currently has an estimated prevalence rate of 12%. In large parts of rural Kenya many sexually active adults are unable to work, and elderly grandparents are left to look after orphaned children (some already infected with HIV), as they struggle to deal with their own grief for the loss of many of their own children. In December 2002 a new government was elected, which gives some grounds for optimism in an otherwise bleak situation.

## Mental health policy and resources

Given the circumstances, it is unsurprising perhaps that mental healthcare was relegated to near oblivion; at present there is no mental health policy. Little or no thought was given to mental health as the country struggled with more life-threatening conditions, including diarrhoeal diseases, measles, malaria and tuberculosis. Commendable efforts are, however, in place to develop a policy with the assistance of the UK's Department for International Development and the Institute of Psychiatry in London, which are now working on a collaborative project with Kenya, Tanzania and Zanzibar.

Existing programmes are hampered by the shortage of commitment, personnel and funds. There is a tangible lack of commitment to mental health in Kenya, reflected in the fact that it receives less than 1% of the Ministry of Health's budget, which is itself less than 7% of the national budget.

Kenya has only 47 psychiatrists for a population of 30 million, although there is the prospect of this number increasing, albeit slowly. More than half of them work in the major urban centres, while the majority of Kenyans live in the rural areas, which makes the relative shortage much worse.

Mathare Hospital started off in 1911 as an isolation unit for people with smallpox and is now a large, poorly resourced traditional mental hospital that houses approximately 750 mainly long-stay patients with psychosis, but it also serves as the forensic referral centre as well as an acute treatment centre. The buildings are in a state of disrepair and require major renovation. This is in marked contrast to the high morale of poorly paid staff, who work tirelessly without complaining and delivering, in their quiet way, a very high-quality service. A newly established drug rehabilitation unit is complemented by a well established occupational therapy department.

The school of nursing, which used to train a high calibre of registered psychiatric nurses, closed some years ago. A disused British army military camp, 100 km from the capital, Nairobi, houses several hundred chronically ill people, who have long since lost contact with their families. Some have been in hospital for more than 30 years.

## Services

Kenya has eight provinces, each of which has a 30-bed psychiatric unit. These units are run by nurses and serve the catchment areas of the large provincial hospitals. Most units can prescribe basic drugs, generally limited to chlorpromazine, benzodiazepines, phenobarbitone and occasionally a tricyclic antidepressant. Although highly motivated, the staff, most of whom have worked in these units for many years, lack reading materials or indeed any contact with new knowledge in mental health practices. They are always keen to receive literature that could inform their practice. Most have no concept of mental health needs beyond psychosis and therefore do not diagnose or treat patients with depression or anxiety-related disorders.

Few people with mental disorders attending primary care clinics receive a psychiatric diagnosis. In one study, 45% of people attending a health centre in Nairobi had some form of psychiatric morbidity. All were misdiagnosed. Misdiagnosis is common because many people with a psychological disorder present with physical symptoms. This leads to frequent and unnecessary drug prescriptions and investigations.

## Training

Although poorly resourced, Mathari Hospital is the main training centre for the University of Nairobi's medical and postgraduate students. A unique feature of the undergraduate training programme is the fact that psychiatry is a fully examinable subject taught to yearly classes of approximately 200 medical students. The department, which has 10 members of staff, also provides supervision and teaching to postgraduate students of paediatrics and internal medicine.

Kenya has had an active postgraduate training programme in psychiatry since the 1980s, and most of the psychiatrists in Kenya have obtained their qualifications (Masters of Medicine) from this programme. Following a period of low enrolment, psychiatry has in the last few years become a popular subject of study and currently there are 20 students in the programme. Significantly, this programme has trained many psychiatrists now working in the region. A postgraduate diploma in psycho-trauma is the most recent addition to the training.

A number of local universities have programmes – both undergraduate and postgraduate – for the training of counselling psychologists, which is a very popular area of study, particularly following the 1998 bombing of the American Embassy in Nairobi, which brought mental health issues to the fore (Njenga et al, 2003, 2004). The tragedy had this one definite benefit to mental health.

A child psychiatry clinic was started by the principal author in 1981 at the Kenyatta National Hospital and now treats approximately 500 children per year. This unit serves as the main training venue for psychiatrists and paramedics in child psychiatry. There are, in addition, active if small programmes in private practice as well as active research in the areas of post-traumatic stress disorder and attention-deficit hyperactivity disorder. There are no formal training programmes in psychotherapy.

# Research

Each postgraduate student of psychiatry at the University of Nairobi is required to conduct original research as part of training. There is a great deal of (unpublished) research data available in the department in all fields of psychiatry. A number of recent publications from the department are, however, indicative of the resurgence of the vibrant academic culture which formerly characterised the department (Othieno et al, 2001; Gatere et al, 2002; Maru et al, 2003). The department is a repository of much high-calibre research, spanning several decades, and any student of psychiatry in Africa would be well advised to consult the department before offering an authoritative opinion on African psychiatry.

Other Kenyan psychiatrists are active in research collaboration with international partners (Jenkins et al, 2002; Kiima et al, 2004). One area into which research is currently being undertaken is drug and alcohol misuse. In addition, an epidemiological survey of mental health disorders in a rural district of Kenya has recently been concluded; this was a unique project bringing together the Kenyan government, the Kenya Psychiatric Association and the Institute of Psychiatry in London (a World Health Organization Collaborating Centre) (Jenkins et al, 2002).

# Meetings

The main event for psychiatrists in East Africa is the annual meeting of Eastern Africa psychiatrists, which has taken place in different cities for the last 7 years; these meetings are always well attended and the presentations of great scientific interest. The last, held in Arusha, Tanzania, was attended by the majority of Kenyan psychiatrists and attracted a large variety of presentations, including ones on drug misuse and AIDS, domestic violence, attention-deficit hyperactivity disorder, policy and service delivery. It attracted presentations from the entire region, as well as from the UK, the USA and South Africa. The organisers are always keen to involve people from others parts of the world, as they continue to struggle with the problem in small communities of 'intellectual inbreeding', whereby younger psychiatrists are exposed to the 'wisdom' and experience only of their seniors, which in turn is limited by their own experiences, idiosyncrasies and areas of interest. Exposure to other senior colleagues is often described as liberating and refreshing.

# Mental Health Act

The current Mental Health Act (1989) provides for the establishment of a mental health board, which in theory regulates mental health services in the country. The Act also provides for voluntary and involuntary admission to those hospitals designated for this purpose under the Act. It also prohibits discrimination by insurance companies against persons with a mental illness. Efforts are currently being made to update the Act, in particular in the areas of safeguarding the human rights of people who have a mental illness. This, however, is low on the list of priorities in Kenya.

# International collaboration

The Royal College of Psychiatrists has a role to play in the promotion of mental health in Kenya, ranging from its participation in exchange programmes (to expose both members and the wider Kenyan public to the strengths and weaknesses of the systems in place in the two countries), as well as in its support of joint research programmes. There is much the North can learn from the South, in particular with regard to the utilisation of meagre resources.

Traditional practitioners have skills that are yet to be researched, while drug trials can take place in (natural) settings in Kenya, where patients previously unexposed to medications are still to be found. Being a largely English-speaking population, and being only 8 hours from London by direct flight (21 a week), Kenya is not only a booming tourist destination but, like the nation's long-distance runners, proposes to capture, in the long run, researchers from the UK and other European capitals. Such adventurers will be met with traditional African hospitality, which includes (these days) a mandatory hunting safari (photographic) to any of the game reserves. Sandy beaches on the coast and the snow-capped Mount Kenya come as extras. As we say in Kenya, 'To go is to see'.

# References

Gatere, N., Othieno, C. J. & Kathuku, D. M. (2002) Prevalence of tardive dyskinesia among psychiatric in-patients at Mathari Hospital, Nairobi. *East African Medical Journal*, **79**, 547–549.

Jenkins, R., Goldberg, D., Kiima, D., *et al* (2002) Classification in primary care: experience with current diagnostic systems. *Psychopathology*, **35**, 127–131.

Kiima, D. M., Njenga, F. G., Okonji, M. M., *et al* (2004) A Kenya mental health country profile. *International Review of Psychiatry*, **16**, 48–53.

Maru, H. M., Kathuku, D. M. & Ndetei, D. M. (2003) Substance use among children and young persons appearing in the Nairobi juvenile court, Kenya. *East African Medical Journal*, **80**, 598–602.

Njenga, F. G., Nyamai, C. & Kigamwa, P. (2003) Terrorist bombing at the US Embassy in Nairobi: the media response. *East African Medical Journal*, **80**, 159–164.

Njenga, F. G., Nyamai, C. N., Kigamwa, P. A., *et al* (2004) Psychological reactions following the US Embassy bombing in Nairobi. *British Journal of Psychiatry*, **185**, 328–334.

Othieno, C. J., Okech, V. C., Omondi, J. A., *et al* (2001) How Kenyan physicians treat psychotic disorders. *East African Medical Journal*, **78**, 204–207.

World Bank (2002) *World Development Report*. Washington, DC: World Bank.

# Malawi

## Felix Kauye and Chitsanzo Mafuta

Malawi is a country with an approximate area of 118 000 km². Its population is estimated at 13 million and the gender ratio (men per hundred women) is 98. The proportion of the population under the age of 15 years is 47% and the proportion above the age of 60 years is 5%. The literacy rate is 75.5% for men and 48.7% for women (World Health Organization, 2005).

For administrative purposes, Malawi is divided into three regions, which are further divided into a total of 28 districts. The capital city is Lilongwe, which is situated in the central region, and the main means of travel between the capital and districts is by road.

The main languages used in Malawi are English and Chichewa. The largest ethnic group is Chewa and the other ethnic groups are Nyanja, Tumbuka, Yao, Nkhonde and Ngoni plus the Europeans, Indians and other foreign nationals. The largest religious groups are Christians followed by Muslims.

## Health indicators

Malawi has high rates of infant and maternal mortality rates. The life expectancy at birth is 40 years for both males and females (National Statistical Office of Malawi).

## Health services

There are very few doctors. Clinical officers, medical assistants and enrolled nurses comprise the backbone of Malawian healthcare, but there are shortages of these health personnel, especially in the rural areas, as people prefer to practise in urban areas.

The smallest health unit in Malawi is the 'health post', which is manned by 'health surveillance assistants' (who have 10 weeks' orientation training). Each health post serves a small number of villages. Next in the referral hierarchy is the health centre, which is usually staffed by medical assistants (who have 2 years' training) and nurses. Patients who cannot be treated at the health centre are referred to the district hospitals, which are present in all but 3 of the 28 districts. There are four general tertiary referral hospitals, distributed in all three regions of Malawi, with two in the southern region, which is the biggest.

# Mental health resources and services

Zomba Mental Hospital, which is situated in the southern region, is the only government tertiary psychiatric referral hospital in Malawi. It has 333 beds and on average admits 1500 patients per year. There is a smaller psychiatric unit in the central region, in Lilongwe, with about 30 beds, and this is run as part of Kamuzu Central Hospital, which is the tertiary referral hospital in the central region. Psychiatric patients from the northern region are usually referred to a missionary hospital, St John of God in the city of Mzuzu, which has 50 in-patient beds and which runs an effective community programme. In total there are therefore just over 400 psychiatric beds for the entire population.

The commonest reasons for admission to Zomba Mental Hospital are schizophrenia, bipolar disorders, intellectual disability, epilepsy, and substance-related and HIV-related conditions (according to hospital statistics for the year 2005). Nearly all patients admitted present with severe forms of these conditions.

Mental health services in all the districts fall under the office of the district health officer and the associated expenditure is included in the district's health budget. As with the other general tertiary hospitals, Zomba Mental Hospital has its own budget.

Public psychiatric services fall under clinical services (curative) within the Ministry of Health. The resources in terms of facilities and staffing at the different care levels are summarised in Table 1.

## Staffing

There is only one psychiatrist for the entire population of Malawi, but since he is based in Zomba, the old capital city, the psychiatrist:population ratio is 0 for the rest of the country.

There are no professional social workers and only one occupational therapist, at Zomba Mental Hospital. There are two clinical psychologists attached to the College of Medicine in Malawi, who teach medical students; they do not do any clinical work in the psychiatric hospitals.

The district psychiatric nurses do weekly outreach clinics, visiting different health centres and health posts within their districts; the management team from Zomba Mental Hospital visits each district twice a year to monitor mental health activities throughout the country.

**Table 1** Government mental health facilities at different healthcare levels

| Level | Facilities | Staffing | Services offered |
| --- | --- | --- | --- |
| Tertiary | Zomba Mental Hospital | One psychiatrist One psychiatric clinical officer Twenty psychiatric nurses Five general clinical workers Four general nursing workers One occupational therapist | Long-stay care Forensic services Hospital day care Acute in-patient care Community services Rehabilitation services Occupational therapy Out-patient care |
| Secondary (district hospitals) | Only two have a psychiatric ward | From one to six psychiatric nurses[a] Variable numbers of general clinical and nursing workers | Acute in-patient care Out-patient care Community services Medium-stay care Outreach clinics Referral to Zomba Mental Hospital |
| Primary (district health centres) | No psychiatric wards | General nurses (sometimes enrolled psychiatric nurses) General health workers (clinical/medical officers) | Minimal out-patient care Referral to district hospitals |

a. Psychiatric nurses are often redeployed to general medical and surgical services, resulting in diminished delivery of mental health activities in the district hospitals.

## *World Mental Health Day*

World Mental Health Day is celebrated publicly every year in a selected district. Posters, T-shirts and leaflets explaining mental health issues are distributed to the public for free at the chosen venue. The public's response to this has always been very encouraging.

# Mental health policy and legislation

The old 2000–04 policy is still being used while it is awaiting review. This policy includes the integration of psychiatric services into the primary healthcare system, the appointment of a national mental health coordinator at the Ministry of Health's headquarters and a human resources development plan.

The Mental Treatment Act was enacted in 1959 and amended in 1968. A Mental Health Bill is awaiting review by stakeholders and later parliamentary amendment; it is anticipated that it will be passed in 2007. It compares well with legislation in countries such as South Africa and Kenya, and includes the formation of a mental health review board, which will monitor the care and treatment of psychiatric patients in hospital. It covers areas such as admissions, the rights of in-patients and the safekeeping of patients' property.

# Training

## Undergraduate medical students

There is one medical school, the Malawi College of Medicine, which is part of the University of Malawi, in Blantyre. As part of their MBBS course, students in the third year have 2 weeks of psychiatry theory and in the fourth year they undergo a 5-week rotation in theory and clinical work.

## Other health workers

The two main health sciences colleges offer training of paramedical staff – the clinical officers, medical assistants and enrolled nurses. Clinical officers can go for further training in specific areas and become psychiatric clinical officers, orthopaedic clinical officers and so on. Plans are being finalised to train district primary health workers in the management of common psychiatric disorders. Currently, most primary health workers lack skills in the assessment and management of psychiatric patients and end up referring all those they come across.

## Postgraduate specialisation

The College of Medicine at the University of Malawi has offered postgraduate training only since 2005 in certain specialties, in conjunction with certain universities in South Africa. This does not include psychiatry, so all psychiatric training at present has to be done outside Malawi.

## Psychiatric nurses

The St John of God College of Health Sciences provides a degree in psychiatric nursing for registered state nurses with a minimum of a university diploma in nursing, and the Malawi College of Health Sciences provides a certificate course in psychiatry for enrolled nurses.

# Research

Mental health in Malawi has been the subject of several research projects. These have included studies in psycho-active substances, the teaching of psychiatry in the colleges and attributions for admissions to Zomba Mental Hospital (MacLachlan et al, 1995). More studies are under way or being developed by Zomba Mental Hospital on, for example:

- community attitudes to and knowledge of mental illness
- the prevalence of HIV and neurosyphilis among in-patients
- district mental health activities in southern Malawi, including what proportions of the district budgets are allocated to mental health
- common causes of relapse and readmission in patients with schizophrenia

- pathways to care for psychiatric patients
- neuropsychological sequalae of cerebral malaria.

At the St John of God Hospital a randomised controlled trial of carer education in schizophrenia and bipolar disorders is under way.

In general, there is not much information on mental health in the Malawian context and this provides opportunities and challenges for research.

## Professional organisations

In the past there was a Mental Health Association of Malawi, but it stopped functioning, for unknown reasons, around 1999. At present, a 'core group' is being formed, comprising: the psychiatrist at Zomba Mental Hospital; the clinical psychologist at the Malawi College of Medicine; the chief nursing officer at Zomba Mental Hospital; and the psychiatric clinical officer at the St John of God Hospital. The main goal of this core group is to develop the preliminary constitution of a new professional association and to recruit members. Some of the functions of the association will be:

- to deal with challenges in mental health
- to act as an advisory body to the Medical Council of Malawi on the registration of mental health professionals
- to develop, review and conduct policy for mental health professionals.

There are at present no non-governmental organisations operating in the mental health field in Malawi.

## Challenges

Notable problems include a critical shortage of trained staff and frequent shortages of drugs owing to procurement problems. The referral system is not very good; neither is follow-up care, as most district psychiatric services seem to be insufficiently well developed.

## References

MacLachlan, M., Nyirenda, T. & Nyando C. (1995) Attributions for admission to Zomba Mental Hospital: implications for the development of mental health services in Malawi. *International Journal of Psychiatry*, **41**, 79–87.

National Statistical Office of Malawi. See http://www.nso.malawi.net/data_on_line/demography/census_98/mortality_measures.htm. Last accessed 23 October 2006.

World Health Organization (2005) *Mental Health Atlas 2005*. See http://www.who.int/globalatlas/predefinedReports/MentalHealth/Files/MW_Mental_Health_Profile.pdf. Last accessed 23 October 2006.

# Mauritius

Mridula S. Naga

The Republic of Mauritius is a group of islands in the south-west of the Indian Ocean, consisting of the main island of Mauritius, Rodrigues and several outer islands, situated 900 km to the east of Madagascar. It has a total land area of 2040 km$^2$ and a population of around 1.2 million. Mauritius has a multiracial population whose origins can be traced mainly to Asia, Africa and Europe. English is the official language but French remains the most widely spoken, along with the local dialect, Creole, which is derived from French. Mauritius is classified as an upper middle income country in sub-Saharan Africa by the World Bank. It has a per capita gross domestic product (GDP) of US$13 200.

## Health resources and statistics

Mauritius spends 2.8% of its GDP on health, 1.9% in the public sector and 0.9% in the private sector.

In 2005, the crude birth rate was 15.2 births per 1000 per year, the death rate was 6.8 per 1000 per year and the infant mortality rate was 14.14 deaths per 1000 live births (Central Statistics Office, Mauritius).

Mauritius provides state health services throughout the country free at the point of use to all its 1.2 million people. It also has a well established private sector. The state health services employ over 650 doctors and the private sector employs over 400 doctors.

## Mental health services

Initially, mental health services were centred at the main psychiatric hospital, named after the renowned Mauritius-born neurologist Charles-Édouard Brown-Séquard. It was renamed the Brown Sequard Mental Health Care Centre (BSMHCC) in 1998. Psychiatric services were decentralised in 1997. Essentially, decentralisation meant opening psychiatric units in each regional hospital, combined with the provision of out-patient services and liaison psychiatry. One or two psychiatrists were attached to each unit, along with medical officers and health officers who had work experience in this field.

There are now 15 psychiatrists nationally, 12 in the public sector. In-patient care was started initially in three hospitals to treat patients with alcohol-related problems, but it had to be discontinued in two centres owing to management problems. Out-patient clinics are also held at a few area health centres. Community care is mostly provided by social workers attached to these hospitals and community rehabilitation workers.

In 2005, a new 250-bed psychiatric hospital was built next to the old hospital. Daily out-patient clinics are held and in-patient care is provided for acutely ill psychiatric patients from all over Mauritius. In addition, a secure unit in the premises caters for patients from courts. Another ward opened in 2006 for in-patient detoxification of intravenous drug users.

The BSMHCC is staffed by six psychiatrists, six medical and health officers, a medical superintendent, three social workers, a psychologist and about 40 psychiatric nurses, general nurses, healthcare assistants, welfare assistants (who are mostly in the old hospital) and other ancillary staff.

Many of the 471 long-stay patients still cared for in the old hospital are institutionalised, having spent over 20 years in the hospital. Vigorous efforts are being made to get alternative care for those who can be relocated.

Patients are treated at the regional hospitals or area health centres as out-patients, but if they need admission or electroconvulsive therapy they are referred to the BSMHCC. After recovery they are referred back to the regions for follow-up. This arrangement will have to continue until the regional units are fully functional. Most psychotropic drugs are available in all centres.

## Mental health statistics

The total number of out-patient attendances (new cases and follow-up cases) at the BSMHCC rose from 1998 to 2003 but thereafter decreased to 2005 (Fig. 1a). At the outstations the numbers increased from 1998 to 2005. These statistics indicate that the total number of patients seeking psychiatric help considerably increased over the period. It is interesting to note that the attendance at the main hospital is still high, despite decentralisation, probably because of the lack of in-patient facilities in the regional units. Many of the patients at the main centre suffer from serious mental illnesses.

However, the number of new cases at the outstations are gradually increasing (Fig. 1b). Attending the main psychiatric hospital is still a taboo. Often people do not come forward to seek help because of the stigma attached to mental illness. The rising number of cases in the outstations is the true indicator of psychiatric morbidity in the island.

The number of in-patients increased slightly from 1998 to 2003 followed by a decline to 2005. In 2004 about 35% of admissions at the BSMHCC were for schizophrenia and other psychotic states. About 51% were due to alcohol-related problems.

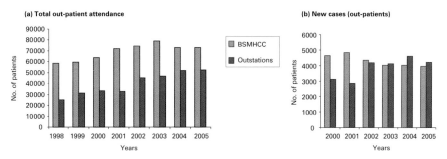

**Fig. 1** (a) Total number of out-patient attendances and (b) numbers of new cases at the Brown-Sequard Mental Health Care Centre (BSMHCC) and regional hospital outstations, 1998–2005.

## Suicide rates

Suicide was on the rise until it reached a peak in 1999 and later declined to 8.1 per 100 000 in 2004.

## Substance misuse

Overall, 41.5% of substances misused were alcohol and 52.9% 'brown sugar' (an adulterated form of heroin).

The National Agency for the Treatment and Rehabilitation of Substance Abusers (NATReSA) is responsible for all demand reduction activities in Mauritius. The National Drug Control Master Plan was formulated in the year 2004 and the Mauritius Epidemiology Network on Drug Use (MENDU) was set up in 2001.

# Legislation and policy

The Mental Health Act was proclaimed in 1998. It deals mainly with involuntary in-patients, although it did make provision for voluntary admission for patients with mental illness. The Act is being amended at present to involve all mental healthcare users and to make provision for community care.

In 2005, a National Strategic Plan for Mental Health was developed and submitted; implementation is awaited. This Plan was developed following a government white paper on health sector development and reform, of December 2002, and in keeping with guidelines from the World Health Organization (WHO). The white paper proposed a National Plan for Mental Health, which was developed in consultation with local specialists and other groups with advice from WHO experts. The National Strategic Plan for Mental Health includes the setting up of fully fledged regional hospitals, community care, rehabilitation services, specialised units (e.g. a child and adolescent unit) and mental health promotion, among other things.

# Health promotion

Health promotion activities have been carried out widely to create awareness regarding mental health in the population, following the National Plan for Mental Health through WHO-funded programmes. A 'focal person' for mental health was appointed who acted as a coordinator for all mental health activities, including health promotion at all levels.

# Training

Training is carried out at different levels.

- Postgraduate training in psychiatry is being given to six doctors with the collaboration of the University of Bordeaux, France. The programme comprises 3 years in Mauritius with regular teaching by visiting French professors and clinical supervision by local psychiatrists followed by 1 year in Bordeaux. After regular assessments and examinations a degree will be awarded. Another batch of six may be trained at a later stage.
- Community physicians and senior medical officers and health officers in the public sector are being given a crash course in psychiatry (under a WHO programme) in order to provide psychiatric services at the primary care level.
- Courses for a diploma in psychiatric nursing are being carried out by the school of nursing.
- House officers are posted for 4 weeks in psychiatric units so as to acquire experience and to try to kindle their interest in this branch of medicine.
- Medical students from the local private medical college are posted for 2 weeks in the psychiatric hospital.
- Community-based rehabilitation workers are given training in psychiatry with the collaboration of the Mauritius Institute of Health.
- A module on psychiatry has been introduced in the training scheme of Non-Communicable Disease (NCD) Staff and Community Nurses, with the ultimate aim of incorporating community psychiatric services in the well established NCD network.
- Occupational therapists and social workers are being trained by the University of Mauritius with psychiatrists also as resource persons.

# Research

## Epidemiological study

An epidemiological study was carried out in the year 2000 by l'Association Septentrionale d'Epidémiologie Psychiatrique (ASEP), the Département d'Information Médicale (DIRM) and l'EPSM Lille Métropole et le Centre Collaborateur de l'Organisation Mondiale de la Santé pour la recherche et la formation en santé mentale de Paris (CCOMS). The Mauritius Institute of

Health and the Ministry of Health and Quality of Life were responsible for carrying out the study locally. The following statistics were presented:

- 22.2% of people interviewed in the study had a mental disorder
- 15% had signs of depression and related disorders
- 10% had signs of neurotic disorders
- 3% had alcohol-related problems
- 3.4% had psychotic states.

## Study on disabilities

A cross-sectional study to detect the number of children with disabilities was carried out in 2003. Of the 2834 children with disability examined, 63.8% had intellectual impairment.

## Joint Child Health Project

A longitudinal study has been carried out in Mauritius from 1972 onwards. Initially it was designed to identify people at risk for schizophrenia and to take preventive measures. Several papers have been published (e.g. Raine *et al*, 2003).

## Study on suicide

In a study on suicide carried out in 1995, the annual suicide rate was reported to be 8 per 100 000 population in the 12- to 20-year age group, 10 per 100 000 for all age groups and 14 per 100 000 in the elderly age group.

# Private sector

Psychiatric services in the private sector are provided by the government psychiatrists on a part-time basis and by three full-time private psychiatrists. There is no provision for involuntary admission in the private sector.

## Non-governmental organisations

There are non-governmental organisations (NGOs) active in the private sector. For example, the only rehabilitation centre for people with serious mental illness is run by an NGO. There are few centres run for people with intellectual disabilities. 'Befrienders' are active and give support to people in distress.

# The way ahead

Psychiatric services have seen tremendous changes in the past 8 years. The Lunacy Act of 1906 was repealed and replaced by the Mental Health Act 1998, which introduced voluntary care for psychiatric patients. With the implementation of the proposed amendments to the law and the dynamic

National Strategic Plan for Mental Health, clear targets have been set. Encouraging public–private partnership is an area to be explored, mainly for rehabilitation and the relocation of long-stay patients. Recruiting the services of relatives as carers with financial incentives is another promising aspect to be looked at, as it will be cost-effective, the state having to spend more to keep the patient in the hospital than in the community. With increased personnel we hope to establish adequate community care and provide comprehensive psychiatric services to the population.

## Sources and references

Raine, A., Mellinghan, K., Lui, J., *et al* (2003) Effects of environmental enrichment on schizotypal personality and antisocial behaviour. *American Journal of Psychiatry*, **160**, 1627–1635.

Republic of Mauritius web portal, http://www.gov.mu (last accessed 19 April 2007).

*US Central Intelligence Agency World Factbook*, https://www.cia.gov/cia/publications/factbook/geos/mp.html (last accessed 19 April 2007).

# Republic of Niger

Julian Eaton, Djibo Douma Maiga and Soumana Pate

The Republic of Niger is a large, landlocked west African country. Around 80% of its vast land mass (1 300 000 km²) is in the Sahara Desert. Its neighbours are Mali, Algeria, Libya and Chad to the north, and Nigeria, Benin and Burkina Faso to the south. The country came under French rule in the 1890s and gained its independence in 1960, but development has been slowed by political instability, lack of natural resources and drought. In 1999, voters overwhelmingly approved a new constitution, allowing for multi-party elections, which were held later that year. An ongoing rebellion in the north makes access to much of the country difficult.

There is a wide diversity of peoples, including nomadic tribes in the north (the Tuareg and Fulani) and settled groups mainly in the south (the Hausa, Zarma and Songhai as well as many others). The majority of the population are Muslim but animist beliefs and ancestor worship are common.

Niger is one of the world's poorest countries, with a gross national income of US$280 per capita in 2007 (World Bank, 2007). The population is estimated at 14.2 million, over half of whom are under 15 years of age (UNICEF, 2008). The majority are subsistence farmers and over 60% of people live on less than US$1 a day. Most of the national export income is derived from uranium mining and cattle-rearing.

Health indicators for Niger are poor. The average life expectancy at birth is 58 years for men and 56 years for women. Niger has the highest fertility rate in the world, with an average of 7.2 births per woman, but infant mortality is also extremely high, and one in four (253/1000) children die before the age of 5 years (UNICEF, 2008). In the year 2000, total health expenditure as a percentage of gross domestic product was 3.7%. Per capita total expenditure on health is US$22, with the government providing US$9 of this total.

## Mental health services

Traditional medicine is the only option available for the majority of the population when they encounter mental or neurological health problems, as there are few modern services outside of the capital city, Niamey. Widely held beliefs that mental illness has a spiritual cause, low levels of literacy, huge distances and poverty are all factors that compound poor access to orthodox psychiatric services.

There are no specialist psychiatric hospitals in the country, but four of the eight regional hospitals have a psychiatry department (Niamey, Tahoua, Zinder and Maradi). There is no specific government budget for mental health other than what is spent in these general hospitals, but even here the budgets for mental health are not fixed. Despite its focus on policy and planning, the World Health Organization (WHO) gives some regular funds for the provision of psychotropic drugs.

Community-based mental health services are currently limited to the activities of one large non-governmental project in Niamey (*Projet de Réadaptation a base communautaire aux Aveugles et autre personnes Handicapées du Niger*, PRAHN). These services mainly consist of occasional outreach 'camps' in remote areas, each requiring several days' travel, rather than a constant presence.

Epilepsy is the most common neuropsychiatric disorder that presents. This reflects the stigma associated with other mental disorders and lack of knowledge about treatability, as well as the positive results of basic treatment for epilepsy.

The availability of psychotropic medication is poor, despite a relatively well organised national medication supply system based on the Bamako initiative (Eaton, 2008). Although in principle this should ensure affordable medication is available, of the basic WHO standard list, only phenobarbital, carbemazepine, chlorpromazine, haloperidol, diazepam, benzhexol and amitriptyline are readily accessible in major hospitals. Beyond these hospitals, only phenobarbital and diazepam are routinely available.

## Human resources

There are five psychiatrists in the country, all of whom work in the general hospital in Niamey. There are around 30 psychiatric nurses and a similar number of psychologists, again mainly in Niamey (WHO, 2005). The psychiatry departments in the other three hospitals are run by nurses, and a few district hospitals have a psychiatric nurse. Some training of general nurses and physicians has taken place but there is anecdotal evidence that people who present with neuropsychiatric disorders are neglected in primary healthcare settings (Cohen, 2001). The basic mental health training for primary care staff is not reinforced by ongoing supervision.

Until recently, all training for doctors and nurses took place outside the country – in Morocco, Senegal or Burkina Faso. Psychiatrists now receive specialist training in a programme based in the Republic of Benin and France, and one is about to finish this training. Four psychiatrists have trained in the past 10 years. Unlike in many surrounding countries, they have generally remained in the country, apart from one who now works for the WHO. A psychiatric nursing school opened in Niger in 2003. Typically, seven or eight specialist nurses graduate from here every 2 years, all of whom are employed in government services.

There is no national mental health professional association, though there are service users' and carers' groups supporting people with epilepsy and intellectual disabilities. There is some professional interaction with other Francophone African countries (e.g. through the West African Health Organisation, WAHO) and French universities have some academic collaboration with Nigerien institutions. The division between Francophone and Anglophone traditions is a significant barrier to accessing information, given that the majority of journals and online resources are in English.

## Research

There has been little systematic epidemiological data collected, but some ethnographic research was carried out in the 1970s and 1980s (Osouf, 1980). A national survey is currently being undertaken by the Ministry of Health as part of the process of policy development and planning.

## National policy and plans

A national mental health policy was formulated in 1993, and a national mental health plan was developed with help from the WHO in 1995, revised in 2000 and 2004 (Ministère de la Santé, 2000). Unfortunately, practical implementation of the plan did not progress beyond some training activities. There has been little long-term impact of the principles of decentralisation of services that formed the core of these policies and plan.

Even with strong advocacy, it is unlikely that there will be adequate funds in the national budget for implementation of a programme unless it is supported by an outside agency. This is in common with other sectors, but the fact that mental health is not specifically mentioned as a Millennium Development Goal makes finding resources more challenging. The integration of mental health as a cross-cutting issue within other areas is one option (Prince et al, 2007), but working towards a specific mental health policy is also important (Jenkins, 2003).

A good relationship is emerging between the government, the WHO country office, and the non-governmental sector (a major healthcare provider in Niger), who are working together to revise the national policy and plan. The ultimate aim of this process is more accessible care, in line with recent international initiatives to scale up services in low- and middle-income countries and to ensure that human rights issues are taken into account (Chisholm et al, 2007). The national plan also incorporates participation of service users and other stakeholders in order to ensure that the process has a meaningful impact on their quality of life.

A pilot programme of service delivery following the latest evidence-based guidelines (Thornicroft & Tansella, 2004) is in development; it integrates a modified community-based rehabilitation model (Chatterjee *et al*, 2003) into primary care. This takes into account the importance of the non-governmental sector in a country like Niger. If successful, the pilot will be replicated nationwide.

# References

Chatterjee, S., Patel, V., Chatterjee, A., *et al* (2003) Evaluation of a community-based rehabilitation model for chronic schizophrenia in rural India. *British Journal of Psychiatry*, **182**, 57–62.

Chisholm, D., Flisher, A. J., Lund, C., *et al* (2007) Scale up services for mental disorders: a call for action. *Lancet*, **370**, 1241–1252.

Cohen, A. (2001) *The Effectiveness of Mental Health Services in Primary Care: The View from the Developing World*. WHO.

Eaton, J. (2008) Ensuring access to psychotropic medication in sub-Saharan Africa. *African Journal of Psychiatry*, **11**, 179–181.

Jenkins, R. (2003) Supporting governments to adopt mental health policies. *World Psychiatry*, **2**, 14–19.

Ministère de la Santé (2000) *Programme National de Sante Mentale* [National Programme of Mental Health.] Ministère de la Santé.

Osouf, P. (1980) Regard sur l'assistance psychiatrique au Niger [On psychiatric assistance in Niger.] *Psychopathologie Africaine (Dakar)*, **16**, 249–279.

Prince, M., Patel, V., Saxena, S., *et al* (2007) No health without mental health. *Lancet*, **370**, 859–877.

Thornicroft, G. & Tansella, M. (2004) Components of a modern mental health service: a pragmatic balance of community and hospital care. Overview of systematic evidence. *British Journal of Psychiatry*, **185**, 283–290.

UNICEF (2008) *Country statistics*. At http://www.unicef.org/infobycountry/niger_statistics.html (accessed 15 December 2008).

World Bank (2007) *World development indicators database*. At http://www.worldbank.org/datastatistics (accessed 15 December 2008).

WHO (2005) *Atlas. Mental Health Resources in the World*. World Health Organization.

# Nigeria

Oye Gureje

Nigeria is a huge country. It covers an area of 924 000 km² on the west coast of Africa. It has a population of about 110 million, which means that every one in six Africans is a Nigerian. It is a country of diverse ethnicity, with over 200 spoken languages, even though three of those are spoken by about 60% of the population. Administratively, it is divided into 36 states and operates a federal system of government, with constitutional responsibilities allocated to the various tiers of government – central, state and local. There are two main religions, Islam (predominantly in the north) and Christianity (predominantly in the south). However, a large proportion of the people still practise traditional religions exclusively or in addition to either Islam or Christianity.

In spite of its abundant natural and human resources, Nigeria is still a poor country, and nowhere is that status indicated better than in its health indices. About 170 out of every 1000 children die before the age of 5 years and life expectancy is 46.8 years for men and 48.2 years for women (World Health Organization, 2000). It spends about 3% of its gross domestic product on health (World Health Organization, 2001) and in a rating of the overall health performance of all 191 member states of the World Health Organization in 2000, Nigeria was ranked 187 (World Health Organization, 2000).

## A brief history

Available records suggest that the first asylum had been established in the southern city of Calabar by 1904. It was followed by the Yaba asylum, also in the south, which was opened in 1907 with 48 patients. Before that, some patients with mental illness were sent to Sierra Leone. However, the seeking of orthodox care for mental illness must have been very uncommon at the time, for a British army physician claimed in 1845 that insanity was rare in Nigeria (Anumonye, 1976). The asylums relied on the services of general medical officers, since there were no psychiatrists and those there were provided essentially custodial management.

When the Aro Mental Hospital was opened in Abeokuta in 1954, it was to respond to the need for improved mental healthcare identified by the British colonial government. Since Dr Thomas Adeoye Lambo had arrived back in the country from England in 1952, the establishment of Aro Mental Hospital was also an opportunity to make the best use of the services of this first Nigerian psychiatrist. The hospital, later to be known as the Aro Neuropsychiatric Hospital, was to play a central role in the development of psychiatry in Nigeria (Asuni, 1967, 1972).

## Clinical practice

From a total of 5 in 1963, 25 in 1975 and 35 in 1981, today there are about 100 psychiatrists working in Nigeria (Jegede, 1981). Most of these are based in departments of psychiatry in the 12 medical schools and the eight psychiatric hospitals in the country. The provision of psychiatric beds amounts to about 0.4 per 10 000 persons, while that of both psychologists and social workers is 0.02 per 100 000 persons (World Health Organization, 2001). Thus, the country is severely underserved in these respects. Psychiatric care is almost entirely located within the public health sector – there is virtually no private psychiatric practice in the country. Since the available resources are also all located in urban centres and predominantly in the southern parts of the country, some sections of the community experience an even worse shortage of resources than others.

Traditional antipsychotic drugs and tricyclic antidepressants are available and relatively affordable. However, the newer formulations are either unavailable or too expensive for most of those in need. For example, a month's supply of risperidone would cost more than twice the minimum monthly wage in the public service.

Traditional healing practices and faith healing, much of which are poorly understood and some of which are quite clearly harmful, are the common resort. The lay view of mental illness is generally still rooted in supernatural beliefs; moreover, given the restricted access to adequate orthodox psychiatric care, few members of the public get even a chance to be convinced of its effectiveness.

## Training

The first generation of Nigerian psychiatrists – those who trained in the early 1960s – received their training almost exclusively in England or Scotland. Most started off with an introduction to the field in Nigeria and, with encouragement and support from Dr Lambo, completed their training in the UK. In later years, Nigerian psychiatrists also trained in places such as North America and Australia (Jegede, 1981).

Most of the psychiatrists currently working in the country received their training locally. The West African Postgraduate Medical College, part of the

West African Health Community, was constituted in 1976. Incorporating Anglophone countries in the West African sub-region (i.e. Nigeria, Ghana, Liberia, Sierra Leone and Gambia), it regulates and conducts postgraduate diploma examinations (termed 'fellowship' examinations) for specialist qualifications. Soon after its inauguration, the West African Postgraduate Medical College was complemented by the National Postgraduate Medical College, which was established by a Nigerian government decree in 1979. The Faculties of Psychiatry of both Colleges run broadly similar courses of training that span a minimum of 4 years. The examinations are conducted in three stages: primary (mainly basic sciences and psychology), part I (consisting of clinical, written and oral examinations) and part II (consisting a supervised research project, the results of which are reported in a bound dissertation and *a viva*). In practice, the average time taken to complete training is 5 years.

Traditionally, attracting doctors to psychiatry had been difficult. Poor conditions of service in the public sector made it unattractive and led doctors to seek specialisation in areas where lucrative private practice could be expected. Psychiatry was and is still not one of these. However, with the recent improvement in the conditions of service for doctors in the public health service, the number of doctors wishing to specialise in psychiatry has increased dramatically in the past few years. Currently, there are about 110 doctors at various stages of training. Whether improved service conditions will also translate into better retention of psychiatrists in the country is not yet clear. Many trainee psychiatrists have obtained training positions overseas (particularly in the UK) in the past and have not shown a willingness to return home to practise after qualifying.

## Research

The contribution of Nigerian psychiatrists to the international psychiatric literature contrasts with their small number on the ground and the general lack of institutionalised support for research in the country. Nigerian psychiatry is known to many for the influential work of Dr Lambo on the Aro village treatment system and his pioneering community epidemiological study (Leighton *et al*, 1963). It is also known for its involvement in such landmark studies as the International Pilot Study of Schizophrenia, the 10-country study of the incidence and manifestations of schizophrenia and, more recently, the Psychological Problems in General Health Care project.

Part of the reason for this is the strong academic orientation of Nigerian psychiatry, with most professionals working at some point in their careers in universities. However, beyond these remarkable achievements, the range of research activities is actually relatively narrow. Most are small-scale surveys and descriptive clinical studies. Many of these address subjects such as drug use in schools and phenomenological studies of psychoses, among others. Intervention studies are rare and cohort studies few. Research addressing special groups such as children and the elderly is very much in its infancy.

# Mental health policy

The first mental health policy for the country was launched in 1991 (Federal Ministry of Health, 1991). Its laudable 14 declarations include:

> The mental health policy shall be based on the national philosophy of social justice and equity.
>
> Individuals with mental, neurological and psychological disorders shall have the same rights to treatment and support as those with physical illness and shall be treated in health facilities as close as possible to their own community. No person shall suffer discrimination on account of mental illness.

It also recommends a revision of laws relating to the mentally ill in Nigerian statutes. The policy is backed with a National Mental Health Programme and Action Plan, which, unfortunately, has hardly been implemented.

The legal provisions in the Nigerian statutes are obsolete. For example, the country still operates within the framework of the Lunacy Act Cap. 112 (Cap. 81 Lagos) of 1916, which in turn was based on the Lunacy Acts 1890–1908 of the United Kingdom. Accordingly, the Act recommends certification for 'lunatics', including 'an idiot or any person of unsound mind'. These provisions fail to recognise the present-day view of severe mental disorders as treatable conditions, or to give special consideration for actions that breach the laws of the land but that are committed when the individual is unable to make a reasoned judgement. However, there is some hope that, in the new democratic political dispensation, there may be some positive changes, as attempts at revising these laws are currently under way.

# Professional groups

The Association of Psychiatrists in Nigeria, formed in 1969 at a meeting in Ibadan attended by seven members, has grown such that there are now over 130 members and associate members. Its annual general and scientific meeting has become an established annual event. The Association was a strong member of the now defunct African Psychiatric Association. Several of its members were also instrumental in the formation and nurturing of the *African Journal of Psychiatry*, which, unfortunately, is also now defunct. Indeed, the involvement of Nigerian psychiatrists in international professional associations started with the organisation in 1961 of the first Pan-African Psychiatric Conference by Dr Lambo. Participants at the conference had come from several African countries, as well as Europe and North America. Currently, Nigerian psychiatrists are fully involved in the activities of the World Psychiatric Association and newly established Association of African Psychiatrists and Allied Workers.

Several Nigerian psychiatrists are members or fellows of the Royal College of Psychiatrists. At present, there is no organised forum for them in which to meet and deliberate on College affairs, even though Nigerian members and fellows are often present at the annual College conference. The story is different for Nigerian psychiatrists working in the UK. Several of these have played active roles in the activities of the College and some have held important leadership positions in training and examination programmes.

# References

Anumonye, A. (1976) *Nigerian Mental Health Directory*. Lagos: LUTH/College of Medicine of the University of Lagos Press.

Asuni, T. (1967) Aro Mental Hospital in perspective. *American Journal of Psychiatry*, **124**, 763–770.

Asuni, T. (1972) Psychiatry in Nigeria over the years. *Nigerian Medical Journal*, **2**, 54–58.

Federal Ministry of Health (1991) *The National Mental Health Policy in Nigeria*. Lagos: Federal Ministry of Health.

Jegede, R. O. (1981) Nigerian psychiatry in perspective. *Acta Psychiatrica Scandinavica*, **63**, 45–56.

Leighton, A. H., Lambo, T. A., Hughes, C. C., *et al* (1963) *Psychiatric Disorder Among the Yoruba – A Report from the Cornell-Aro Mental Health Research Project in the Western Region, Nigeria*. Ithaca, NY: Cornell University Press.

World Health Organization (2000) *The World Health Report 2000*. Geneva: WHO.

World Health Organization (2001) *Atlas: Country Profile of Mental Health Resources*. Geneva: WHO.

# Uganda

Fred Kigozi

Uganda is a landlocked developing country in East Africa with an estimated population of 24.8 million people (2002 census). At independence (in 1962) Uganda was a very prosperous and stable country, with enviable medical services in the region. This, however, was destroyed by a tyrant military regime and the subsequent civil wars up to 1986, when the current government took over the reigns of power.

The 2000/2001 Uganda Demographic and Health Survey (UDHS) and the 2002 census report revealed several poor demographic and health indicators. The data showed a high population growth rate (in excess of 3% per annum) due to the high fertility rate, estimated at seven children per woman. The age structure is therefore young, with about half the population below 15 years of age. The infant mortality rate was 88 per 1000 live births and maternal mortality rate 50.4 per 10000 live births. Life expectancy was 43 years. Gross domestic product (GDP) per capita was around US$300.

By the mid-1980s, the economy had been destroyed and many of the medical personnel had left the country. The net effect was the current low GDP and poor health indices, which, however, have gradually improved over the last decade or so. The continuing civil wars in the north and north-eastern parts of the country continue to drain valuable national resources, and the affected areas have very poor socio-demographic and health indices. The net effect has been a dilapidated infrastructure and psychosocial problems, mainly manifesting as post-traumatic stress disorders.

Uganda is one of the countries in sub-Saharan Africa that was hard hit by the HIV/AIDS epidemic; however, with a sound government strategy and a timely response, HIV infection has been reduced from a prevalence of 20–28% in the mid-1980s to the current 5.6%. Uganda stands as one of the few developing countries that has succeeded in reversing the tide of the HIV epidemic (UNAIDS, 2004).

## Health reforms

The government has developed a new health policy (1999) and health sector strategic plan (2000), for which primary healthcare (PHC) was the basic philosophy and strategy for national health development, so that equitable services could be offered to the population. The policy emphasises a strong partnership approach between the public and private sectors, non-governmental organisations (NGOs) and traditional practitioners, while safeguarding the identity of each stakeholder. Under the health policy, a basic minimum healthcare package was formulated, in which mental health was a key element, to be delivered at all levels of the health service.

Brief history of mental health services

Uganda has been offering some care for people with a mental illness since the 1920s. Initially these were rudimentary services based on custodial confinement in the south-western part of the country. Better care was started in the capital, Kampala, in the 1930s, followed by modern psychiatric services at the then newly built national referral psychiatric hospital, Butabika Hospital, on the outskirts of the capital in the mid-1950s.

## Mental health programme and services

The current challenges to Ugandan psychiatry and the delivery of mental health services include the continued civil wars in the north and north-eastern parts of the country (where the prevalence of post-traumatic stress disorders is very high) and the psychosocial effects of HIV/AIDS (Boardman & Ovuga, 1997). There is rapid migration of people to urban areas but no corresponding job opportunities. The poverty levels and illiteracy rates are high as well. Consequently, the country experiences a high burden of psychosocial problems in addition to traditional mental health disorders. However, the government attaches great importance to improving mental health services so as to address the burden of mental health problems.

The mental health programme was formulated in 1996 and revised in 2000, following the above health reforms. Its main objective is to provide improved access to primary mental health services for the entire population and to ensure ready access to quality mental health referral services at district, regional and national levels. The strategy incorporates both a remodelling of the infrastructure and the provision of the required human resources through the training of specialists and retraining of general health workers.

Mental health services have been decentralised and also integrated within the general healthcare delivery systems and primary healthcare. The result has been a structure that promotes equity of access by all Ugandan citizens to some mental health interventions, including preventive and rehabilitative services. The process encourages orderly referrals from village level (health centre I), through parish (health centre II), sub-county (health centre III) and county (health centre IV) to district hospitals and regional referral hospitals up to the national referral teaching hospitals at Butabika and Mulago.

At the lower levels (up to the district hospital), clients requiring mental health services are generally managed together in an integrated way, with all other patients, at both out-patient and in-patient facilities. Specialisation and separation begin at the regional referral hospitals, where both physicians and psychiatric clinical officers are usually available. At the regional referral hospitals, 22–32 beds are available, as are an out-patient department and community outreach services.

At the apex of mental healthcare delivery are Butabika and Mulago hospitals, and the Division of Mental Health at the Ministry of Health. Butabika Hospital is the national referral mental hospital, and therefore offers tertiary mental health services. These include curative, preventive and rehabilitative psychiatric services. Mulago is the national referral general hospital. It has a 50-bed psychiatric ward run by the department of psychiatry, which offers active in-patient and out-patient care. There is also a consultation–liaison psychiatric service in the general wards. The Division of Mental Health at the Ministry of Health headquarters, headed by a principal medical officer, coordinates all the mental health activities in the country.

There is, though, an imbalance in the deployment of specialist personnel. All 18 psychiatrists are deployed in the capital city, save for one at Mbarara University. The situation is the same for the few psychologists and psychiatric social workers in the country. This is in the process of being revised: a policy has been developed to post those psychiatrists and social workers who are about to complete their postgraduate courses to all 11 regional mental health units.

In addition to the above government structure is a large support system throughout the country based on NGO health facilities (hospitals and dispensaries) as well as non-facility NGOs. These are encouraged and supported to offer mental health services within their catchment areas, such as supportive psychotherapy and counselling services, in addition to the usual treatment programmes.

All psychiatric patients seen in the public sector receive free psychiatric services, including the basic psychiatric drugs.

Because of stigma and discrimination in the past, many Ugandans had been denied mental healthcare by their relatives or carers and the system, which was not welcoming. This is no longer tolerated. Mental health advocacy is offered by several consumer organisations, and this is gradually coming to play a significant role, though its effect is still generally seen only in urban areas.

## Psychiatric education and research

Psychiatric education in Uganda started in the early 1960s, with the training of psychiatric nurses initially at enrolled level and later at registered level. This was done at Butabika Hospital, to which the School of Psychiatric Nursing was attached. In the late 1960s, the University department of psychiatry was started at Makerere Medical School, where much research was undertaken. The education of undergraduate medical students has, since then, continued with guided transformation. Psychiatric postgraduate training started in 1974. Recently, a new medical school was opened in western Uganda and its department of psychiatry offers undergraduate psychiatric teaching.

Undergraduate training at the universities offers opportunity for students undertaking the MB ChB degree to learn behavioural sciences in the first and second years, and theoretical and practical psychiatry in the third year to fifth years, with 10 weeks' resident clerkship during the fourth year. The clerkship offers clinical skills training, with supervised interviews, case presentations, ward rounds, tutorials and so on. Administrative psychiatry and the management of psychiatric problems within primary healthcare are also covered.

Postgraduate training in psychiatry has been ongoing at Makerere Medical School but with relatively few enrolments, as most resident doctors have preferred to specialise in other branches of medicine. This situation has begun to change in recent years. Enrolment is open to holders of the MB ChB degree, who must have completed their internship and had at least one year's experience as a practising doctor. Postgraduate training is a 3-year full-time programme leading to the award of a master of medicine degree in psychiatry (MMed Psych). It is designed to produce skilled specialists who are able to offer specialised mental health services. It also teaches students to provide leadership skills in community mental health services.

The postgraduate programme is organised in semesters. There are two semesters per year, and there are recess semesters in the first and second years. Much of the training involves clinical apprenticeship, whereby each student is required to carry out psychiatric interviews, do investigations, and to offer treatment and psychotherapy under supervision. The other methods of teaching are lectures, tutorials, interactive discussions and individual study, assignments, seminars and case presentations. Courses are offered in: advanced anatomy, neuropathology, and psychopharmacology, as well as experimental psychology, medical sociology and anthropology, clinical neurology, and health systems management. Also taught are child and adolescent psychiatry, critical skills appraisal, clinical skills and phenomenology. Courses are also offered in psychological therapies, forensic/administrative psychiatry, organic psychiatry, old age psychiatry, addiction psychiatry, community psychiatry, general adult psychiatry and consultation–liaison psychiatry. Research methods and epidemiology are also taught.

The child and adolescent psychiatry course for postgraduates teaches clinical description, aetiology, recognition, diagnosis and specialist management of the various psychiatric disorders encountered among children and adolescents. The course covers practical skills, including investigations, psychotherapy, drug treatment and mental health promotion in children and adolescents.

The course on psychological therapies teaches the principles and practice of psychological methods of treatment in general terms, but also highlights specific psychotherapies found to be relevant to Uganda (i.e. behavioural therapy, marital therapy, family therapy, supportive psychotherapy and child psychotherapy). Classical psychoanalysis is covered theoretically.

Research in psychiatry has been undertaken over the years in epidemiology, clinical psychiatry and social psychiatry. Current research areas include the epidemiology of suicide in Uganda, prenatal depression, psychosocial effects among the displaced population in northern Uganda, and alcohol and drug use among the secondary-student population in the central region of Uganda (to mention but a few). There is also collaborative research being undertaken in HIV/AIDS with Case Western Reserve University.

## Psychiatric association

The Uganda Psychiatric Association (UPA) has been in existence since 1996 and members have regularly met at its scientific congresses, sometimes with other regional associations. Membership includes all psychiatrists practising in Uganda, while other mental health workers, such as psychiatric clinical officers, psychologists and psychiatric social workers, have been accorded associate membership status. The UPA carries out a number of education activities and anti-stigma programmes, in collaboration with mental health consumer groups and NGOs, such as Mental Health Uganda, the Uganda Epilepsy Support Association and the Uganda Schizophrenia Fellowship.

The UPA is a member of the World Psychiatric Association (WPA) and its current President is also the WPA representative for Zone 14 (Eastern and Southern Africa) to the WPA executive committee.

## Mental health law reform

Uganda has had a Mental Health Act since independence in 1962; it was revised in 1964. The main emphasis was custodial care, safeguarding the security of patients and the public, and the protection of the property of people who have a mental illness. The Act is currently being reviewed by a select ministerial committee, to bring it in line with modern mental health legislation. Two members of this team attended a series of workshops on mental health legislation organised by the World Health Organization (WHO) in North Africa and Geneva. The new Bill has as its guiding principle the human rights of those who are mentally ill, including privacy, consent to treatment and conditions for involuntary admission. It gives experts a bigger role in decision making based on professional psychiatric assessment, without compromising the rights of the patient. It establishes an independent mental health tribunal, a national mental health coordination committee and district mental health coordinating committees. The role of the judiciary and the police is clearly defined. The passing of this Bill will greatly enhance psychiatric care and safeguard the rights of people who are mentally ill.

# Conclusions

- Uganda is a low-income country that has recently begun to emerge from decades of civil strife and wars.
- It has a high level of poverty and low literacy rates, as well as a high proportion of young people.
- There is a significant burden of mental health problems, worsened by the psychosocial effects of civil wars and the HIV/AIDS pandemic.
- Health reforms in the past 5 years or so, together with formulation of the national mental health policy, have led to a sizeable investment in education and training as well as infrastructure in the mental health sector.
- The challenges that remain concern: the integration of mental health into primary healthcare, which has to overcome some resistance and issues of stigma; the inadequate number of specialists (psychiatrists, clinical psychologists, psychiatric social workers); the limited availability of newer psychiatric drugs; mental health promotion and prevention; improved education and training in psychiatry; and the limited awareness of mental health consumers of their rights.

# References and further reading

Boardman, J. & Ovuga, E. B. L. (1997) Rebuilding psychiatry in Uganda. *Psychiatric Bulletin*, **21**, 649–655.

Bolton, P., Bass, J., Neugebauer, R., *et al* (2003) Group interpersonal psychotherapy for depression in rural Uganda: a randomized controlled trial. *Journal of the American Medical Association*, **289**, 3117–3124.

Kigozi, F., Kinyanda, E. & Kasirye, R. (1999) Street children in Uganda: a product and a high risk group for HIV/AIDS. *Southern African Journal of Child and Adolescent Mental Health*, **2.**

Kinyanda, E. (1998) Frequency with which psychiatric disorder is associated with a positive HIV-1 serostatus as seen in persons attending a TASO clinic in Mulago. *South Africa Medical Journal*, **88**, 1178.

Kinyanda, E. & Musisi, S. (2001) War traumatisation and its psychological consequences on the women of Gulu district. In *Medical Interventional Study of War Affected Gulu District, Uganda*. Kampala: ISIS-WICCE.

Kinyanda, E., Hejelmeland, H. & Musisi, S. (2004) Deliberate self-harm as seen in Kampala, Uganda: a case–control study. *Social Psychiatry and Psychiatric Epidemiology*, **39**, 318–325.

Musisi, S. & Kinyanda, E. (2000) *Psychiatric Problems of HIV/AIDS and Their Management in Uganda. A Book for Primary Health Care Workers*. Kampala: STIP/Ministry of Health.

Musisi, S., Kinyanda, E., Leibling, H., *et al* (1998) The psychological consequences of war traumatisation on women of Luwero district, Uganda. In *Short Term Intervention of the Psychological and Gynaecological Consequences of Armed Conflict in Luwero District*. Kampala: ISIS-WICCE.

Musisi, S., Tugumisirize, J., Kinyanda, E., *et al* (2001) Psychiatric consultation liaison at Mulago Hospital, Kampala Uganda. *Makerere University Medical School Journal*, **35**, 4–11.

UNAIDS (2004) *4th Report on the Global AIDS Epidemic*. Geneva: UNAIDS.

# Zambia

## Jedrin Ngungu and Julian Beezhold

Zambia, previously called Northern Rhodesia, was a colony of Great Britain until 1964, when it gained independence and changed its name. It is a landlocked country located in southern Africa and shares its borders with Zimbabwe, Namibia, Botswana, Mozambique, Malawi, Tanzania, Congo and Angola. It has an area of 752 612 km², about three times the size of Britain, but a population of only 12 million.

The country is divided into nine provinces for administrative purposes, each with a provincial headquarters. Although there are 72 languages spoken in Zambia, there are seven main ones: Nyanja, Bemba, Lunda, Luvale, Kaonde, Lozi and Tonga. The official language is English, which is spoken by most citizens. Zambia is largely a youthful country, with 90% of its population less than 45 years old; only 2% are over 65.

## Policy and legislation

Since 1992, the country has had five national development plans; the latest was the Fifth National Development Plan (FNDP) in 2006. In the first four plans, there was no mention of mental health. There is only a casual mention in the FNDP, in which the health agenda is dominated by infectious diseases (HIV, tuberculosis, malaria and diarrhoeal diseases) followed by child health and reproductive health. The strategy for mental health is less than coherent.

Zambia still uses the 1951 Mental Disorders Act in which patients are referred to as idiots, imbeciles and invalids. Since the early 2000s, there has been some effort to reform the Act and this reached the stage of a parliamentary draft bill in 2006. However, the draft bill is far from perfect as it is not based on the United Nations human rights charter, which is the bedrock of most current mental health legislation. The limited availability of mental health professionals to spearhead this agenda has contributed to the lack of progress. It has to be said, however, that there is almost no recourse to the Act in clinical practice, as most people are too ignorant to challenge their detention for treatment against their will.

## Personnel

Zambia has only three psychiatrists for a population of 12 million. Two of these are not in clinical practice but are attached to the local university. There are no graduate psychologists, occupational therapists or mental health social workers. The bulk of the work in mental health is carried out by clinical officers, who are specially trained medical assistants (see below).

## Infrastructure and services

Zambia has only one psychiatric hospital, Chainama Hills Hospital, which is based in the capital city of Lusaka. It was opened in 1962 as a national referral centre. It has a capacity of 500 beds, divided into 380 general adult and 120 forensic. It is modelled after the asylums that characterised English mental healthcare more than 50 years ago. The wards are large halls with many patients in each. The beds are usually just mattresses placed on the floor.

Apart from Chainama, there are smaller units, called annexes, in seven provincial headquarters: Ndola, Mansa, Kasama, Kabwe, Chipata, Mongu and Livingstone. These provide a few extra beds and are staffed by clinical officers and psychiatric nurses.

In Zambia, therapy almost exclusively comprises the use of psychotropics; talking therapies are non-existent. However, this is not as problematic as it might be, given that almost all admissions are for psychotic illness (mostly acute psychotic episode, followed by schizophrenia and bipolar disorders). It is rare to see patients with depression unless they have psychotic symptoms as well. The country has no specific forensic, drug and alcohol or children's services.

## Education and training

The University of Zambia's School of Medicine is the country's only medical school. It produces 40 graduates every year, half of whom never practise locally but leave the country. Whereas there is postgraduate training in surgery, medicine, paediatrics and obstetrics and gynaecology, there is no such training in psychiatry. To become a psychiatrist, one has to go abroad and herein lies one of Zambia's problems: the few who go for such training rarely return. (There are at least six Zambian psychiatrists working abroad.)

Similarly, there is no graduate training for psychologists, social workers or occupational therapists. What is available is training for psychiatry clinical officers and nurses. This is based at Chainama Hills College of Health Sciences, which is located in Lusaka just adjacent to Chainama Hospital. Clinical officers are the mainstay of mental health services in Zambia. These are medical assistants who spend 3 years studying medicine before graduating to work in general medicine. After about a year, some of the clinical officers return to Chainama College for an extra year, to become psychiatry clinical officers.

# Challenges and way forward

## Government policy and legislation

While some progress has been made in putting forward the mental health agenda for government policy, much remains to be done to convince not only government but also parliament of the importance of a robust mental health policy and infrastructure. Successful lobbying cannot be achieved by locals alone but requires the help of international partners such as the World Health Organization and the World Psychiatric Association.

## Human resources

There is a serious deficit of trained personnel in the medical field. This is even more pronounced in mental health. Zambia needs more psychiatrists just to help build capacity in the mental health services, let alone to run such services. There is also a need for other mental health professionals, including psychologists and occupational therapists. To address this deficit, local training must be developed. Training people overseas, as has been proved over the years, is not a viable option. The establishment of training facilities will be expensive, nonetheless.

## Infrastructure

There is a need to have mental health beds in every district. Every district has a general hospital and, to keep costs down, some of these could be allocated to psychiatry.

## Stigma

High levels of stigma exist not only against those who are mentally ill but also against their families and those working in the mental health services. Many patients are disowned by their families. Most long-stay patients in Chainama Hospital have no contact with their family members. The 'out of sight out of mind' mentality is prevalent.

Public awareness campaigns are needed. These could be targeted at schools, colleges, workplaces and other public areas. One or two charities are trying but, with limited capacity, little is being achieved. The government may decide to make this one of the priorities for mental health. It is certainly an achievable goal which, unlike the above, does not require massive funding.

# Sources

Haworth, A. (1988) Psychiatry in Zambia. *Bulletin of the Royal College of Psychiatrists*, **12**, 127–129.

Mayeya, J., Chazulwa, R., Mayeya, P. N., *et al* (2004) Zambia mental health country profile. *International Review of Psychiatry*, **16**, 63–72.

Mwanza, J., Sikwese, A., Banda, M., *et al* (2008) *Phase 1 Country Report. Mental Health Policy Development and Implementation in Zambia: A Situation Analysis*. WHO. Available at http://www.who.int/mental_health/policy/development/Zambia%20Country%20report.pdf (last accessed January 2009).

# Zimbabwe

## Walter Mangezi and Dixon Chibanda

Zimbabwe is a landlocked country which has recently emerged from some marked political and socioeconomic challenges. Against this background, mental health has fallen down the priority list, as matters such as food shortages and the AIDS scourge have taken precedence. Zimbabwe is in southern Africa; Zambia and Botswana lie to the north, Namibia to the west, South Africa to the south and Mozambique to the east. Its population is 11.4 million. The capital city is Harare, which has a population of 1.6 million.

## Recent health service history

Zimbabwe had centralised health services prior to 1980. In 1984 a project was set up to decentralise health services by upgrading the infrastructure. Each of the country's nine provinces had a provincial hospital built or refurbished. The provinces are subdivided into districts, and district hospitals were also built or refurbished. In each district there are smaller hospitals, called health centres. In the community, local clinics were built within a radius of 10 km of all households. A referral system was put in place where patients accessed treatment at clinics and were referred via the different levels of services up to the central hospitals. Unfortunately, there was pressure to reduce public spending and the projects had to be abandoned before completion. Each of the provincial hospitals was supposed to have a psychiatric unit and the district hospitals psychiatric beds. The project was abandoned before this could be achieved. The problem was made worse with the political and socioeconomic crisis which began in 2000. Psychiatric nurses began to emigrate in large numbers and health services gradually became centralised again. Mental health services were once free for all but this became unsustainable as the country's economy contracted. Social workers were then used to determine who had the means to pay hospital fees and who would be given permission to access free mental health services. The country's economy is now showing signs of stability and the process of decentralisation is being re-implemented. Mental health services are free again in all government facilities.

# Mental health services

There are six public institutions with psychiatric beds: Harare Hospital Psychiatric Unit, Parirenyatwa Hospital Annexe, Ingutsheni Hospital, Mpilo Hospital Psychiatric Unit, Ngomahuru Hospital and Mutare Hospital Sakubva Unit. In addition, three facilities provide forensic psychiatry services: Mlondolozi Special Institution, Harare Central Prison and Chikurubi Special Institution. The facilities available are not suitable for children or the elderly. Parirenyatwa Hospital Annexe and Harare Hospital Psychiatric Unit are the only institutions with a psychiatrist.

The staff of Zimbabwe's mental health services comprise: a deputy director, a mental health manager and nine provincial mental health coordinators, plus seven psychiatrists – one working for the government, two for the medical school and the others in private practice. They all work in Harare. The country welcomes any foreign English-speaking psychiatrists on condition they are registered and licensed with the Zimbabwe Medical and Dental Council. The only challenge is the low remuneration. Foreign psychiatrists can assist the university by identifying a project sponsored by a donor or research project.

The country has one child psychiatrist, who is in the private sector. All the psychiatrists belong to the Zimbabwe College of Psychiatrists, which discusses issues related to mental health in the country and administers continuing medical education (CME) for psychiatrists and other medical practitioners. The College has no formal links with other psychiatric associations in the region or further abroad, but works with the Zimbabwe Therapist Association, whose membership comprises psychologists and counsellors.

The primary healthcare clinics serve psychiatric patients. They screen psychiatric patients, refer them to the psychiatric hospitals and are involved in follow-up (mainly resupply of medication).

In addition, some non-governmental organisations (NGOs) offer mental health services. The main one is the Zimbabwe National Association for Mental Health (ZIMNAMH), which represents the interests of people with mental illness. It was founded in 1981 and has been the main vehicle for advocacy for mental health services. The Association has been involved in rehabilitation; its main project is based at Tirivanhu Farm. Amani Trust is an organisation which helps torture victims and promotes human rights. There are also organisations that look at the psychosocial issues of HIV/ AIDS.

In the informal sector, the Zimbabwe National Traditional Healers Association (ZINATHA) has a big role in the management of psychosomatic and anxiety disorders. ZINATHA has attempted to educate its members in the referral of patients with mental health problems to the formal sector. Unfortunately, there has not been much collaboration between the formal and informal sectors. Psychiatrists could do more in the training of traditional healers.

## Training

There is one medical school, at the University of Zimbabwe. The Department of Psychiatry teaches undergraduate medical students and offers a 1-year tertiary diploma in mental health and a 3-year masters degree in psychiatry. Normally, the diploma has four students and the masters degree has up to two candidates in each year (currently there is one student in the first year, none in the second year and two in the third year). Psychiatry is the least popular of the medical specialties because the remunerations in private practice are the lowest. Psychiatric nurses are trained at Ingutsheni Hospital. The programme is 18 months' long and normally has approximately 12 students.

## Mental health disorders

In Zimbabwe in-patients typically present with schizophrenia, substance-induced psychosis, bipolar affective disorder (mania), epilepsy or the psychiatric complications of HIV. In the psychiatric out-patient clinics and private practice, depression, substance dependency and anxiety disorders are also typical. Eating disorders and personality disorders are diagnoses rarely made among the Black population. The reason for this might be a poor detection rate by health personnel. Research on the prevalence of personality disorder would be an area of interest.

## Mental health policy

Zimbabwe's mental health policy was introduced in 1999 and has attempted to decentralise services. Coordinators have now been established in each province. The economic downturn has slowed the establishment of community mental health centres. An important emphasis of the policy is to incorporate mental health within the national HIV/AIDS programme.

## Mental health legislation

The Mental Health Act of 1976 was repealed in 1996. The country now uses the Mental Health Act 1996 No. 15, which safeguards the rights of a patient but still emphasises institutionalisation of those who are mentally ill. An extensive mental health training programme focusing on the rights of offenders with mental disorders was provided for officers of the courts between 2006 and 2008. This led to a substantial decline in the incarceration of people who are mentally ill when brought before the courts for minor offences.

## Publications and research

The country does not have a psychiatric journal. Most research work is being done into the psychosocial aspects of HIV and depression. Earlier research has, however, led to the development of indigenous screening tools for common mental disorders. There is currently a move to incorporate use of the validated Edinburgh Postnatal Depression Scale into the routine 6-week postnatal visit at primary postnatal clinics. At primary city health clinics, lay health workers since 2006 have screened for common mental disorders using the Shona Symptom Questionnaire (SSQ-14), an indigenous screening tool. The lay health workers then provide structured problem-solving therapy. There is a need to carry out a randomised controlled trial of this intervention delivered by lay health workers.

## Conclusion

In Zimbabwe, mental health services have come a long way. The harsh socioeconomic environment slowed the process of decentralisation which was embarked on when the Mental Health Act and policies were reviewed. The central structures are now in place and services are being brought to the people. As socioeconomic conditions improve, the country can increasingly focus on the setting up of community mental health services; it also needs to encourage more medical and nursing students to train in mental health and to arouse greater interest in mental health research.

## Sources

World Health Organization (2009) See http://www.afro.who.int/en/zimbabwe/who-country-office-zimbabwe.html (accessed July 2010).

Zimbabwe Ministry of Health and Child Welfare (2009) See http://www.mohcw.gov.zw (accessed July 2010).

# Asia

# Afghanistan

Peter Ventevogel, Ruhullah Nassery, Sayed Azimi
and Hafizullah Faiz

Afghanistan's historic strategic position between the great civilisations of India, Persia and Central Asia has made it from the very beginning both a crossroads for trade and cultural exchange and an almost continuous battlefield. In the years since the Soviet invasion in 1979 the country has become the stage of an ongoing complex humanitarian emergency. The period of Soviet occupation was characterised by massive human rights violations. The Soviet army and its allies were involved in indiscriminate bombardments and targeted executions, while the mujahedeen were involved in guerrilla warfare. The USSR was forced to withdraw in 1989 and the remnants of Afghanistan's communist regime were defeated in 1992.

Rivalry among the mujahedeen groups in the early 1990s led to the destruction of large parts of the capital, Kabul, and divided the country into different regions belonging to different ethnic groups.

The rise of the fundamentalist Islamic Taliban movement was accompanied by a period of harsh rule, in which individual freedom was curtailed and the rights of women were severely restricted. In November 2001 the Taliban were ousted from power by the former mujahedeen, supported by a US-led multinational coalition. The situation has stabilised since, but violence is not over yet, with continued insurgent activities targeting government officials, schools for girls, non-governmental organisations and United Nations agencies.

## Effects on health

The effects of 25 years of violence in Afghanistan on the physical and human infrastructure have been enormous. The war caused an estimated 1 million deaths (Human Rights Watch, 2003). At the height of the crisis, the total number of Afghan refugees in Iran and Pakistan reached 3.7 million, amounting to 15% of the total population of Afghanistan, which is estimated at between 21 and 28 million. Afghanistan is one of the countries most severely affected by mines and other types of unexploded ordnance (International Campaign to Ban Landmines, 2001).

Decades of war and violence are reflected in Afghanistan's health statistics, which are among the poorest in the world. Life expectancy at birth is 43 years (World Bank, 2004), the mortality rate for children under 5 years of age is 257/1000 (fourth highest in the world) and the maternal mortality rate is 1900/100000 (second highest in the world) (UNICEF, 2005).

## Mental health status

The few publications from the pre-war period about mental health and mental healthcare in Afghanistan give the impression that Afghanistan was not very different from any other developing country in the region (Waziri, 1973).

Little is known about the effects of the war on the mental health status of the Afghans during the Russian occupation and the armed resistance of the mujahedeen. In the refugee camps in Pakistan, clinicians reported that they saw many patients with anxiety and depressive symptoms (Dadfar, 1994).

The Taliban policy of extreme gender segregation and the denial of basic human rights to women led to increased rates of depression and anxiety. A study conducted in 2000 by the organisation Physicians for Human Rights compared the mental health of women living in a Taliban-controlled area with that of women living in a non-Taliban-controlled area, and found that major depression was far more prevalent among the women exposed to Taliban policies (Amowitz *et al*, 2003).

The fall of the Taliban regime has not resulted in dramatic improvements in the mental health status of the population. A nationwide survey (Lopes Cardozo *et al*, 2004) and an in-depth survey in Nangarhar province (Scholte *et al*, 2004) both found persistently high prevalence rates of depression and anxiety, in particular among women, with elevated scores on depression questionnaires in around two-thirds of all women (58.4% and 73.4% in the two studies respectively) and anxiety symptoms in four-fifths of all women (78.2% and 83.5%). The studies found a clear relationship between the number of traumatic events and the likelihood of developing psychopathology. The prevalence figures mentioned here must be interpreted with caution, since there are several possible sources for bias from the use of self-report questionnaires (Bolton & Betancourt, 2004).

## Use of opiates and other drugs

Afghanistan is the largest producer of opiates in the world. Despite efforts to control poppy cultivation, in 2004 the country produced 87% of the world's opium (Todd *et al*, 2005). No reliable epidemiological data about the prevalence of opiate misuse among the Afghan population are available. The use of all intoxicants (nasha-i-mawad) in Islam is forbidden (haram), and in Afghanistan the Taliban have left a legacy of severe punitive measures for drug users (UNODC, 2003). None the less, it is estimated that Kabul alone has at least several tens of thousands of opiate users. Injection drug use appears to be a relatively new phenomenon and is thought to be on the increase, in particular among former refugees from neighbouring countries. Afghanistan has a Ministry of Counter Narcotics, which has drafted a national strategy for narcotics (2003, revised in 2005), a demand reduction policy (2003) and a harm reduction policy (2005). At present, harm reduction and drug treatment programmes are available only on a small scale. In Kabul the psychiatric hospital has a maximum of 20 beds for patients with substance misuse. Some Afghan non-governmental organisations (NGOs) have limited treatment facilities (10–20 beds) for heroin users in Kabul and provinces such as Kandahar and Paktya.

The prevalence of cannabis use is significant, especially in rural areas of the country, where it is not considered harmful. No data are available on the use of alcohol.

## Mental healthcare facilities

In the 1980s the Department for Mental Healthcare in the Ministry of Public Health attempted to decentralise mental healthcare and develop community mental health services. This resulted in four community mental health centres being established in Kabul, but the process was halted in other parts of the country by the rising civil war. Much of the qualified workforce and technical expertise have left the country. Currently, a mental healthcare system hardly exists outside Kabul. The mental health hospital in Kabul was so severely damaged in the course of fighting in the capital that the building was eventually demolished. A newly built psychiatric hospital in Kabul with a total of 60 beds opened in 2004. Small in-patient facilities for psychiatric patients exist in Jalalabad and Mazar i Sharif. A few provincial capitals have asylums (marastoon), whose main function is to provide shelter and food for homeless people, drug addicts and psychiatric patients with severe behavioural disturbances who have no family support.

Many people with mental disorders medicate themselves with psycho-pharmacological drugs or seek refuge in traditional religious shrines (van de Put, 2002).

## Mental health in primary care

The new health authorities have declared mental health a priority (Fatimi, 2004). In 2005 a department for mental healthcare within the Ministry of Public Health started to function again, and a beginning was made to integrate mental health into general health policies. The government, backed by major international donors, has decided to contract NGOs for health service delivery in the most underserved parts of the country.

The Ministry of Public Health has developed a 'Basic Package of Health Services' (BPHS) that defines the medical interventions to be made available in all districts of the country (Government of Afghanistan, 2003). The BPHS drafts the necessary interventions in seven priority areas: maternal and newborn health, child health and immunisation, public nutrition, communicable diseases, disability, essential drugs, and mental health. It is a novelty for a low-income country to give mental health such a high priority. The Afghan government justifies this by pointing at the clearly felt need for mental healthcare by its population after decades of war and internal conflict. Besides, this mirrors developments in international health policy.

The creation of available, accessible, affordable and acceptable mental health facilities in Afghanistan can be accomplished only through a major policy shift away from hospital-based psychiatry and towards integration of mental health into primary care services (Ventevogel *et al*, 2002). In the past few years the government, with the assistance of NGOs, the World Health Organization (WHO) and donors, has started to integrate mental health into primary care (Ventevogel & Kortmann, 2004).

## Psychosocial assistance

The need for psychosocial programmes is obvious (Baingana *et al*, 2005; Bolton & Betancourt, 2004). Several NGOs have developed focused psycho-social programmes for children (De Berry, 2004) and for women who have been subjected to violence. Others offer psychological assistance through counselling centres in different parts of Kabul or through community-based psychosocial services linked to the primary care system.

## Specialist education

Recent data collected by the WHO and Ministry of Public Health for the Assessment Instrument for Mental Health Systems (AIMS) demonstrated once more the paucity of human resources. The country has only two trained psychiatrists, one working in the WHO and the other in private practice. About 60 doctors work in mental healthcare but their training varies from almost nothing to some in-service training or short courses in institutes abroad. In 1999 a 3-month diploma course was held in northern Afghanistan to train 20 doctors in psychiatry (Mohit *et al*, 1999). Because of ongoing violence this initiative could not be followed up.

There is no postgraduate training in psychiatry and mental health is hardly represented in the undergraduate curricula for medical doctors, nurses or midwives. Psychologists at Kabul University are trained but there are no training institutes for clinical psychology, psychiatric nursing or social work.

## Conclusion

The unmet mental health needs of the Afghan people are enormous. The challenge to increase the capacity of the mental health sector will remain huge over the coming years. Sustained efforts of government, NGOs, institutional donors and United Nations bodies are needed to expand the coverage of basic mental healthcare and psychosocial services to the whole population of Afghanistan.

# References

Amowitz, L. L., Heisler, M. & Iacopino, V. (2003) A population-based assessment of women's mental health and attitudes toward women's human rights in Afghanistan. *Journal of Women's Health*, **12**, 577–587.

Baingana, F., Bannon, I. & Thomas, R. (2005) *Mental Health and Conflicts: Conceptual Framework and Approaches*. Washington, DC: World Bank.

Bolton, P. & Betancourt, T. S. (2004) Mental health in postwar Afghanistan. *Journal of the American Medical Association*, **292**, 626–628.

Dadfar, A. (1994) The Afghans: bearing the scars of a forgotten war. In *Amidst Peril and Pain. The Mental Health and Well-being of the World's Refugees* (eds A. J. Marsella *et al*), pp. 125–139. Washington, DC: American Psychological Association.

De Berry, J. (2004) Community psychosocial support in Afghanistan. *Intervention*, **2**, 143–151.

Fatimi, M. A. (2004) *Health priorities in the coming five years*. Statement by the Minister of Public Health. Kabul: Ministry of Public Health.

Government of Afghanistan (2003) *Basic Package of Health Services*. Kabul: Ministry of Public Health.

Human Rights Watch (2003) *Killing You Is a Very Easy Thing For Us*. Human Rights Abuses in Southeast Afghanistan. New York: HRW.

International Campaign to Ban Landmines (2001) *Landmine Monitor Report 2001*. Available at http://www.icbl.org/lm/2001/report

Lopes Cardozo, B., Bilukha, O. O., Crawford, C. A., *et al* (2004) Mental health, social functioning, and disability in postwar Afghanistan. *JAMA*, **292**, 575–584.

Mohit, A., Saeed, K., Shahmohammadi, D., *et al* (1999) Mental health manpower development in Afghanistan. *A report on a training course for primary health care physicians. Eastern Mediterranean Health Journal*, **5**, 373–377.

Scholte, W. F., Olff, M., Ventevogel, P., *et al* (2004) Mental health problems following war and repression in eastern Afghanistan. *Journal of the American Medical Association*, **292**, 585–593.

Todd, C. S., Safi, N. & Strathdee, S. A. (2005) *Drug use and harm reduction in Afghanistan*. Harm Reduction Journal, 2, 13. Available from http://www.harmreductionjournal.com/content/2/1/13

UNICEF (2005) *State of the World's Children 2005*. New York: United Nations Children's Fund.

UNODC (2003) *Community Drug Profile 5: An Assessment of Problem Drug Use in Kabul City*. Kabul: United Nations Office for Drugs Control. Available at http://www.unodc.org/pdf/afg/report_2003-07-31_1.pdf

van de Put, W. (2002) Addressing mental health in Afghanistan. *Lancet*, **360 (suppl.)**, S41–S42.

Ventevogel, P. & Kortmann, F. (2004) Developing basic mental health modules for health care workers in Afghanistan. *Intervention*, **2**, 43–54.

Ventevogel, P., Azimi, S., Jalal, S., *et al* (2002) Mental health care reform in Afghanistan. *Journal of Ayub Medical College*, Abbottabad, **14** (October–December), 1–3.

Waziri, R. (1973) Symptomatology of depressive illness in Afghanistan. *American Journal of Psychiatry*, **130**, 213–217.

World Bank (2004) *World Development Report*. New York: Oxford University Press.

# Armenia

Armen Soghoyan, Arega Hakobyan, Harutyun Davtyan, Marietta Khurshudyan and Khachatur Gasparyan

Armenia is a landlocked mountainous country between the Black Sea and the Caspian Sea, in the southern Caucasus. It shares borders with Turkey to the west, Georgia to the north, Azerbaijan to the east, and Iran and the Nakhchivan exclave of Azerbaijan to the south. Its total area is 29 743 km$^2$. A former republic of the Soviet Union, Armenia is a unitary, multi-party, democratic nation state with an ancient cultural heritage. Armenia prides itself on being the first nation formally to adopt Christianity (in the early 4th century).

According to the census of 2001, the population of Armenia is 3 219 200 but the July 2009 estimate is 2 967 004. The population of Armenia is homogeneous – Armenians form 97.9% of the population. The spoken language is Armenian. The main religious group is Armenian Apostolic (94.7%). The age structure is as follows: 14 years or under, 18.2% (male 289 119, female 252 150); 15–64 years, 71.1% (male 986 764, female 1 123 708); 65 years and over, 10.6% (male 122 996, female 192 267) (2009 estimates). The population growth rate is estimated to be 0.03% per year, the birth rate per 1000 population to be 12.53 and the death rate 8.34 per 1000. The infant mortality rate is 20.21 per 1000 live births. Life expectancy at birth is 72.68 years (69.06 years for males, 76.81 years for females) and healthy life expectancy at birth 66.7 years. A majority of the population (64.2%; 2 066 700 persons) resides in urban areas. Most adults (99.5%) are literate.

## Healthcare system

As a post-Soviet state, the Republic of Armenia inherited a health system organised according to the Semashko model, with guaranteed free medical assistance and access to a comprehensive range of medical care for the entire population. The system was highly centralised, with vertical management dominating. Financial and other allocations were based on national norms and failed to take account of population health needs. There was an emphasis on structural and quantitative indicators, resulting in the expansion of physical capacity, an oversupply of health personnel and a surplus of hospital beds, along with an unequal distribution of resources.

Since independence, the health system in Armenia has undergone numerous changes. Following the decentralisation of public services, the ownership of health services has been devolved to local and provincial governments.

The population, especially those in need, has limited access to health services. The services delivered are sometimes of questionable quality. Many health facilities, especially in rural areas, lack modern medical technology and human resources.

Armenia is increasingly engaged in changing the system from one that emphasises the treatment of disease and response to epidemics to one that emphasises prevention, family care and community participation. Although the emphasis of reform has been on increased state budgets and more efficient use of resources, the majority of financing is still derived from out-of-pocket payments, both formal and informal. The shift towards an orientation on primary care is noticeable, with gradually increased roles for health workers to influence the determinants of health (Hakobyan *et al*, 2006).

## Mental health legislation

After 1991, when Armenia became independent, Parliament passed a few laws on public health and healthcare but no law on mental health, until comparatively recently. Up until 2004, mental healthcare in Armenia was regulated by an order of the Minister of Health of the USSR, although the order did not have power of law. In September 1998, the Board of the Mental Health Foundation began to draft a mental health law and to publish a series of materials on mental health legislation. In January 1999, a draft Bill was presented to the Minister of Health and mental health is now regulated by the Law on Psychiatric Care, adopted on 25 May 2004. This regulates involuntary treatment, the civil and human rights of people with mental disorders, and other mental health issues. The Law was amended in 2006.

The criminal law also has a bearing on mental health, mainly in relation to involuntary treatment.

Amendments to the Law on Psychiatric Care have been proposed by the National Assembly of the Republic of Armenia. These focus on treatment facilities and service structures as well as human rights. It would also be useful if future revisions could address areas of potential conflict between mental health specialists and other service providers and patients' interests. For example, the terms of voluntary and involuntary admissions have not been clearly defined within the legislation. A maximum duration of involuntary admission is fixed by criminal law but is not stated in the Law on Psychiatric Care. Similarly, the rights of family members and other carers are not stated.

Policy on mental health is still not well developed and there is no governmentally approved and adopted mental health programme in Armenia. General approaches to mental health require modernisation, as some strategies and practices have been retained from the Soviet period.

Another concern is that there is no emergency/disaster preparedness plan for mental health (WHO Regional Office, 2007).

# Mental health services

Because of the country's transition from the Soviet period, the mental health system in Armenia has changed significantly over the past two decades.

Mental health services in Armenia are lacking and those available are poorly integrated into the primary care system. The current system focuses on in-patient care. There is a lack of trained social workers and other mental health professionals, which limits the potential for service provision at community level. Essentially, psychiatric care is still exclusively provided in specialised mental health institutions, including hospitals and social psychoneurological centres. Currently, only 3% of the overall public healthcare budget is given to mental health. In turn, around 88% of the mental health expenditure is on mental hospitals.

The essential psychotropic medicines are provided free of charge to all registered patients. In addition, all severe and some mild mental disorders are covered by social insurance schemes under which patients get free treatment. Also, those who are recognised to have chronic disorders get financial support from the government in the form of a disability pension.

There are 135 hospitals in Armenia with 13 100 beds: 99 hospitals with 8732 beds are in the public sector (that is, under the management of the Ministry of Health), 27 are private and 9 are run by other governmental bodies or departments. An overcapacity of in-patient beds leads to the unnecessary admission of individuals with chronic illness who would better be treated in out-patient settings. Unfortunately, there is no systematic approach to developing community mental health services except for some small-scale pilot projects, usually supported by international organisations (Hakobyan *et al*, 2006).

There are 467 primary healthcare clinics in Armenia, of which 380 are physician-based in the public sector and 69 physician-based in the private sector; the other 18 are under other governmental bodies or departments.

Psychosocial rehabilitation is underrepresented in the mental hospitals and few patients receive psychosocial interventions. In contrast, psychotropic medicine is highly accessible in in-patient mental health facilities. All mental hospitals have available at least one psychotropic medicine of each therapeutic class (antipsychotic, antidepressant, mood stabiliser, anxiolytic, or anti-epileptic).

There are only five out-patient mental health facilities. All of them are organisationally integrated with mental hospitals; two are for children and adolescents only. There are 1311.5 users per 100 000 general population in these out-patient facilities. Of these out-patients, 29% are female and 2% are children and adolescents. Of all those treated in out-patient facilities, 28% have a primary diagnosis of schizophrenia or schizotypal and delusional disorders.

Three mental health facilities provide day care, all for adults only (there are no day treatment facilities for children and adolescents). Day treatment mental health facilities treat 9.5 users per 100 000 population.

In general, in Armenia mental health and mental disorders in children and adolescents are not regarded with anything like the same importance as their physical health. Although some programmes have been initiated recently concerning general mental health, there are no plans that would include children and adolescents.

## Training, education and research

In 2008, per 100 000 population, 11.1 medical doctors (not specialised in psychiatry) graduated in Armenia, as did 50 nurses (not specialised in psychiatry). There are no psychiatrists, psychologists or nurses and social workers with more than 1 year of training in mental healthcare. Around 20% of psychiatrists emigrate to other countries within 5 years of the completion of their training.

In 2008, no mental healthcare staff received more than 2 days of refresher training in the rational use of drugs, psychosocial interventions or child and adolescent mental health issues. The major problem for mental health education, as in the field of public health in general, is that there is no regular provision of continuous medical education for psychiatry and clinical psychology. The government supports training for professionals once in every 5 years, but even then this training is generally formal and psychiatrists are not satisfied with it.

International exchange experience is lacking at governmental level. This means that new trends in treatment and drugs are neglected. There are some donor organisations supporting international exchange for a few professionals, and others try to participate in internationl conferences and workshops using their personal resources.

Mental health research is underdeveloped and lacks governmental support. There is, though, some research based on the interests of individual investigators or some priorities suggested by donor organisations. This tends to be focused on epidemiological studies in community samples, epidemiological studies in clinical samples, biology and genetics, policy, programmes, financing/economics, and pharmacological, surgical and electroconvulsive interventions.

## Sources

Hakobyan, T., Nazaretyan, M., Makarova, T., *et al* (2006) Armenia: health system review. *Health Systems in Transition*, **8(6)**, 1–180.

National Statistical Service of the Republic of Armenia, at http://www.armstat.am (accessed May 2009).

Soghoyan, A. (2003) Psychiatric care in Yerevan. *Mental Health Reforms*, **1**, 16–19.

Van Baelen, L., Teocharopoulos, Y. & Hargreaves, S. (2005) Mental health problems in Armenia: low demand, high needs. *British Journal of General Practice*, **55**, 64–65.

WHO Regional Office (2007) *Evaluation of Emergency/Disaster Preparedness Capacities of Armenia*. WHO.

# Azerbaijan

## Fuad Ismayilov

Azerbaijan is a nation with a Turkic population which regained its independence after the collapse of the Soviet Union in 1991. It has an area of approximately 86000 km². Georgia and Armenia, the other countries comprising the Transcaucasian region, border Azerbaijan to the north and west, respectively. Russia also borders the north, Iran and Turkey the south, and the Caspian Sea borders the east. The total population is about 8 million. The largest ethnic group is Azeri, comprising 90% of the population; Dagestanis comprise 3.2%, Russians 2.5%, Armenians 2% and others 2.3%.

The gross domestic product (GDP) per capita in 2002 was US$755 and 0.9% of the GDP was allocated to health. The proportion of the national budget spent on the overall health system is 6.6% and mental health expenditure is 0.33% of the total national budget. The numbers of physicians (of all specialties), paramedical staff and beds per 10 000 population are, respectively, 36.3, 74.6 and 86.0 (State Statistical Committee, 2002).

Azerbaijan is one of the first republics of the former Soviet Union to face a large-scale refugee problem. At present there are 819 000 refugees and internally displaced people, who had to leave their homes owing to the 1988–93 armed conflict with Armenian military forces in Nagorno-Karabakh (Ismayilov & Ismayilov, 2002).

## Current mental health system

In line with the old Soviet model, mental healthcare in Azerbaijan is oriented to the institutional approach, but the conditions within the psychiatric institutions do not meet basic standards. Primary care for people with mental illness is not well developed, although almost all kinds of service are available at the level of specialist care. The principal mental healthcare providers are psychiatric hospitals, psychiatric dispensaries and psychiatrists in private practice.

There are 5.0 psychiatrists per 100000 population. Each administrative district of the country has an out-patient clinic with a consulting room for a psychiatrist. Moreover, eight cities have inter-regional psychoneurological dispensaries (PNDs), with out-patient and in-patient facilities. In the city of Baku there are two PNDs: one of them provides services to children, the other to adults (Aliyev, 1999).

In-patient treatment is provided by nine psychiatric hospitals. In addition, there are psychosomatic departments in two large general hospitals and psycho-neurological departments in the military hospitals. The total number of beds is 5670, or 71 per 100 000 population. Some metropolitan districts, such as Baku, Soumgait and Gandja, are able to provide round-the-clock psychiatric teams working in an ambulance service.

The main restriction on mental healthcare in Azerbaijan is financial. A doctor's salary is around US$10–20 a month. As a rule, physicians also demand a fee for their services, and there is therefore little difference between the private and public sectors. Illegal demands for payments are often made for mental health services, as well as for drugs, and food in hospital. In fact, most people are not able to afford hospital treatment, which costs on average US$200–250, and most patients do not wish to go into hospital even if they are financially secure. The other disadvantages of the existing system are the over-centralisation of services and a paternalistic approach towards people with mental illness. Community care and rehabilitation are carried out by a few non-governmental organisations involved in local mental health projects (Akhundov, 2001).

Since the arrival of the large number of refugees, the national government has passed several acts related to privileged services for refugees. One of the first of them was Order 145, which simplifies the process for the admission of refugees to psychiatric institutions, regardless of their place of residence and the availability of referral from a primary care institution. In addition, some special pharmacies that supply medicines free of charge to refugees were established.

# Epidemiology

Systematic epidemiological studies have not been performed in Azerbaijan. According to official statistics (Ministry of Health, 2001), the number of patients with a first psychiatric diagnosis in 2001 and the total number of psychiatric patients registered in PNDs per 100 000 population were 85.8 and 1034.5, respectively. (These figures relate to severe mental disorders only.)

Despite a relatively low rate of suicide, of 2.7 per 100 000, there is a consensus among mental health professionals that the prevalence of depressive, anxiety and somatoform disorders has dramatically increased recently (Ismayilov, 2000). Also evident is an increase in alcoholism and drug misuse (presently with a prevalence of 274.4 and 191.3 per 100 000, respectively).

# Training in psychiatry

At undergraduate level, psychiatric education is available at the Azerbaijan Medical University. In the fourth and fifth years of their course, medical students are obliged to study psychiatry (including medical psychology); this involves about 150 hours of academic work at the Department of Psychiatry. At this level the training programme is divided in two sections – a series of lectures on the theoretical foundation to the subject, and workshops on general psychiatry (psychiatric disorders). Additionally, medical students have to acquire skills in the interviewing and assessment of psychiatric patients.

A medical graduate who wishes to become a psychiatrist spends one year as an intern at a psychiatric hospital and after passing the special examination can start working independently. The intern programme is focused on obtaining initial experience in diagnostics and treatment. Such training is insufficient and the administration of the Medical University, jointly with the Ministry of Health, has planned a four-year programme of training, which is due to be implemented from 2005.

Every five years psychiatrists have to have four months' training at postgraduate level at the Department of Psychiatry of the Azerbaijan State Doctors' Advanced Training Institute. Unfortunately, because of the obsolete training programmes and old-fashioned approaches, this continuing education is not particularly effective. There are no subspecialty programmes (e.g. in child and adolescent, geriatric or forensic psychiatry or psychotherapy). Before the collapse of the USSR, mental health professionals from Azerbaijan could be trained at the accredited Soviet scientific centres, generally those in Moscow and St Petersburg. At present the country does not have bilateral arrangements with other countries for training in psychiatry.

A two-year programme is provided for the training of nurses. This includes a 32-hour combined course on psychiatry and neurology. Psychiatric nurses need not have any specialist psychiatric training and can start working as soon as they leave nursing school. Psychiatric nurses do, however, receive 192 hours of specialist training once every five years. This continuing education is formally encouraged by linking it to further qualifications; if a further degree is obtained, this is rewarded by an increase in salary (although this increase amounts only to US$2–3 per month). However, it has to be said that most mental health professionals are not satisfied with the standard of this continuing education for psychiatric nurses.

In 1999 a training programme for clinical psychologists was launched at Baku State University; however, their official involvement in the provision of mental health services has not yet been established. There are at present no training programmes for other mental health professionals, such as psychiatric social workers and occupational therapists.

# Azerbaijan Psychiatric Association

Over the past five years the Azerbaijan Psychiatric Association (AzPA) has worked in partnership with the World Psychiatric Association, the Association of European Psychiatrists and the Geneva Initiative on Psychiatry to improve mental healthcare in the country. One initiative of the AzPA has been to translate important documents, including ICD–10, guidelines on ethics in psychiatry and the Madrid Declaration, into the Azeri language and to distribute them among mental health professionals. More than 50 members of the AzPA have participated at international scientific meetings. Also several members of the Association were involved in the ANAP Project (Attitudes and Needs Assessment in Psychiatry) conducted in six countries of Central and Eastern Europe.

# Mental health reform

One of the first steps towards reform of the mental health services resulted in the adoption of the Mental Health Law by the Azerbaijan parliament on 29 June 2001. Derived from Western standards of mental healthcare, the Law is focused on the protection of the civil and human rights of mentally ill people and it regulates mental health service provision. With the help of international organisations (including the Geneva Initiative on Psychiatry and the International Consortium for Mental Health Policy and Services) a working group has been established to draft documents on mental health policy and a national mental health programme. This working group has indicated that the main priority is a programme of deinstitutionalisation, with the simultaneous development of community services; also required are an improvement in the financing and distribution of services, and the establishment of effective links between the different sectors involved in mental health (Musabayova & Zeynalova, 2000; Manuchery-Lalei, 2000; Ismayilov, 2001).

Collaborative efforts should be undertaken to prevent stigma and to involve users in the planning and evaluation of services. Finally, the priority for any mental health policy must be to improve the system of training. The training of psychiatrists should meet contemporary standards of professional education, and specialist training programmes in clinical psychology, psychiatric social work, psychiatric nursing, occupational therapy and so on need to be developed.

# References

Akhundov, N. G. (2001) Basic principles of psychosocial rehabilitation of refugees and internally displaced children in places of their temporary residence. *Azerbaijan Psychiatric Journal*, **4**, 58–63.

Aliyev, N. (1999) Organisation of mental health services in Baku and perspective on their development. *Azerbaijan Psychiatric Journal*, **1**, 66–69.

Ismayilov, N. (2000) Treatment of somatoform disorders related to social stress. *Azerbaijan Psychiatric Journal*, **3**, 28–35.

Ismayilov, F. (2001) Mental health services: evaluation and research. *Azerbaijan Psychiatric Journal*, **4**, 13–21.

Ismayilov, N. & Ismayilov, F. (2002) Mental health of refugees: the case of Azerbaijan. *World Psychiatry*, **1(2)**, 121–124.

Manuchery-Lalei, A. (2000) Concept of community care and its perspectives in Azerbaijan. *Azerbaijan Psychiatric Journal*, **3**, 20–25.

Ministry of Health (2001) *Medical Statistics – Annual Report*. Baku: Ministry of Health.

Musabayova, G. & Zeynalova, N. (2000) Rehabilitation in a children's psycho-neurologic dispensary. *Azerbaijan Psychiatric Journal*, **3**, 91–93.

State Statistical Committee (2002) *Independent Azerbaijan*. Baku: State Statistical Committee

# Bahrain

## M. K. Al-Haddad and Adel Al-Offi

The Kingdom of Bahrain is an archipelago of 33 islands, located in the Arabian Gulf, covering 2400 km². The main island, Manama, is the nation's capital. The total population stands at 742 562, 62.3% of whom are local Bahrainis and the remaining 37.7% expatriates (Central Statistics Organisation Directorate, 1991). Bahrain first entered the historical stage around 3000 BC, and for almost 2000 years was the centre of the old Dilmun civilisation (Bibby, 1969). Dilmun was perceived as a sacred land by the Sumerians and Babylonians; it was a burial ground for their dead, and Bahrain has over 100 000 burial mounds each containing 200–250 bodies. In the old Babylonian epic of Gilgamesh, which antedates Homer's *Iliad*, Dilmun is described as a paradise where the worthy enjoy eternal life (Clarke, 1981).

## Psychiatric services

Al-Haddad & Al-Offi (1996) provide a history of Bahraini psychiatric services. Before 1930, no institution cared for psychiatric patients in Bahrain. Left to look after an ailing relative, families often devised their own form of therapy. One of the most common remedies was conducting a Zar ceremony, which was thought to help rid a person of the demons or jin believed to be responsible for mental ailments. Other forms of treatment included reciting verses from the Holy Quran, as well as cautery applied on either the occipital or parietal regions of the head.

In 1930, Charles Belgrave, the English counsel to Bahrain's ruler, suggested the creation of a place for local 'lunatics' which would safely put them under the direct supervision of the Municipal Council. In 1932 a small house was rented in the capital to host 14 patients (12 male, 2 female). The residence was named the 'Mad House' and psychiatric patients were looked after by 'attendants' (who were essentially labourers rather than nursing staff). The Municipal Council continued supervision of the asylum until 1948, when responsibility was transferred to the Department of Health. A report by Dr Snow, chief of the Department of Health at the time, illustrates improvements to the asylum; the building was refurbished and newly painted with pleasant colours, and patients were encouraged to spend more time outside their cells.

In 1964 Dr Butler, an English internist, started to run regular daily psychiatric out-patient clinics, recruited trained psychiatric nurses from India and Lebanon, and introduced the first drug (chlorpromazine) for the treatment of mental illness.

The 1970s witnessed many changes, such as the establishment of a child and adolescent out-patient unit (1975), community psychiatric services and a day hospital (1979), and an 88-bed unit for both chronic patients and psychogeriatric patients (1979). In the same year, a liaison service was established with Bahrain's main general hospital, which hosted two general admission units for psychiatry, with a capacity of 48 beds divided equally between males and females. In 1984 a new out-patient complex with lecture halls, teaching facilities and office space was built. In 1987 an alcohol and drug rehabilitation unit was separately developed, with an initial capacity of 17 beds, which had reached 29 beds in 2008.

## Current mental health services

Today, there is still only one dedicated psychiatric hospital in Bahrain. Private general hospitals employ psychiatrists who mainly work with out-patients, although they do occasionally admit non-psychotic patients, but there are no private beds specifically for psychiatry. The psychiatric hospital has 296 beds for all psychiatric specialties, divided into general psychiatry (114 beds), long-term and rehabilitation (104 beds), psychogeriatrics (10 beds), drug and alcohol rehabilitation (29 beds), adolescents (15 beds), children (12 beds) and forensic psychiatry (12 beds). The same community and day hospital service (in existence since 1979) covers the entire adult and elderly population via three community teams. There are two specialised out-patient clinics, one for anxiety disorders and one for intellectual disability..

The hospital employs 49 full-time psychiatrists, 14 consultants, 11 chief residents, 9 senior residents and 15 residents. There are in total 276 trained psychiatric nurses, 12 occupational therapists, 7 social workers, 4 clinical psychologists, and 2 physiotherapists. There are also 9 consultant-level psychiatrists working in the private sector and a further 2 in the Bahrain Defence Force Hospital. Thus in total there are 60 psychiatrists.

For the past 20 years, psychiatric services have been successfully incorporated within primary care services in Bahrain. Family physicians are also afforded access to psychiatric medications. This is the first such initiative in the Arab world.

### Resources

The Royal College of Psychiatrists' (2002) recommended consultant norms are: 5.4 per 100 000 population for general psychiatry, 1 consultant per 10 000 for the elderly population, 1.5 per 100 000 for children and adolescents, 0.9 per 100 000 for substance use, 8 per 1 000 000 for forensic psychiatry and 1 per 600 general beds for liaison psychiatry. These norms can be applied to Bahrain's population of 742 562. The population above 65 years is 18 756, and so requires 2 psychiatrists, but there is in fact only one consultant in psychogeriatrics. The child and adolescent population has reached 202 565, and so requires 3 consultants, which there are now. The general adult population is 521 238, requiring 28 consultants but there are only 11 consultants currently working in the field. The registered substance misuse population is 4270, covered by 3 consultants instead of the recommended 4.6. In forensic psychiatry the need is for nearly 6 consultants, but there is only 1 practising. For liaison psychiatry there are 2 consultants serving 1714 public sector beds, and another 323 beds are covered by psychiatrists working in the private sector; there is a need for a further 3 consultants in that field.

## Mental health programme

A 12-year mental health programme was drafted in 1988, covering Bahrain up to the year 2000 (Al-Haddad, 1988). More than 95% of the set targets were achieved ahead of time. Accordingly, another plan was drafted in 1997 with an ambitious set of 88 objectives (Al-Haddad, 1997).

## Mental health legislation

Over the past 20 years, many attempts have been made to pass a mental health act in Bahrain. This has still not been achieved. Currently, psychiatrists work within the limited rules related to psychiatry made available in court regulations; some of these date back to when Bahrain was a British protectorate.

# Training

The psychiatric hospital runs a 4-year training programme leading to qualification with the Arab Board of Psychiatry. After qualifying with the Arab Board a further 2 years of clinical training in the UK or USA in general psychiatry or subspecialties is required.

# Research and publications

Many local psychiatrists are actively involved in research. The establishment of the Medical School as part of the Arabian Gulf University in 1984 was an important catalyst in promoting this. To encourage research, the Ministry of Health stipulates a minimum of two publications for doctors to obtain a consultant post.

# Service development

Progress has been achieved in three key areas:

1 In February 2007 the Parliament passed legislation to establish a separate centre for the treatment and rehabilitation of substance misusers. The number of drug users registered in the drug rehabilitation unit is 4270. A 10-year follow-up study found a 100% relapse rate among them (Derbas & Al-Haddad, 2001). The seroprevalence rate of HIV among drug users was 21.1% (Al-Haddad *et al*, 1994).

2 The Ministries of Education and Health agreed in 2007 to appoint a psychiatrist with a team of nurses, social workers and psychologists in public school health services to provide counselling and treatment for school children with intellectual disabilities or psychiatric problems.

3 One of the unachieved objectives of the 1997 mental health programme was to establish independent specialist teams of psychiatrists, nurses and social workers in the areas of affective disorders, schizophrenia and other subspecialties. The plan was to establish a separate admission area for each and to encourage research and specialised management. However, a specialist neurosis team and clinic have been established, and have been active since 1998.

There are four areas of service in which further progress is needed:

1 The current day hospital is under the management of the community team and it renders its services to adult populations only. Other categories of psychiatric patients needing such services are the elderly, people with an intellectual disability and adolescents.

2 Another challenge is the establishment of sheltered employment for all categories of psychiatric patient. The Bahraini labour law stipulates that 5% of the working population's employment opportunities should be allocated to people with special needs. In a competitive job market this is difficult to attain, making sheltered employment a challenging but helpful solution.

3 Both community and day patient facilities still need to be expanded.

4 Improvement is still needed in psychiatric services in primary care (by furthering family physicians' training in psychiatry).

# References

Al-Haddad, M. K. (1988) *Bahrain Mental Health Programme Till the Year 2000*. Ministry of Health.

Al-Haddad, M. K. (1997) *Mental and Psychological Health Plan*. Ministry of Health.

Al-Haddad, M. K. & Al-Offi, A. (1996) History of psychiatric services in Bahrain. *Journal of the Bahrain Medical Society*, **8**, 127–131.

Al-Haddad, M. K., Khashaba, A. S., Baig, B. Z., *et al* (1994) HIV antibodies among intravenous drug users in Bahrain. *Journal of Communicable Diseases*, **26**, 127–132.

Bibby, G. (1969) *Looking for Dilmun*. New American Library.

Central Statistics Organisation Directorate (1991) *Bahrain in Figures*. Government of Bahrain.

Clark, A. (1981) *The Island of Bahrain*. Historical and Archeological Society, Bahrain.

Derbas, A. & Al-Haddad, M. K. (2001) Factors associated with relapse among opiate addicts in Bahrain. *Eastern Mediterranean Health Journal*, **7**, 473–480.

Royal College of Psychiatrists (2002) *Model Consultant Job Descriptions and Recommended Norms (occasional paper OP55)*. RCPsych.

# Bangladesh

M. Rezaul Karim, Fakhruzzaman Shaheed
and Siddhartha Paul

The People's Republic of Bangladesh is located in South Asia. The total land area of Bangladesh is 147570 km². Its total population in 2001 was about 123 million. The population growth rate is 1.47%; of the total population, 75% live in rural areas and 25% in urban areas (Bangladesh Bureau of Statistics, 2000).

## Health indicators

Life expectancy at birth in 1998 was estimated to be 61 years for both sexes. The infant mortality rate was 57 per 1000 live births in 1998. The number of hospital beds is 43143 and the number of registered physicians is 30869 (Bangladesh Bureau of Statistics, 2000).

## History of psychiatric services in Bangladesh

In what is now Bangladesh, there were no mental health facilities until 1947, when India was divided. (Psychiatric patients had to go to the Central European Asylum in Ranchi, which was too far away for many people.) In that situation the government (of what was then East Pakistan) decided to establish a mental hospital, and in 1957 one was opened in Pabna, a district town 175 km from the capital, Dhaka. Initially it was a 50-bed hospital, but it grew to become today a 500-bed hospital. In 1974 Dhaka Medical College introduced a mental health service. This service was then extended to the Institute of Postgraduate Medicine and Research (now Bangabhandu Sheikh Mujib Medical University, BSMMU) and other medical colleges, as well as to the Institute of Mental Health and Research. This service included both out-patient and in-patient departments. At present, all 13 government medical colleges and hospitals and some of the non-government medical college hospitals provide psychiatric services, both out-patient and in-patient.

# Prevalence of psychiatric disorder

Psychiatric disorder is common in Bangladesh, as in any other country, but the psychiatric service at present is confined to Pabna Mental Hospital, the Institute of Mental Health, the BSMMU and the medical college hospitals (Islam *et al*, 1993). Although the results of a recent national survey of psychiatric morbidity are yet to published, the evidence from smaller surveys suggests that psychiatric disorder is prevalent in both the urban and rural communities. In a survey of the rural population of Dasherkandi (a village near Dhaka) it was found that 29 per 1000 people suffered from psychiatric disorder, and an additional 36 per 1000 had both a psychiatric and a physical disorder (Chowdhury *et al*, 1981).

In another study it was found that 29% of patients seen in a medical general practice during the course of 1 year were suffering from a purely psychological or emotional disorder (Alam, 1978).

At the medical out-patient department of the Institute of Postgraduate Medical Research, it was found that 31% of patients had a purely psychological condition and an additional 15% had a condition with both organic and psychogenic features (Chowdhury *et al*, 1975).

In a study of 600 patients attending a psychiatric clinic in Chittagong city, schizophrenia and affective disorder were found in 30% and 25% of patients, respectively. Neurosis and personality disorder in combination were found in 30%. Organic disorder and learning disabilities were found in 7% and 3% respectively (Ahmed, 1978).

# Medical education

## *Undergraduate education*

Psychiatry is included in the undergraduate curriculum. The course comprises 15 lectures (1 hour each) and 15 days of clinical clerkship in the fourth-year MBBS class, which is mandatory for all students. In the MBBS, 12.5% of marks are allotted to mental health in the written final examination.

## *Postgraduate education*

Postgraduate courses in Bangladesh include fellowship and membership of the Bangladesh College of Physicians and Surgeons (FCPS and MCPS), master of philosophy (MPhil) and doctor of medicine (MD). The FCPS course is run by an autonomous body following the curriculum of the MRCPsych. It has part I and part II examinations and also requires 2 years of full-time clinical experience. There have been 34 fellows to date. The MD course is run by the BSMMU. It has had one successful student complete the course and another 11 are currently taking it. The MD is a 5-year course, which includes 3 years of training. The MPhil course is run by both the BSMMU and Sylhet MAG Osmani Medical College. It is a 3-year course, including 1 year of residential training. So far 25 students have gained the

MPhil and 18 students are presently on the course. At the end of both the MD and the MPhil courses, students have to submit a thesis, and FCPS students have to submit a dissertation.

# Training

The BSMMU, the Institute of Mental Health and Research and the 13 government-run medical colleges provide postgraduate training in psychiatry. Doctors interested in psychiatry work as 'indoor' medical officers, assistant registrars or honorary medical officers. The institutes do not pay the non-government doctors, who work as honorary medical officers. The training is full time and residential.

# Child psychiatry

Child psychiatry has not been developed in Bangladesh, although there is a child psychiatry wing at the BSMMU and another child psychiatry department at the Institute of Mental Health and Research. The country has only three psychiatrists trained (abroad) in child psychiatry.

# Psychotherapy

Psychotherapy (which is still in a rudimentary state) is mostly done by psychiatrists. In the University of Dhaka there is a clinical psychology department. Students are trained in psychotherapy at the psychiatry department of the BSMMU.

# Research

Research is mainly epidemiological, although some research into different disorders and on drug misuse, suicide and child psychiatry is ongoing. The Bangladesh Association of Psychiatrists publishes journals.

# Mental health professionals

There are 73 psychiatrists nationally. The Institute of Mental Health and Research is training medical graduates and primary health workers throughout the country. In total, 2048 doctors and some 4000 health workers have been trained in psychiatry.

# Mental health services in Bangladesh

As the number of psychiatrists is low relative to the size of the population, psychiatric patients are taken care of by psychiatrists, doctors trained in psychiatry, doctors practising relevant specialties and general practitioners.

There is no formal referral system, although patients are referred by other health professionals to psychiatrists for proper management.

Many patients attend psychiatrists after 'referral' from people in their local community. Some patients are now referred to psychiatrists by traditional healers, faith healers and unqualified medical practitioners (so-called 'village doctors'). There are approximately 800 beds sanctioned for psychiatric patients in government hospitals. In non-government sectors, there are about 1000 psychiatric beds, most of which are occupied by drug misusers, whereas in the government sector people with a psychosis occupy almost all the beds. There is one government drug addiction treatment centre, with 75 beds, situated in Dhaka.

Doctors who have been trained in psychiatry work mostly in primary care centres. They are supposed to take care of the psychiatric patients in their areas, but there are no statistics regarding the patient care undertaken by these doctors. Also, there are no refresher courses for these trained doctors, so they are not in touch with recent advances in psychiatry.

## Mental health legislation and policy

Still there is no mental health act in Bangladesh. The Indian Lunacy Act 1912 (modified in 1957 and 1973) is generally followed. A draft mental health policy has been formulated by the Ministry of Health in collaboration with the World Health Organization and the Bangladesh Association of Psychiatrists; this policy is presently at the Law Ministry for finalisation.

## Human rights

As mentioned above, a large number of psychiatric patients receive treatment from traditional and faith healers, local religious leaders and practitioners of indigenous medicine. They believe that illness is related to supernatural influences, and so many patients are reluctant to consult practitioners of modern allopathic medicine. The non-medical healers are less concerned about the human rights of patients and people generally are not conscious of the proper rights of those with a mental disorder. In some special circumstances, for example when these patients are the focus of stories in the news media, then human rights activists often come forward to help them. Practising psychiatrists and the Association of Psychiatrists have very little influence in maintaining the human rights of psychiatric patients in the community, but in hospital settings psychiatric patients are treated as general patients.

## Associations

There are two psychiatric associations: the Bangladesh Association of Psychiatrists (BAP), of which all psychiatrists practising in Bangladesh are members; and the Forum of Psychiatry, which has emerged only recently.

# Overview

Education and services in psychiatry are gradually increasing, but still psychiatrists and psychiatric services tend to be available only in big cities. Most of the psychotropic medications are available in Bangladesh. On the other hand, psychotherapy is not widely available. Bangladesh lacks a mental health act. The BAP has been struggling to have an act passed and to expand psychiatric services in remote areas.

# References

Ahmed, S. U. (1978) Analysis of the epidemiological data of 600 psychiatric patients. *Bangladeshi Medical Research Council Bulletin*, **4**, 43–48.

Alam, M. N. (1978) Psychiatric morbidity in general practice. *Bangladeshi Medical Research Council Bulletin*, **4**, 38–42.

Bangladesh Bureau of Statistics (2000) *Statistical Yearbook of Bangladesh 2000*, pp. 5–10. Dhaka: Bangladesh Bureau of Statistics.

Chowdhury, A. K. M. N., Selim, M. & Sakeb, N. (1975) Some aspects of psychiatric morbidity in the out-patient population of a general hospital. *Bangladeshi Medical Research Council Bulletin*, **1**, 51–59.

Chowdhury, A. K. M. N., Alam, M. N. & Keramat, S. M. (1981) Dashkerkandi project studies: demography morbidity and mortality in rural community of Bangladesh. *Bangladeshi Medical Research Council Bulletin*, **7**, 22–39.

Islam, H., Mullick, M. S. I. & Khanam, M. (1993) Sociodemographic characteristics and psychiatric morbidity of out-patients in the Institute of Mental Health and Research. *Journal of the Institute of Postgraduate Medicine and Research*, **8**, 69–78.

# Brunei Darussalam

## Reehan Sabri and Ajmal-Khan Kudlebbai

Brunei Darussalam occupies a sliver of land on the north-west coast of the island of Borneo with a geographical area of just 5765 km$^2$ (Government of Brunei, 2004). It is divided into the four districts: Brunei-Muara, Temburong, Tutong and Belait. Two-thirds of the land is covered by lush tropical rainforest and the climate is perpetually warm and humid. It is ruled by Sultan Hassan Al-Bolkiah, the head of a dynasty which has governed Brunei for 650 years.

The population of 374 000 (United Nations Population Fund, 2005) enjoys one of the highest standards of living anywhere in the world, thanks to the discovery of oil in 1929, but the economy remains almost entirely dependent on oil and gas. The Bruneian population is 66% ethnic Malay and 15% ethnic Chinese; the rest are a mixture of indigenous and other races, such as the Ibans, who were once the feared headhunters of Borneo. There is also a large population of expatriate workers from the Indian subcontinent, South-East Asia, Australasia and Europe.

## Religion and culture

The different cultural groups in Brunei have interesting beliefs about physical and mental health (Kumaraswamy, 2007). These often present a challenge to medical practitioners and psychiatrists in particular. In spite of the official state adoption of Islam, many Malays adhere to beliefs that are a mixture of Islam, misunderstandings of Islam, animism and Hinduism, and this religious stance is a major influence on their beliefs about health. The Chinese and indigenous communities also have their superstitions and forms of traditional medicine.

Unsurprisingly, therefore, the first line of help for any kind of ailment among Bruneians, particularly psychiatric, is the Malay shaman or Bomoh. Bomohs practise a type of folk medicine under the veneer of Islam but their heretical practices are frowned upon by the religious authorities. Their knowledge is passed from generation to generation (Abdul Kadir, 2006) and their treatments include calling upon spirits as well as the prescription of herbs, spells and charms. Three-quarters of all Malay psychiatric patients will have consulted a Bomoh before resorting to mental health services (Salleh, 1989).

# Healthcare in Brunei

Brunei has an extensive primary healthcare network, with accessible local clinics in most parts of the country. There is one hospital in each of the four districts, although most specialist services are provided in the capital city, Bandar Seri Begawan. There are a few individual private medical practitioners and one major private hospital.

# Psychiatric services

There are two psychiatric departments in Brunei: one in the country's main hospital, Raja Isteri Pengiran Anak Saleha (RIPAS) Hospital in Bandar Seri Begawan, and a smaller department in Suri Seri Begawan (SSB) Hospital, in the town of Kuala Belait, in Belait District. There is significant stigma associated with mental illness and a certain amount of justified fear of psychiatric services. Before RIPAS Hospital was built, in 1984, there was a psychiatric unit in the old hospital known as 'Ward 5', which, by all accounts, was a classic asylum-style ward. The legacy of this unit continues to haunt Brunei's present-day mental health services. Even today, locals often refer to the hospital's modern mental health unit (MHU) as 'Ward 5' and recount with horror tales of screams and the sight of restrained patients.

There are four consultant psychiatrists (or 'specialists' as they are known in Brunei) in RIPAS Hospital and one in Kuala Belait. Although the specialists have expertise in different subspecialties, there are no formal subspecialist services.

The RIPAS MHU is a 20-bed ward with a virtually constant occupancy rate of at least 100%. At any one time, almost half the patients are 'bed-blockers' with chronic mental illness, abandoned by their families and so lacking any appropriate discharge destination. In Brunei, there are no residential facilities for people who are mentally ill. The RIPAS MHU also doubles up as a day hospital but activities and the interventions of the highly able occupational therapists are severely limited by a lack of space. SSB Hospital has a handful of long-term in-patients. There is a nascent community psychiatric service based at RIPAS Hospital which administers depot antipsychotic medication in patients' homes and follows up some of the difficult-to-engage patients.

Electroconvulsive therapy is available and there is a reasonable array of modern antipsychotic drugs. However, the range of antidepressants is limited and hopelessly outdated. Drugs not on the formulary, such as clozapine and venflaxine, can be acquired on a named-patient basis, but delays of, on average, 3 months are usual. Their clinical usefulness is, hence, severely limited. Another curious problem is the highly variable supply of drugs. It is not uncommon to run out of stock without any prior warning.

Until recently, there was a single trained clinical psychologist, in RIPAS Hospital. With his recent departure and the absence of a successor, there is no effective alternative to pharmacotherapy, which exacerbates the problem of limited supplies and types of psychotropic drugs. However, there is a day centre for the rehabilitation of those with chronic mental illness, which has succeeded in helping a number of individuals back to employment.

## Mental health legislation

The Lunacy Act 1929 (Attorney General's Chambers, 2004) allows for the detention of persons suspected of having a mental illness who are at risk. Unfortunately, the text of the Act is rather brief and imprecise. In practice, the relatives of any person suspected of having a mental illness may approach a magistrate and obtain a court order that authorises the involuntary detention of their family member. There is no right of appeal for the patient. Neither psychiatrists nor social workers are involved in this process; hence, there is potential for abuse of the law.

One of the laudable social welfare developments in Brunei is the Mental Health Allowance, which is a modest sum of money given monthly to those who are long-term mentally ill and incapable of working. The children of such individuals also receive an allowance. Furthermore, the Religious Department's treasury or 'Bait ul-Maal' distributes charitable donations to the needy members of Bruneian society, including those with psychiatric disorders and, in the case of converts to Islam, it also provides housing. Hence, it is unusual to see the type of grinding poverty often seen in Western countries among those who are mentally ill.

## Types of mental illness

There are no documented prevalence studies of psychiatric disorders in Brunei, but the common illnesses which psychiatrists are familiar with are assessed and treated by the mental health services. Notably, suicide is virtually unheard of, as are cases of eating disorder. As one may expect, given the country's prohibition of alcohol, alcohol-related psychiatric disorder is uncommon, although not absent, since supplies are smuggled from across the border with Malaysia and small quantities can be legitimately brought into the country by non-Muslims, for personal consumption. Perhaps for the same reason, violence is also uncommon in Bruneian society. Any form of aggression often causes great consternation and may lead to a referral to psychiatric services.

One very worrying trend is the widespread use of methamphetamine, or Syabu (pronounced 'shaboo') as it is known locally. Despite severe laws on drug trafficking, there is anecdotal evidence of a pending methamphetamine epidemic among Bruneian youth. Consequently, people with methamphetamine-induced disorder are frequently admitted. Other common drugs of misuse include cannabis and solvents.

## Future developments

Brunei Darussalam faces a number of challenges over the next few years, all of which are likely to affect its mental health services. Perhaps the most significant issue is the effect of the country's depleting oil reserves. The economy has not significantly diversified; if the prosperity dries up along with the oil wells, foreign workers are likely to leave. An exodus of Brunei's expatriates would be devastating for the mental health services, whose medical staff is composed entirely of foreigners. Psychiatry remains an unpopular choice of career with Brunei's small number of medical graduates, who are mostly trained in the UK, where they usually have a few weeks' exposure to psychiatry as undergraduates. A handful of Bruneian junior doctors are currently training as psychiatrists in nearby countries, but it is unlikely that a fully trained Bruniean psychiatrist will emerge for a number of years.

The mental health services face a number of tasks. The priorities are to raise the profile and understanding of psychiatry, as well as to undertake epidemiological research. There are plans to expand specialist services but these developments are already facing paralysing bureaucracy. Furthermore, there is a need for psychological treatments as well as better and newer drugs to be made available. The most ominous of unmet needs, however, is the establishment of drug treatment services. Finally, a new Mental Health Act is being drafted; it is hoped that it will afford greater protection to patients and will take account of the opinion of psychiatrists in the process of involuntary detention.

## References

Abdul Kadir, A. H. (2006) Of roots, barks, paracetamol and EDTA. *Malaysian Journal of Medical Sciences*, **13**, 1–6.

Attorney General's Chambers (2004) *Lunacy Act 1929: Selected laws of Brunei*. See http://www.agc.gov.bn/HTML/cap48.htm (accessed 30 August 2007).

Government of Brunei Darussalam (2004) *Land and People*. See http://www.brunei.gov.bn/about_brunei/land.htm (accessed 25 August 2007).

Kumaraswamy, N.( 2007) Psychotherapy in Brunei Darussalam. *Journal of Clinical Psychology*, **63**, 735–744.

Salleh, R. S. (1989) The consultation of traditional healers by Malay patients. *Medical Journal of Malaysia*, **44**, 3–13.

United Nations Population Fund (2005) Brunei Darussalam. *UNFPA Worldwide: Population, Health and Socio-Economic Indicators*. See http://www.unfpa.org/profile/brunei.cfm (accessed 25 August 2007).

# Cambodia

## James MacCabe, Ka Sunbaunat and Pauv Bunthoeun

Cambodia is a low-income country in south-east Asia. It covers an area of 181 035 km$^2$ and has a population of 14.5 million, of whom 42% are less than 15 years old. Life expectancy is 56.8 years and 36% of the population live on less than US$0.50 per day. Cambodia experienced a brutal civil war and genocide in the 1970s under the Khmer Rouge regime, during which approximately 1.7 million Cambodians were killed (Chandler, 1999) and the social and medical infrastructure was almost completely destroyed. No mental health services existed throughout the conflict and subsequent Vietnamese occupation, despite the incalculable impact of the Khmer Rouge regime on Cambodians' mental health. The current political situation is more stable, although there remain concerns about human rights abuses (Khan, 2005).

## Historical perspective

From 1935 to 1975, all psychiatric care was provided by a single psychiatric hospital located about 9 km to the south of Phnom Penh. By 1975, the patient population of the 800-bed hospital had grown to around 2000. Under the Khmer Rouge, the psychiatric hospital was destroyed and it is likely that all the patients were murdered. Across the country most professionals of all types were also killed – only 43 doctors survived, none of whom were psychiatrists (Savin, 2000). Between 1975 and 1994, there were no statutory psychiatric services and no mental health training in Cambodia.

### Revitalisation of psychiatry in Cambodia

In 1994, a cohort of 10 junior doctors joined the Norwegian-funded Cambodian Mental Health Training Programme; they graduated in 1998. A second cohort of 10 completed training in 2001 and, in addition, 40 psychiatric nurses have now been trained in Cambodia. The first out-patient department was opened in Phnom Penh in May 1994. The present mental health service situation in Cambodia is summarised in Box 1.

---

**Box 1** Current public sector mental health services in Cambodia

Staffing:

- 26 psychiatrists
- 40 psychiatric nurses
- about 150 medical doctors have been trained in basic mental healthcare
- about 170 registered nurses have been trained in basic mental healthcare.

Services:

- 3 in-patient units for emergency assessment
- 18 psychiatric out-patient departments at provincial level (in general hospitals)
- 13 psychiatric units at health-centre level
- 1 child psychiatric out-patient department at national level
- day-care centre at national level.

---

Paradoxically, the complete destruction of the former mental healthcare system presented a unique opportunity to introduce community-based mental health services, as the often difficult tasks of reintegrating institutionalised patients into community settings and retraining staff who are accustomed to a custodial model of care were obviated in Cambodia.

## Cambodian beliefs about mental health

Considerable stigma and fear surround mental illness. The majority of Cambodians with mental health problems are cared for by their families, neighbours, friends or traditional healers. Common complaints include tiredness, 'thinking too much', 'feeling very insecure' and flashbacks or disturbing dreams of traumatic events.

Under traditional belief systems, psychiatric disorders are typically attributed to witchcraft, possession by spirits or curses that pass from one generation to the next within a family. Some syndromes recognised by traditional healers approximate Western conceptions of mental illness, including alcohol dependence, postnatal depression and psychosis. Referral rates from traditional healers to mainstream services were thought to be low, but there is some evidence that they may be increasing.

## Mental health policy and services

The Mental Health Subcommittee of the Cambodian Ministry of Health, now known as the National Programme for Mental Health (NPMH), was given responsibility for developing mental health services in Cambodia in 1992. It is helped by the World Health Organization and collaborates closely with foreign aid organisations. Considering the paucity of central government funding, the NPMH has had considerable success in developing community psychiatric services in Cambodia.

Government mental health clinics are now operating in 23 of the 24 provinces and cities of Cambodia, although, because of the poor transport infrastructure, patients commonly have to travel for several days to reach help. Consultation and initial medical treatment are subsidised by the government, but patients are expected to pay for ongoing treatment themselves and this is frequently beyond their means. In some settings, brief psychological interventions are offered, usually in groups. Home visits by psychiatric nurses are occasionally available in some areas. There are small in-patient units at the main psychiatric clinic in Phnom Penh and in two provinces; these are used exclusively for brief assessments, usually for 24 hours or less.

Under a pilot scheme in the province of Battambang, mental health services have been integrated into the existing system of 13 community health centres, which operate at the village level. The NPMH hopes to extend this model into other provinces.

There is no legislation relating to the involuntary detention of patients in hospital.

## Voluntary and charitable organisations

In addition to the statutory services, a number of non-governmental organisations (NGOs) are working in mental health in Cambodia. Probably the largest is the Trans-cultural Psychosocial Organisation (TPO Cambodia), which was set up in 1995 by its parent organisation, TPO Amsterdam. TPO focuses on raising awareness of mental health issues and the training of local health professionals, volunteers, religious leaders and traditional healers in the detection and treatment of psychiatric disorders. It now employs over 60 staff, including two psychiatrists, six psychologists and six social workers. Another NGO, the Centre for Child Mental Health, established Cambodia's only child mental health service. The Social Services of Cambodia, another NGO, has been working on community mental health projects since 1994.

## Patient mix and referral patterns

A survey undertaken by K.S. and P.B. of clinic attenders at the main psychiatric out-patient department in Phnom Penh in 1996 found that around two-thirds were female. Nineteen per cent were diagnosed with psychotic disorders, 40% with mood disorders and 33% with anxiety disorders. Around a third had initially sought advice from traditional healers, a third had consulted general medical services and the remaining third had not consulted previously for their presenting problem.

# Training and research

Psychiatry is now part of the undergraduate curriculum for both doctors and nurses, and is taught in all regional training centres. There are plans for a basic 3-month training programme to be made available to doctors and nurses, as well as plans for a 2-week mental health course for general practitioners and registered nurses working at health-centre level.

In order to attract investment in mental health, there is a need for research into the health needs and illness behaviour of Cambodians with mental health problems. In addition, the tragic recent history of Cambodia and the post-conflict situation make the country a potentially important resource for research into the individual and collective psychiatric sequelae of genocide and other traumatic events. Some foreign universities are collaborating in research and training in Cambodia, including the Institute of Psychiatry in London, but there is little research infrastructure within Cambodia itself.

# Conclusion

Mental health services in Cambodia have progressed at an impressive rate in the past 10 years, but there is much that remains to be done. So long as the political situation remains relatively stable, and foreign aid continues at current or increased levels, the hard work of the mental health professionals in Cambodia should continue to reduce the gap between the need for and the provision of mental health services.

# References

Chandler, D. (1999) *Voices From S21: Terror and History in Pol Pot's Secret Prison.* University of California Press.

Khan, I. (2005) *Open letter on the occasion of International Human Rights Day 2005 raising concern about the state of freedom of expression in the Kingdom of Cambodia.* Amnesty International. Public statement ASA 23/006/2005. See http://www.amnestyusa.org/countries/cambodia/document.do?id=ENGASA230062005. Last accessed 8 February 2007.

Savin, D. (2000) Developing psychiatric training and services in Cambodia. *Psychiatric Services*, **51**, 935.

# Hong Kong

Eric F. C. Cheung, Linda C. W. Lam and Se-fong Hung

Hong Kong was a UK colony before 1997 but has since been a Special Administrative Region of the People's Republic of China. It is located in southern China and has an area of 1104 km². Approximately 95% of Hong Kong's population is ethnic Chinese. Hong Kong is a developed capitalist economy, with a gross domestic product of US$301.6 billion (2009 estimate), of which about 5.5% is spent on healthcare and about 0.24% on mental health (World Health Organization, 2005). Despite the relatively low level of spending on healthcare, Hong Kong nevertheless has one of the longest life expectancies in the world (79.2 years for men; 84.8 years for women) and a very low infant mortality rate (2.93 per 1000 live births) (Central Intelligence Agency, 2010).

## Mental health policy and legislation

There is no specific mental health policy in Hong Kong. Instead, mental health services are subsumed within the overall health service of the territory, which is directed at the Hong Kong government level by the Food and Health Bureau. The lack of a coherent mental health policy has resulted in a lack of coordination between the medical sector, which provides assessment and treatment of mental disorders, and the social sector, which provides rehabilitation and ensures reintegration and support for people recovering from mental disorders (Hong Kong College of Psychiatrists, 2007).

On the other hand, a specific mental health ordinance was enacted in Hong Kong as early as 1906, in the form of the Asylums Ordinance, which underwent several major revisions and amendment in 1950, 1960, 1988 and 1997 (Lo, 1988; Cheung, 2000), during which process it became the Mental Health Ordinance of Hong Kong, largely based on the UK Mental Health Act 1983. In its current form, this ordinance contains provisions for: the management of the property and affairs of mentally incapacitated persons; the reception, detention and treatment of patients; guardianship; the admission of persons with a mental disorder who are involved in criminal proceedings; mental health review tribunals; and issues related to consent for medical and dental treatment for persons who are mentally incapacitated.

## Mental health service delivery

Hong Kong has a mixed medical economy. A small proportion of specialist psychiatrists practise in the private sector. There is a lack of coverage of mental disorders by most medical insurance schemes. Consequently, the majority of mental healthcare in Hong Kong is provided by the public sector through the Hospital Authority (HA), a statutory body that manages all public hospitals in Hong Kong. Because of the relatively underdeveloped primary care system in Hong Kong, the mental health service has to take care of virtually all Hong Kong citizens who manage to access the public system with a mental health problem. To cope with the ever-increasing demand as the population becomes more aware of mental health problems, the service has evolved, over time, into a highly efficient system, characterised by high service throughput and efficient management of patients, but with a focus on risk aversion rather than personalised care.

The typical in-patient setting is an institutional one that ensures efficiency of management of a large number of patients; the total number of in-patients treated in 2008/09 was 15 887. A typical out-patient clinic is characterised by long waiting lists and a short consultation time per patient; the total number of out-patients served rose by 19% between 2003 and 2009. In 2009, a total of 151 259 out-patients were registered with the public system.

Since the year 2000, a number of small-scale initiatives and pilot programmes to reform the public mental health service have begun. These have concerned:

- the development of an early-intervention programme for young people with a first episode of psychosis
- the gradual down-sizing of large psychiatric hospitals – the total number of in-patient beds in Hong Kong decreased from 4730 in 2003/04 to 4000 in 2008/09
- funding to provide new psychiatric drugs for patients
- the gradual development and enhancement of community psychiatric services
- the development of community old-age psychiatric services, including outreach to institutions and a suicide prevention programme.

Although effective in their own right, most of these programmes were implemented only in selected areas of Hong Kong. After intensive lobbying by the Hong Kong College of Psychiatrists and other organisations, in 2009 the government announced that it would commit substantial resources in 2010 to two key areas: the implementation of a multidisciplinary case management approach in caring for patients with severe mental illness in the community; and the deployment of resources to develop shared care for common mental disorders with primary care practitioners.

The HA is also in the process of developing a Mental Health Service Plan that outlines the various strategies for mental health service development in the medical sector until 2015. This was the subject of consultation with various stakeholders in 2010.

# Psychiatric training

## Undergraduate medical training

Hong Kong has two medical schools, at the University of Hong Kong and the Chinese University of Hong Kong. The language of instruction in both universities is English and both medical schools have introduced problem-based learning, which has largely superseded traditional didactic teaching. Within the 5-year medical undergraduate course, psychiatry is taught in phases in the last 2 years. Medical students are expected to develop basic competencies in managing individuals with mental health problems through a combination of lectures, small-group tutorials and clinical bedside teaching.

## Postgraduate training in psychiatry

Postgraduate training in psychiatry in Hong Kong is governed by the Hong Kong College of Psychiatrists, a constituent college of the Hong Kong Academy of Medicine, which is the statutory body responsible for overseeing the provision of specialist training and continuous medical education in Hong Kong. Historically, psychiatric training in Hong Kong has closely followed the UK system and most psychiatrists in Hong Kong obtained the Membership of the Royal College of Psychiatrists (MRCPsych) as part of their postgraduate training. Since the mid-1980s, psychiatric training in Hong Kong has been structured and accredited by the Royal College of Psychiatrists and the Hong Kong Training Scheme formally became a recognised training scheme for the MRCPsych examination.

After the formation of the Hong Kong Academy of Medicine in 1993, postgraduate training in psychiatry underwent further reform and became a 6-year programme. The first 3 years of basic training incorporate the pre-MRCPsych training scheme, giving the trainee the opportunity to take the MRCPsych examination or the Part II of the Fellowship Examination of the Hong Kong College of Psychiatrists (FHKCPsych). After this milestone, a further 3 years of higher training is required before a trainee is eligible to take Part III of the FHKCPsych, in which the submission and the successful oral defence of a research dissertation is required before the trainee can become a specialist in psychiatry in Hong Kong (Hong Kong College of Psychiatrists, 2008).

Postgraduate training for research in psychiatry is also available in the psychiatric departments of the two universities. Mental health professionals with an interest in pursuing postgraduate research training have opportunities to enrol on masters and doctoral programmes.

More recently, the Hong Kong College of Psychiatrists has embarked on the development and preparation of formal subspecialisation by forming clinical divisions in general adult psychiatry, old age psychiatry, child and adolescent psychiatry, psychotherapy, addiction psychiatry, rehabilitation psychiatry and learning disability.

# Research

Despite its small size and lack of research funding, Hong Kong has a vibrant research scene in which multidisciplinary research addressing both neurobiological and psychosocial aspects of mental health takes place. The psychiatric departments of the two medical schools are the major research centres for psychiatry in Hong Kong. Particular areas of excellence include behavioural and statistical genetics, neuroimaging, research into early psychosis, sleep disorders, suicide and old-age psychiatry. In addition, applied and clinical research projects, such as clinical trials and service evaluations, are regularly conducted in HA hospitals throughout the territory.

Over the years, Hong Kong has also developed close research collaborations with major academic centres in mainland China, particularly in the area of psychosis, suicide and epidemiology.

# Links with mainland China

Since the hand-over of Hong Kong in 1997, links between Hong Kong and mainland Chinese psychiatrists have gradually developed. Joint scientific conferences, exchanges and clinical attachments for psychiatrists are regularly organised between the two sides. In the past 3 years, a tripartite training scheme jointly organised by the Chinese University of Hong Kong, the University of Melbourne and local psychiatric institutes has facilitated the training of a large number of mainland psychiatrists and mental health workers. This has centred on imparting the knowledge, skills and practical information to implement community psychiatric care for patients with severe mental illness.

# Future directions and conclusion

The mental health service in Hong Kong is undergoing tremendous change. With a firm foundation in education, training, legislation and research in psychiatry, despite meagre public spending on mental healthcare, Hong Kong has developed a highly efficient mental health service that addresses the basic mental health needs of its citizens with a hospital-based secondary and tertiary care model. However, this system is becoming unsustainable, because of the increasing pressure of demand. In the last 10 years or so, a gradual reform of the mental health service has begun. It is hoped that the service will be transformed from a system characterised by the efficient management of patients to a system that delivers personalised care to patients, informed by the cutting edge of psychiatric research.

# References

Central Intelligence Agency (2010) *The World Factbook: Hong Kong*. Available at https://www.cia.gov/library/publications/the-world-factbook/geos/hk.html (last accessed April 2010).

Cheung, H. K. (2000) The new mental health ordinance 1996 to 1997 – a reference guide for physicians and mental health workers. *Hong Kong Journal of Psychiatry*, **10**, 3–13.

Hong Kong College of Psychiatrists (2007) *Submission of the Hong Kong College of Psychiatrists to the Food and Health Bureau on Mental Health Policy in Hong Kong*. HKCP.

Hong Kong College of Psychiatrists (2008) *Education, Training and Examination for Fellowship*. HKCP.

Lo, W. H. (1988) Development of legislation for the mentally ill in Hong Kong. *Journal of the Hong Kong Psychiatric Association*, **8**, 6–9.

World Health Organization (2005) *Mental Health Atlas*. WHO.

# India

## Vikram Patel and Shekhar Saxena

India is a low-income country that is characterised by huge diversity within and between its 35 states and union territories. For example, the infant mortality rate (per 1000 live births) ranges from a low of 16.3 in Kerala to a high of 86.7 in Uttar Pradesh, over a fivefold difference (International Institute for Population Sciences & ORC Macro, 2001). This considerable variation is evident in virtually every aspect of human development in India, and any summary figures are likely to be unrepresentative of most parts of the country. Within the scope of this short article, this important limitation of averages must be recognised at the outset.

The latest population figures for India show that the population has now crossed the 1 billion mark and is continuing to grow, although at a gradually slower pace than before. The substantial epidemiological evidence base in relation to mental disorders shows that severe and common mental disorders are at least as common as in the developed world. The social and economic risk factors for mental disorders are on the rise in many parts of the country and there has been a reduction in the already pitiful level of spending by the Government on health and social welfare (5.2% of gross domestic product). There is evidence that a substantial proportion of healthcare in India is delivered in the private sector; some estimates put this at above 75% of all health consultations.

## Mental health resources

There are an estimated 4000 psychiatrists in India, which represents a ratio of approximately one psychiatrist for 250000 people (WHO, 2001). However, as mentioned earlier, this rate varies hugely between urban and rural areas, and between more developed and less developed states. Thus, in some states the ratio falls to one psychiatrist for more than one million people. The majority of psychiatrists work in urban areas, and in the private sector. The number of other mental health professionals, such as psychologists or psychiatric nurses, is even lower: there is one nurse for every 10 psychiatrists and one psychologist for every 20. There are an estimated 25 000 psychiatric beds in the country, or one bed for every 40 000 people. About 80% of these beds are situated in mental hospitals, where the quality of care has been found to violate even basic human rights (National Human Rights Commission, 1999).

If one considers that the estimated number of persons with schizophrenia alone is 10 million, it is obvious that the vast majority of persons with mental disorders will not have access to a mental health professional in India. The numbers of professionals in specialised areas of psychiatry, such as child, substance misuse or elderly mental health, cannot even be estimated because, barring in a few academic centres, these specialities do not exist (the provision is within general services). Thus, it may be fair to say that the primary provider of mental healthcare in India is the primary health sector, with its wide (though uneven) network of primary health centres and general hospitals, in both the private and public sectors.

The traditional and complementary medical sector is also a vibrant player in mental healthcare. This sector includes an array of religious, spiritual and alternative healing systems such as Ayurveda, faith-healing and unani medi¬cine. Recently, there has been a renaissance of traditional systems of health promotion, such as yoga.

The non-governmental sector is also playing a key role in mental healthcare, in particular by filling in niche areas of need such as child mental healthcare, and by developing innovative community-based models of care (Patel & Thara, 2002).

A large, mostly indigenous, pharmaceutical industry ensures that most psychotropic drugs are available in India, often at a fraction of their cost in high-income countries; however, this low cost does not translate into consistent availability in Government-run primary and general healthcare settings.

## Mental health education and qualifications in psychiatry

India has about 125 medical colleges, most of which have departments of psychiatry; about a quarter of these departments are recognised by the local universities for higher training in psychiatry. The most common qualifications are the MD (doctor in medicine), which is different from the MD in the USA (in that it is a specialist qualification) and that of the UK (in that a research dissertation is only one component; the other components include written and clinical examinations). The MD requires a residency of three years, followed by another three years of senior residency training to become a consultant.

Other qualifications include the Diploma in Psychological Medicine (DPM), which requires a two-year residency, and the Diplomate of the National Board, administered by the National Academy of Medical Sciences, which is an all-India examination styled along the lines of the Membership of the Royal College of Psychiatrists.

# Government policies and programmes

Mental health has been receiving increasing attention in national health policy and programming; this is best illu¬strated by a specific mention of mental health as a priority area for the new National Health Plan drafted for the coming decade. The National Mental Health Programme was formulated in 1982 with the objective of ensuring the availability and accessibility of basic mental healthcare, particularly to the most vulnerable and under-privileged sections of the population. The programme, though visionary in its conceptualisation, made slow progress, mainly because of a lack of dedicated finances. It is implemented at present in 22 districts (out of 593) and will be extended to over 100 districts in the next few years. The key approaches used are the training of primary healthcare personnel, the provision of neuropsychiatric drugs in peripheral institutions, the establishment of psychiatric units at the district level, with streamlined referrals, and the encouragement of community participation. However, it is worth noting that, despite this programme, less than 1% of the total health budget is devoted to mental health.

# Psychiatric associations

The flagship psychiatric association is the Indian Psychiatric Society, established in 1947. The Society holds an annual conference and organises continuing medical education; it also publishes the Indian Journal of Psychiatry. The Society has five regional zones, which all hold annual conferences; some also publish their own journals.

There are several other associations in India, including the Indian Association for Child and Adolescent Mental Health, the Indian Association for Social Psychiatry, Indian chapters of world associations, such as the World Association for Psychosocial Rehabilitation, and, most recently, the Indian Association for Private Psychiatry.

# Research and journals

India has a substantial research base in mental health. A recent review of the contribution of various non-Western countries to the international psychiatric literature found that 14% of the papers published over three years in six high-impact journals were from India, a figure second only to Japan (Patel & Sumathipala, 2001).

The requirement that every MD in psychiatry must complete a research dissertation means that about 100 research projects are completed each year; many, however, suffer from methodological problems as a result of inadequate supervision and research skills (Patel, 2001). Another problem is that the research often consists of drug trials funded by industry, with the primary purpose of meeting the national regulations for the introduction of new medicines. Health services and public health research is conspicuously missing.

The research infrastructure in India centres on medical school departments of psychiatry and national centres for higher research, such as:

- the National Institute for Mental Health and Neurosciences (NIMHANS) in Bangalore
- the All India Institute for Medical Sciences (AIIMS) in New Delhi
- the Post-graduate Institute for Medical Education and Research (PGIMER) in Chandigarh.

Research is also being conducted by non-governmental organisations; some of the best-known studies on schizophrenia in India, for example, have been the result of research by the Schizophrenia Research Foundation (SCARF) in Chennai (Thara & McCreadie, 1999).

There are more than 10 journals in psychiatry and allied specialities in India, the best-known being the *Indian Journal of Psychiatry* and the *NIMHANS Journal*. However, despite a continuous publication record of several decades, the *Indian Journal of Psychiatry* is still not indexed on major international citation databases, and this limits its impact on world psychiatry. Not surprisingly, some of the best scientific studies from India still go to international journals.

## Mental health legislation

The Mental Health Act of 1987 replaced the Indian Lunacy Act of 1912. The Act has provided new definitions, simplified admission and discharge procedures, introduced licensing of psychiatric hospitals, set up central and state mental health authorities and promoted human rights for people with mental illnesses (WHO, 2001). However, the implementation of this law has been very uneven across the states. Courts in India have provided much support to the mental health field by repeatedly asking the Government to provide better care, within the framework of basic human rights. Another key piece of legislation has been the Persons with Disabilities Act, which includes mental disabilities, and which provides access to social welfare and employment schemes. The Narcotic Drugs and Psychotropic Substances Act (amended in 2001) deals with the prevention, treatment and rehabilitation of people with drug-dependence.

## Role of Indian members of the Royal College of Psychiatrists

India has a considerable human resource base for mental health initiatives, but this base is very inadequate to meet the mental health needs of the population. The key to closing the treatment gap is to use the resources available (for example, including private psychiatrists and non-governmental organisations in mental health pro¬grammes), strengthening services in primary care, providing more effective referral systems and building the research evidence on cost-effective health service interventions. Members of the College can play a number of important roles by strengthening links with Indian associations and organisations. In our view, the key priorities for such collaborations are:

- to build research capacity through collaboration on specific research projects and strengthening research training opportunities
- to share models of training for primary and general healthcare practitioners in mental health interventions
- to share models for the development of community care, in particular for severe mental disorders, learning disabilities and mental disorders affecting children and the elderly
- to facilitate the training of general psychiatrists in specialist areas such as substance abuse, child psychiatry and forensic psychiatry
- to facilitate the process of reforming mental hospitals in India by enabling hospital staff to improve the physical, social and therapeutic environment of the hospital.

# References

International Institute for Population Sciences & ORC Macro (2001) *National Family Health Survey – 2, 1998–99*. Mumbai: International Institute for Population Sciences.

National Human Rights Commission (1999) *Quality Assurance in Mental Health*. New Delhi: NHRC.

Patel, V. (2001) Research in India: not good enough? *Indian Journal of Psychiatry*, **43**, 375–377.

Patel, V. & Sumathipala, A. (2001) International representation in psychiatric literature. *Survey of six leading journals. British Journal of Psychiatry*, **178**, 406–409.

Patel, V. & Thara, R. (2002) *Meeting Mental Health Needs in Developing Countries: NGO Innovations in India*. New Delhi: Sage.

Thara, R. & McCreadie, R. G. (1999) Research in India: success through collaboration. *Advances in Psychiatric Treatment*, **5**, 221–224.

WHO (2001) *Atlas Country Profiles of Mental Health Resources*. Geneva: World Health Organization. See http://mh-atlas.ic.gc.ca/

# Iran

## Majid Sadeghi and Gholamreza Mirsepassi

The Islamic Republic of Iran is located in the Middle East between the Caspian Sea and the Persian Gulf. Iran's total land area is 1 648 000 km². Its total population in 2003 was about 68 920 000 (UNICEF, 2003). The population growth rate is 1.41%. Of the total population, 60.4% live in urban and 39.6% in rural areas (Yasamy *et al*, 2001).

## Health indicators

Life expectancy at birth in the year 2002 was estimated to be 66.5 years for males and 71.7 years for females (World Health Organization, 2003). The mortality rate for infants (under 1 year) was 33 per 1000 live births in the year 2003 (UNICEF, 2003). Iran has a rather young population: roughly 40% are under 15 years and only 4.5% are aged 65 years or more (Iran Centre of Statistics, 2003).

The rate of suicide is estimated to be 6.2 per 100 000 per year in both males and females.

## History of psychiatry in Iran

In Iran, the history of psychiatry is as old as the history of medicine. In the middle ages, when in the West people with a mental illness were typically punished and tortured as witches or were looked upon as being possessed, the main approach to their care in the Islamic world, including Iran, generally involved kindness and some form of counselling, combined with herbal, aroma and music therapy and custody in special asylums.

Rhazes (Muhammad ibn Zakariya al-Razi, 865–925) and Avicenna (Abu Ali Ibn Sina, 980–1037), two great Iranian physicians and philosophers, in their writings described such mental disorders as melancholia, mania and delirious states. They also prescribed psychotherapy for their patients and described the effects of emotions on the cardiovascular system.

Modern psychiatry in Iran begins with the foundation of Tehran University in 1934. In 1937 the department of psychiatry at the medical school began teaching students. The first teachers at the department were mainly French-educated, among them the late Professor Abdolhossein Mirsepassi and Professor Hossein Rezai, who were pioneers of psychiatry in Iran.

There had been some asylums for the custody of psychiatric patients since the 19th century in Tehran and other major cities of Iran; these were mainly managed by the municipalities, and were mostly in an unfavourable condition. Roozbeh Hospital was founded in 1946 as the first modern psychiatric teaching hospital in Iran. This hospital has since trained many generations of psychiatrists and still is the leading centre in psychiatric education, treatment and research (Kermani, 1966).

## Prevalence of psychiatric disorders

Various studies have estimated the point prevalence of all psychiatric disorders to be in a range from 11.9% (Bash & Bash-Liechti, 1969) to 41.1% (Motamedi *et al*, 1998). In a recent study about a fifth of interviewees (25.9% of the women and 14.9% of the men) were rated as likely 'cases'. Symptoms of depression and anxiety were more prevalent than somatisation and social dysfunction. The rates of learning disability, epilepsy and psychosis were 1.4%, 1.2% and 0.6%, respectively (Noorbala *et al*, 2004).

## Substance misuse in Iran

Opium and its natural and synthetic components (especially heroin) are the most widely used substances in Iran, although other substances, notably cannabis, amphetamine-like drugs and to a lesser extent cocaine, seem to be used increasingly, especially by adolescents.

An estimated 2.8% of the Iranian population over the age of 15 years used opiates in 2001 (International Narcotics Control Strategy, 2003).

One study found that 93% of opiate addicts in Iran were male, with a mean age of 33.6 years, and 1.4% were HIV positive (Yasamy *et al*, 2001).

Methadone maintenance and HIV prevention programmes are expanding, although HIV infection in the prison population is a serious problem (Hashemi Mohammad Abad & London, 2003).

## Healthcare beliefs

Despite a significant decrease in discrimination and stigmatisation in recent years, it seems that attitudes towards mental health remain a major challenge in Iran. In a recent (unpublished) study of the families of 300 patients with schizophrenia, major depressive disorder and bipolar disorder, 49%, 30% and 51% of these respective groups reported stigma and humiliation (further details from the first author on request).

As in many other developing countries, emotional problems are frequently expressed in somatic form. Beliefs that illness may be caused by a person with the 'evil eye' (i.e. who can harm others merely by looking at them) or an imbalance in 'hot/cold' temperaments or foods are common and coexist with more medical concepts (Sadeghi, 2003).

In general, there is less verbalisation of emotions, especially depression and anxiety. Feelings of guilt are seldom expressed spontaneously. Hypochondriasis and somatic complaints are frequent (Sartorius *et al*, 1983).

Traditional healers still have a major role. One study found that 16% of patients had visited traditional healers and used alternative medicine before their first psychiatric visit (Omidvari *et al*, 2001).

# Mental health facilities

There are currently 8950 psychiatric beds distributed among 23 psychiatric and general hospitals, and 825 psychiatrists are practising throughout the country, of whom 30 are child psychiatrists (National Research Centre of Medical Sciences, 2003; Ministry of Health and Medical Education, 2003).

The therapeutic modalities in Iran are mainly pharmacotherapy (the most widely used), psychotherapy and electroconvulsive therapy (ECT). Although many newer psychotherapeutic drugs are available in Iran they are generally too expensive for the average patient. Psychiatric rehabilitation facilities in general are scanty and insufficient.

# Psychiatric non-governmental organisations in Iran

The Iranian Psychiatric Association was founded in 1966 and is a member of the World Psychiatric Association (WPA). The Child and Adolescent Psychiatric Association was founded in 2001.

There are also other non-governmental organisations (NGOs) active in mental heath, including the Association for the Support of Schizophrenic Patients and Narcotic Anonymous (NA), a self-support group for ex-addicts.

# Education

## Undergraduate

The duration of general medical training in Iran is 6–7 years. Medical students have a 1-month course in psy¬chiatry, which covers theoretical aspects, and a 1-month internship during which psychiatric history taking and interviewing skills are taught.

## Postgraduate

Postgraduate psychiatric training is a 3-year course covering the theoretical and practical aspects of psychiatry, including in-patient and out-patient adult psychiatry, psychiatric emergencies, psychotherapy (especially cognitive–behavioural and/or analytical approaches), consultation–liaison psychiatry, child psychiatry and rotations in forensic psychiatry and neurology. Every psychiatric resident has to conduct a supervised research project during his/her training as a prerequisite for participation in written and oral board certification examinations set by the National Board Examiners' Committee.

The only subspecialty training is child and adolescent psychiatry, which is a 2-year course.

## Research

The publication of papers in international journals has seen considerable growth during recent years: from about four in 1973 to more than 90 in 2001. However, because none of the 23 mental health journals published in Iran are indexed in international databases, the output of Iranian researchers in branches of medicine related to mental health is less than may appear to be the case.

## Mental health promotion and policies

The National Programme of Mental Health, which seeks to integrate mental healthcare within primary healthcare, was started in 1989 as a pilot study in two rural areas (Yasamy & Bagheri Yazdi, 2004). In 1995 it was jointly evaluated by the World Health Organization and the Tehran Psychiatric Institute. The programme was recognised as one the most successful in the region (Murthy, 2002).

The aim is to establish a hierarchical, pyramid-like referral system. At the base of the pyramid there are health workers known as Behvarz, who are mainly local residents of each primary healthcare area; they are trained to recognise, refer and follow psychiatric cases to the higher level, which comprises rural health centres (Fenton, 1998). Currently, 21.7% of the urban population and 82.8% of the rural population is covered by the National Programme of Mental Health (Yasamy et al, 2001).

## Future of psychiatry in Iran (opportunities and threats)

The advancement of psychiatric education and the promotion of mental health policies in the past decade have profoundly affected psychiatric services. At present, it seems that there are enough psychiatrists in major cities throughout the country, and most psychotropic medications are available in Iran. All psychiatric hospitals are equipped with modern ECT machines.

On the other hand, non-biological treatments are not extensively available, being mainly limited to four or five major cities in the country. Iran lacks a practical and comprehensive mental health act. Limited coverage of mental health expenses by insurance companies has affected psychiatric care in both the private and the governmental sectors. Despite a dramatic increase in recent years, the mental health budget still remains highly insufficient. The Mental Health Bureau of the Ministry of Health and the Iranian Psychiatric Association have been struggling to increase the budget.

# References

Bash, K. W. & Bash-Liechti, J. (1969) Studies on the epidemiology of neuropsychiatric disorders among the population of Shiraz, Iran. *Social Psychiatry*, **9**, 163–171.

Fenton, W. S. (1998) *In Mental Health in Our Future Cities* (eds D. Goldberg & G. Thornicroft). Maudsley Monograph 42. Philadelphia, PA: Psychology Press.

Hashemi Mohammad Abad, N. & London, M. (2003) Psychiatric practice in Iran and the UK. *Psychiatric Bulletin*, **27**, 190–191.

International Narcotics Control Strategy (2003) *Report released by the Bureau for International Narcotics and Law Enforcement Affairs.*

Iran Centre of Statistics (2003) *Annual Report.* Tehran: Iran Centre of Statistics.

Kermani, E. J. (1966) Psychiatry in Iran. *American Journal of Psychiatry*, **122**, 949–952.

Ministry of Health and Medical Education (2003) *Statistics on Psychiatric Beds in Iran.* Tehran: Ministry of Health and Medical Education.

Motamedi, S. H., Yasami, M., Karbasi, H., *et al* (1998) Determination of the prevalence of mental illnesses in two rural areas of Kerman. *Journal of the Kerman University of Medical Sciences*, **5**, 31–36.

Murthy, R. S. (2002) Mental health in the Islamic Republic of Iran. *Andishe Va Raftar*, **7** (**suppl. 4**), 40–57.

National Research Centre of Medical Sciences (2003) *Statistics on Psychiatric Beds in Iran.* Tehran: National Research Centre of Medical Sciences.

Noorbala, A., Bagheri Yazdi, S. A., Yasamy, M. T., *et al* (2004) Mental health survey of the adult population in Iran. *British Journal of Psychiatry*, **184**, 70–73.

Omidvari, S., Bina, M. & Yassemi, M. T. (2001) Pre-hospitalization pathways among psychiatric patients in Imam Hussain Hospital in 1999. *Andishe Va Raftar*, **6**, 4–12.

Sadeghi, M. (2003) Iran. In *Handbook of Cultural Health Assessment* (ed. C. D'Avanzo). St Louis, MO: C. V. Mosby.

Sartorius, N., Davidian, H., Emberg, G., *et al* (1983) *Depressive Disorders in Different Cultures. Report on the WHO Collaborative Study on Standardized Assessment of Depressive Disorders.* Geneva: World Health Organization.

UNICEF (2003) *At a Glance: Iran (Islamic Republic of) Statistics.* New York: UNICEF.

World Health Organization (2003) *The World Health Report, Country Profiles, Iran (Islamic Republic of).* Geneva: WHO.

Yasamy, M. T. & Bagheri Yazdi, S. A. (2004) *National Programme of Mental Health.* Tehran: Ministry of Health and Medical Education.

Yasamy, M. T., Shahmohammadi, D., Bagheri Yazdi, S. A., *et al* (2001) Mental health in the Islamic Republic of Iran: achievements and areas of need. *Eastern Mediterranean Health Journal*, **7**, 381–389.

# Iraq

Sabah Sadik and Abdul-Monaf Al-Jadiry

Iraq is known to be the cradle of civilisation – a country with a rich history. Present-day Iraq occupies the greater part of the ancient land of Mesopotamia, the plain between the Euphrates and Tigris rivers. Some of the world's greatest ancient civilisations arose in this area, and Iraq possesses a huge number of historical monuments and archaeological sites.

Modern Iraq has a geographical area of just under 440 000 km² and a population of just over 27 million. The main languages spoken in the country are Arabic, Kurdish and Turkman. The two main religions are Islam and Christianity. The country is in the lower middle-income group (according to World Bank criteria).

The proportion of the population under the age of 15 years is 41% and the proportion of those over 60 years is 5%. Life expectancy at birth is 59.1 years for males and 63.1 years for females. Healthy life expectancy at birth is 49 years for males and 52 years for females. The literacy rate for men is 54.9% and for women is 23.3%.

The healthcare system in Iraq is centralised and provided free of charge at the point of delivery. The Minister of Health is supported by three deputies and a number of directors and advisors, each having responsibility for a directorate. There is a plan for the new Iraq to look at devolution, with the governorates having some form of independence, as well as looking at private–public partnerships. Social services are provided by the Ministry of Labour and Social Affairs, and there is a close working relationship between the two ministries to provide social care alongside healthcare.

## History of mental health services

Pioneers like Al-Razi (865–925) and Ibn-Sina (Avicenna, 980–1037) established the first mental hospitals and applied humane treatments. Indeed, the first mental hospital in the world was built in Baghdad in 705. The region then entered the dark ages and it was not until the middle of the 20th century that modern psychiatric services appeared in Iraq. In the early 1950s, Dr Jack Aboud and Dr Ali Kamal led in establishing Al-Rashid and Al-Rashad mental hospitals (the former was later replaced by Ibn Rushid State Hospital). The 1960s and 1970s saw the development of mental health centres and units in general hospitals, school mental health programmes and public awareness campaigns. Strategic short-term and long-term plans were established. However, from the mid-1980s onwards mental health services experienced a significant deterioration, with an exodus of psychiatrists, due to a poor (even intimidating) working environment, shortages of medication, lack of information systems and a lack of educational opportunities. This situation was compounded by three disastrous wars, 12 years of sanctions and the recent fall of the regime, followed by the continuing violence. In addition, there was widespread looting of medical facilities.

In the past, mental health planning was run within the Primary Care Directorate of the Ministry of Health by a physician, who was supported by an advisory committee of four psychiatrists, although they had very little influence. The group ran limited activities of public education, refresher courses for general practitioners and lectures for school teachers in an attempt to increase public awareness.

## Recent developments: governance and accountability

In July 2003 the East Mediterranean Regional Office (EMRO) of the World Health Organization (WHO) held a meeting in Cairo as one of the WHO initiatives to support mental health in Iraq (see WHO, 2003). The new Iraqi government was appointed in September 2003. The Minister for Health declared that mental health was a priority, and appointed a National Advisor, who, with the support of colleagues, formed the National Mental Health Council (the first in the history of Iraq). The Council included representation from all relevant ministries and non-governmental organisations (NGOs) and there are plans to include service users. The Council had its inaugural meeting in March 2004. In June 2005 the Minister approved the structure for the National Advisor's office shown in Fig. 1.

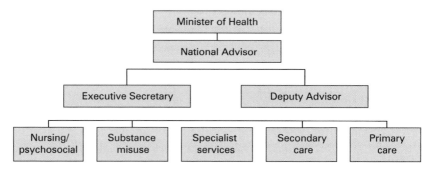

**Fig. 1** The approved structure for the National Advisor's office.

The National Advisor, with members of the National Council, has conducted field visits to oversee developments in mental health across Iraq as well as to lend support to colleagues.

## National Strategy for Mental Health and Mental Health Act

The first priority the National Council set for itself was to draw up the National Strategy for Mental Health (a copy is available on request). Previous attempts by colleagues to do so over the past 20 years were blocked by the previous regime. Those attempts were revived and the National Council held a workshop to discuss and finalise the Strategy on 21 and 22 June 2004. The Mental Health Act was approved by the Cabinet in October 2004. A draft Code of Practice is out for consultation and is awaiting final approval.

# Facilities

Iraq has two mental hospitals, both in Baghdad: Al-Rashad, with 1200 beds, and Ibn Rushid, with 70 beds. There are also four units in general hospitals in Baghdad and eight more units in other governorates. All facilities have limited resources. Multidisciplinary working is not practised.

The National Council has established ten outreach clinics and psychosocial support centres in Baghdad.

# Workforce

In December 2005 the National Mental Health Council, in partnership with the WHO, completed the Assessment Instrument for Mental Health Systems (WHO, 2005). This showed that there were 1.6 professionals in mental health facilities, including private practice, per 100000 population. Table 1 breaks this down further according to profession.

The National Council engineered the return to work of psychiatrists, psychologists and social workers who had been unemployed or dismissed for political reasons, and those who had left their jobs in the past because of poor pay and working conditions.

**Table 1** Total numbers of workers in mental health facilities

| Discipline | Percentage of workforce | Number |
| --- | --- | --- |
| Psychiatrists | 33 | 91 |
| Other medical doctors (i.e. non-psychiatrists) | 2 | 7 |
| Nurses | 53 | 145 |
| Psychologists | 5 | 16 |
| Social workers | 9 | 25 |
| Other mental health workers | 47 | 128 |

The National Council, with the support of the Japan International Cooperation Agency and the WHO, ran training programmes for Iraqi nurses, held in Egypt (two 6-week courses in September and November 2004 for 40 senior nurses). Another 2-month course started in Bahrain in April 2006.

## Academic activities

The National Council has organised a number of multidisciplinary educational activities for mental health workers. Dr Sadik has been appointed Visiting Professor in Psychiatry at Baghdad University and has become a member of the Iraqi Scientific Council for Postgraduate Studies and the Arab Board in Psychiatry.

### Research and publications

Fifteen pilot studies have now been completed and a full research programme was expected to be concluded in April 2006, when reports on individual projects were to be submitted for publication.

A special issue on Iraq of the *Muslim Mental Health Journal* was planned for October 2006.

## Drug misuse

A National Council for Drug Misuse was re-established in 2004 but in February 2006 it joined the National Council for Mental Health to become the National Council for Mental Health and Substance Misuse. It is chaired by the Minister of Health and has representatives from the Ministry of the Interior, the Ministry of Social Welfare and other committees within the Ministry of Health.

A programme to address drug misuse has been agreed in collaboration with the regional WHO team (a copy is available on request) and a drug control law has been submitted to the Cabinet for approval. Iraq is now a member of the United Nations Office on Drugs and Crime.

## Child mental health

The National Council supported the formation of a multidisciplinary Child Mental Health Association. Registered with the Arab Psychiatric Association (APA) and the World Child Mental Health Association, the Iraqi Child Mental Health Association has been asked to lead on educational activities as well as to draw up a strategy for child mental health.

## Non-governmental organisations

The National Council has supported various activities headed by NGOs, including:

- the Heartland Alliance's Integrated Torture Treatment project
- a psychosocial support project for children in Baghdad, run by MOVIMONDO of Italy
- a psychosocial support project for children and families in Babylon, run by the organisation 'Together' from Slovenia – this has now been extended to Baghdad
- a psychotherapy service with a focus on children, provided by Diaconia, a Swedish organisation that operates offices in Dahouk, Erbil and Suleymania (the Heartland Alliance has collaborated with staff from Diaconia to deliver Heartland Alliance training in Dahouk)
- the rehabilitation of Ibn Rushid Hospital, supported by the Japanese government
- the rehabilitation of Al-Rashad Hospital, funded by the Red Cross.

# World Health Organization

The EMRO of the WHO has supported the planning and training activities of the National Council. This included finalising the National Strategy. More recently, the National Mental Health Council in partnership with the WHO completed the Assessment Instrument for Mental Health Systems mentioned above. Further work has now started on a national screening programme for mental health.

In collaboration with the WHO, the following activities have been approved for funding, to start in the near future:
- a needs assessment workshop (as part of a national mental health survey, which was due to start in June 2006)
- rebuilding of mental health facilities (work on 12 units has already been completed)
- building of new mental health units in general hospitals (six in total: two have been completed, work has begun on two and work is yet to start on the remaining two; in addition, approval for another six units has recently been given)
- a national epidemiological survey with the Composite International Diagnostic Interview (CIDI) (this has just started).

# Partnerships

The National Council has established a working partnership with the US Substance Abuse and Mental Health Services Administration (SAMHSA), through regular teleconferencing as well as participation in stakeholder events. A planning group formed of international experts connecting with SAMHSA's support has been invaluable in securing training curricula and opportunities, service development and planning and drawing in international expertise.

With the support of the SAMHSA, the WHO, the UK Department of Health and the World Bank, the First Action Planning Iraq Mental Health Conference was held in Amman, Jordan, in March 2005 (a copy of the proceedings is available on request). A second conference was held in March 2006 in Cairo, Egypt.

The WHO has been instrumental in supporting all of the above activities and developments.

The Royal College of Psychiatrists has supported:

- the Iraqi Mental Health Forum (IMHF) in the UK
- representation of Iraqi mental health professionals at its annual and regional meetings
- the formation of a subcommittee of the Board of International Affairs to address and support Iraqi mental health services and training needs.

The UK Department of Health has provided financial support to address service development and training needs.

In a recent meeting of Iraqi psychiatrists a committee was elected to prepare for and oversee fair and free elections for the Iraqi Psychiatric Association. Close liaison continues with:

- the American Psychiatric Association
- the International Institute for Mental Health
- the Kent and Medway NHS and Social Care Partnership Trust
- the United Nations Office on Drugs and Crime.

## Challenges

The potential to achieve a high standard of comprehensive community-based mental health services in Iraq is a reality. However, the ongoing violence and poor security, coupled with bureaucracy and political instability, have hindered progress. Progress has been very slow on developing an efficient and effective information system, in establishing performance management and in applying healthcare standards. The distribution of medicines and equipment, the movement of staff and the organising of training events remain high-risk activities. Recent improvements in the pay and conditions for staff working in higher education have led many health service professionals to switch to teaching. Furthermore, physical threats to doctors have forced many to leave the country.

In spite of these difficulties, the achievements of the National Council for Mental Health and Substance Abuse in such a short period and its continuing activities have been a landmark in Iraq's recent health services history.

## References

World Health Organization (2003) *Report of a Consultation on Mental Health and Rehabilitation of Psychiatric Service in Post-conflict and Complex Emergency Countries*. EMRO/MNH/22. Geneva: WHO.

World Health Organization (2005) *AIMS Country Report for Iraq*. Geneva: WHO.

# Israel

Itzhak Levav and Alexander Grinshpoon

Israel is a multicultural society in a state of permanent change. The population, of about 6.5 million, comprises the following religious groupings: Jews (77.5%), Muslims (15.3%), Christians (2.1%), Druzes (1.7%) and others (3.4%). The organisation of and the approaches used by the country's health services have been determined by this socio-cultural plurality, and also by a continuous influx of immigrants (among whom, 882 600 and 44 200 arrived from countries of the former USSR and Ethiopia, respectively, between 1990 and 2001), as well as by the precarious security situation (the country has seen several wars with its neighbours in addition to the long-standing conflict with the Palestinians). The patterns of care of the population reflect both Western psychiatry and traditional systems. Because of such complexity, the present brief overview is necessarily selective.

## Health indicators

The description of mental health services that follows will be better understood against a background of selected public health indicators and socio-demographic variables. Mean life expectancy in the year 2000 was 76.7 years for men and 80.9 for women. The infant mortality rate was 5.1 per 1000 live births in the year 2001. The coverage for immunisation for poliomyelitis reached 93% during the first year of life (1998 figure). The chief causes of mortality are the chronic disorders, an area of health that calls for closer linkage with the mental health professions. With regard to age, 28.5% of the population are under 15 years and 9.8% are 65 years old or more. The median time spent in education for people aged 15 and over was 12.3 years by the year 2000. All these figures refer to the combined Israeli population; however, there are some notable differences between specific population groups (Central Bureau of Statistics, 2002).

## National health insurance

By law, all residents are insured for healthcare and contribute to a national fund according to income. Most of the population is served by one of the four health maintenance organisations, the largest of which was established in the pre-State years (before 1948) by the labour unions.

Importantly, the law that established this health system did not include either psychiatric care or geriatric and nursing services. In 2002, the government decided to transfer all responsibility for mental healthcare (see below) to the health maintenance organisations; implementation of this decision is expected in 2005.

Care provided by a general practitioner is free. A visit to a specialist (other than a psychiatrist) carries a nominal fee (less than US$5). Visits to a psychiatric clinic, care in a psychiatric hospital or hostel, and certain specified drugs are free of charge. Preventive maternal and child health services are provided free by the municipalities and by the Ministry of Health.

## Policy principles guiding the provision of mental healthcare

Israel has not yet developed a national mental health plan, but the first steps are being taken and the political will exists to formulate one. Once adopted, the plan will be based on the following policy objectives, which are endorsed by almost all stakeholders:

- to promote the mental health of the population
- to integrate mental healthcare within the general health system
- to ensure equity of access to services in all parts of the country
- to provide high-quality evidence-based and cost-effective care to persons with mental disorders
- to promote the psychosocial rehabilitation of persons with mental disability
- to strengthen and expand community-based care and reduce both hospital admission rates and length of stay
- to ensure the availability of emergency and crisis services, specially in security-related situations.

## The organisation of mental healthcare

The government is responsible for the overall planning, budgeting and monitoring of the mental healthcare provided to all the population. Two multi-sectoral national advisory councils, one on mental health and the other on community-based mental health rehabilitation, assist the government in this.

The national fight against addictions, including health promotion and prevention activities, is the responsibility of an autonomous council. The services, such as methadone supply, however, are the responsibility of the Ministry of Health, in association with the welfare system.

The Ministry of Health allocates 5.9% of its budget to mental health services (2002 figure). This is not all the budget available for public mental healthcare, since this percentage does not include sums from other public-sector organisations. As noted above, curative care is provided by the government, although some services are offered by the health maintenance organisations. The responsibility for psychosocial rehabilitation services is shared with the welfare services and, especially, with the National Insurance Institute (see section on legislation, below).

Any inhabitant can freely access any mental health curative service (Feinson *et al*, 1997). Although referral by a general practitioner is preferable, any resident can attend mental health services directly, without such a referral. The country has 114 clinics and day-care centres, 12 psychiatric wards in general hospitals and 20 mental hospitals.

Since the early 1950s, Israel has run a psychiatric case register. All admissions and discharges are cumulatively entered into a database. Of late, this database has incorporated additional sources of information (e.g. clinic-originated information). The confidentiality of the database is specifically protected by law (Department of Information and Evaluation, 2002).

Table 1 highlights some statistics relating to in-patient care in Israel. The rates of hospital admission per 1000 are lowest for Muslims (men 2.50, women 1.19), intermediate for Christian Arabs (2.48 and 1.69, respectively) and highest for Jews (3.49 and 2.50, respectively). Similarly to most countries, 51.8% of admissions are for schizophrenia or delusional disorders. Five per cent of psychiatric beds are in general hospitals. The number of beds has fallen over time.

## Consumer and family organisations

These organisations are highly visible and active in both advocacy and mutual support. (A special issue of the *Israel Journal of Psychiatry*, vol.

**Table 1** In-patient psychiatric services, 2001

| | |
|---|---|
| Beds (number per 1000 persons aged 15 and above) | 1.17 |
| Annual rate of first admission, per 1000 persons aged 15 and above | |
| Total | 0.92 |
| Jews | 0.99 |
| Muslim Arabs | 0.70 |
| Others | 0.34 |
| Annual rate of readmissions per 1000 persons aged 15 and above | 2.96 |
| Annual admission rate per 1000 persons aged 15 and above to in-patient and hospital-based day care | |
| Men | 3.4 |
| Women | 2.3 |
| Average length of hospital stay (days) | 131 |
| Proportion of all admissions that are voluntary | 74.2% |

39, no. 3, 2002, was wholly devoted to the consumers of mental health services.) They have representation on the national councils and have a strong voice in the efforts leading to the transfer of mental healthcare to the health maintenance organisations. The Ministry of Health recognises their important role in the humanisation and democratisation of mental healthcare by contributing to their support. These organisations were consulted in the process of drafting the laws alluded to below and their representatives take part in the quality-control activities that have recently been initiated.

In addition, several non-government organisations are active in mental healthcare, such as ERAN, which offers telephone first-aid assistance nationally, and another that provides initial guidance to foreign workers.

## Legislation on psychosocial rehabilitation

Perhaps the single most important piece of legislation that facilitates the ongoing – but slow – process of psychiatric reform is that adopted in 2000. This is the Community-Based Rehabilitation of the Mentally Disabled Act, whereby all consumers whose degree of mental disability reaches 40%, as established by the National Insurance Institute, are fully entitled to receive a set of rehabilitation services in the community. This law has enabled the mental hospitals to discharge people who would otherwise remain merely for custodial reasons and to promote their social reintegration. Funds have thus become available to contract out to private and social enterprises running hostels with different levels of supervisory services for their clients. To avoid recreating the atmosphere of mental institutions, these hostels are periodically inspected by staff from the Ministry of Health.

The range of rehabilitation services is wide: they include dental care, for example – an item often neglected in psychiatric health plans – and supported education. With regard to the latter, special efforts are being made to help consumers to complete their educational cycle within the regular system of education for adults.

## Health services and the security situation

The unstable security situation has led the country to devote considerable resources (in services, research and teaching) to help the civilian population overcome the stress resulting from both open warfare and acts of terrorism. This section alludes to the 1991 Gulf War, when areas of the country were subjected to missile attack by Saddam Hussein's Iraq, and to the current second Intifada, which began in October 2000.

In the Gulf War, studies covered a number of health issues among adults, such as mortality (the early elevated cardiovascular mortality rate that was found was presumably linked to the use of gas masks and extended stays in sealed rooms – Kark *et al*, 1995); self-appraisal of physical health (worsened health status); health behaviour (increased smoking, diminished physical activity, changed eating habits); and psychological distress (higher in the exposed areas) (Nakar *et al*, 1996; Soskolne *et al*, 1996). Other studies explored reactions in children (Laor *et al*, 1996) and among the elderly (Solomon & Prager, 1992), and acute stress in evacuees (Solomon *et al*, 1993).

Soskolne *et al* (1996), in addition to the measures noted above, enquired into the use of tranquillisers and the use of services. They found higher use of tranquillisers compared with the preceding month but no differences in service utilisation.

Nakar *et al* (1996) compared the 2-week consulting load in a family practice of an area that was highly exposed to SCUD missile attack with the equivalent period during the previous year. The authors reported that the total rate of visits was cut by half, but with a relative and absolute increase in psychological consultations and a decrease in consultations for infectious and respiratory conditions. Apparently, worries about the attacks led to a reduction in consultations for trivial disorders, but to an increase in the anxiety level of the population.

During the second Intifada, the Ministry of Health and several non-governmental organisations have established mental health activities that are provided as early as possible in the emergency rooms and wards of general hospitals that treat casualties. The Ministry has trained several teams of eight mental health specialists, who are attached to a general hospital. Half of them are trained to care for children and adolescents, and half for adults. Immediately following an attack (or other disaster), they are expected to report to their hospital. Their task is to examine all persons who are lightly injured and those suffering from a stress reaction. Following first-aid treatment, everyone is transferred to another area near the emergency room for individual and group intervention. The intervention includes an explanation about the nature of psycho-trauma, the provision of emotional support and the giving of information about psychological and social security assistance. This information is offered in five languages – Hebrew, English, Russian, Arabic and Amharic. An additional role of the mental health team is to provide emotional support to doctors and nurses who are involved in the care of the wounded.

Hospital social workers are responsible for meeting the family members and friends of the injured, and helping them to locate the casualties, assist with their grief, and accompany the family members to the hospital morgue to identify victims.

The Ministry of Health's system for emergency intervention and treatment with regard to psychological trauma also includes activities that take place at the community level. Trained personnel in out-patient clinics are entrusted with the care of persons affected by acute stress disorders or post-traumatic stress disorder. At the time of a national emergency, these out-patient clinics are open 24 hours a day.

# Research

Much mental health research has been and is being conducted both in the universities and in the services. National and international funding sources support Israeli research. For the sake of brevity, the main areas of research are briefly summarised below. The studies cited here are merely examples – a national database is available at www.szold.org.il.

## Epidemiology

Studies have been conducted with regard to the mental health of communities both in peace and in war. Currently, the national authorities are conducting household surveys of the young and adults, the latter as part of epidemiological studies in a number of countries, run jointly by the World Health Organization and Harvard University. A large survey exploring emotional distress (common mental disorders) among Arabs and Jews has concluded relatively recently. The fact that many early immigrants were

Holocaust survivors provided the substance for studies on the mental health status of first- and second-generation immigrants (Levav, 1998).

## Social psychiatry

The cultural mosaic of Israel has prompted investigators to explore the knowledge, attitudes and practices of different Arab and Jewish groups of the population.

## Health services research

The Ministry of Health supports a relatively large staff, who are entrusted with the responsibility of providing data for planning, monitoring and evaluation. These efforts are buttressed by studies conducted by university staff and students.

## Biological psychiatry

This area, in consonance with the current psychiatric zeitgeist, is flourishing and making significant contributions in a number of respects, particularly with regard to schizophrenic, obsessive and depressive disorders and post-traumatic stress disorder.

# Training

Graduate, postgraduate and in-service education is a vibrant area. The country trains all the range of mental health professionals (clinical psychologists, nurses, etc.). There are 16.4 psychiatrists per 100 000 population. The register of the Child and Adolescent Society numbers about 150 specialists (Apter, 1998). In addition, there are approximately 200 residents in training. To be recognised as a specialist, the resident has to complete four years of postgraduate education in a variety of services and pass two examinations.

# Looking back, moving forward

Throughout the country's history, the mental health services in Israel have had to face the challenge of how to provide care to persons from very different cultural and religious backgrounds – Jewish, Muslim, Druze and Christian – see Al-Krenawi (1999) and Al-Krenawi & Graham (1999) with regard to the Arabs, and Bilu & Witztum (1997) and Greenberg & Witztum (2001) with regard to different Jewish Israeli groups, who emigrated from 70 or so countries, wherein many had endured severe persecution and the traumatic loss of their significant others, and whose lives since the dawn of the State have been punctuated by war and terrorism.

A judgement on how well the services have performed is beyond the scope of this report. However, it is fair to say that mental healthcare is increasingly recognised by decision makers and the public as an important link in the chain of efforts that the health system makes towards the health of the nation. Mental health services are free and open to all, and the service users and their families are being sought as natural partners of mental health professionals.

In the field of research, Israel is contributing its share to the global pool of scientific knowledge, as has been noted by Patel (2002).

Admittedly, not all is well. Psychiatric reform, which involves deinstitutionalisation, community-based care and the humanisation of services, is progressing more slowly than is wished by many. Mental hospitals still remain the main axis of care, command an unusual amount of power and authority, and consume most of the mental health budget. A large proportion of their personnel, although less fearful of community-based care than they were, remain ambivalent at best about the psychiatric reform that is leading to the transfer of mental healthcare to the health maintenance organisations. Despite the free access to care, equity has not been achieved, and the barriers to care for foreign workers, particularly those without papers, have not been lowered. Child and adolescent mental health services and services for the elderly, although available, are probably less than are needed (an ongoing survey will identify needs among the young). A last limitation worth noting is that the services have yet to balance their efforts in care and rehabilitation with health promotion and illness prevention.

In conclusion, the Israeli mental health services are genuinely attempting to upgrade the mental healthcare for the whole population. To overcome the remaining and still formidable obstacles, both internal and external, to the system, will require, much as in other nations, the support of many stakeholders, and a successful blend of political and social will, the application of scientific and technical know-how, the involvement of service users and their families, and the dedication and commitment of mental health workers.

# Acknowledgement

Bella Ben-Gershon, BA, provided information on the emergency preparedness programme.

# References

Al-Krenawi, A. (1999) Explanation of mental health symptoms by the Bedouin-Arabs of the Negev. *International Journal of Social Psychiatry*, **45**, 56–64.

Al-Krenawi, A. & Graham, J. R. (1999) Gender and biomedical/traditional mental health utilization among the Bedouin-Arabs of the Negev. *Culture, Medicine and Psychiatry*, **23**, 219–243.

Apter, A. (1998) Child psychiatry in Israel – towards the millennium. *Israel Journal of Psychiatry*, **35**, 251–252.

Bilu, Y. & Witztum, E. (1997) The mental health of Jews inside and outside Israel. In *Ethnicity, Immigration, and Psychopathology* (eds I. Al-Issa & M. Tousignant), pp. 235–256. New York: Plenum.

Central Bureau of Statistics (2002) *Statistical Abstract 2001*. Jerusalem: Government of Israel.

Department of Information and Evaluation (2002) *Mental Health in Israel*. Statistical Annual 2002. Jerusalem: Ministry of Israel.

Feinson, M. C., Lerner, Y., Levinson, D., *et al* (1997) Ambulatory mental health treatment under universal coverage: policy insights from Israel. *Milbank Quarterly*, **75**, 235–260.

Greenberg, D. & Witztum, E. (2001) *Sanity and Sanctity*. New Haven, CT: Yale University Press.

Kark, J. D., Goldman, S. & Epstein, L. (1995) Iraqi missile attacks on Israel: The association of mortality with a life-threatening stressor. *Journal of the American Medical Association*, **273**, 1208–1210.

Laor, N., Wolmer, L., Mayes, L. C., *et al* (1996) Israeli preschoolers under SCUD missile attacks: A developmental perspective on risk-modifying factors. *Archives of General Psychiatry*, **53**, 416–423.

Levav, I. (1998) Individuals under conditions of maximum adversity. In *Stress, Adversity and Psychopathology* (ed. B. P. Dohrenwend). New York: Oxford University Press.

Nakar, S., Kahan, E., Nir, T., *et al* (1996) The influence of SCUD missile attacks on the utilization of ambulatory services in a family practice. *Medicine, Conflict, and Survival*, **12**, 149–153.

Patel, V. (2002) *Research Environment in Developing Countries: Making It Happen*. Cape Town: World Health Organization.

Solomon, Z. & Prager, E. (1992) Elderly Holocaust survivors during the Persian Gulf War: a study of psychological distress. *American Journal of Psychiatry*, **149**, 1707–1710.

Solomon, Z., Laor, N., Weiler, D., *et al* (1993) The psychological impact of the Gulf War: a study of acute stress in Israeli evacuees. *Archives of General Psychiatry*, **50**, 320–321.

Soskolne, V., Baras, M., Palti, H., *et al* (1996) Exposure to missile attacks: the impact of the Persian Gulf War on physical health behaviors and psychological distress in high and low risk areas in Israel. *Social Science and Medicine*, **42**, 1039–1047.

# Japan

## Tsuyoshi Akiyama

During the Edo period in Japan (1603–1867), people with mental illness were not excluded from society. Upon the introduction of European psychiatry around the 1870s, Japanese society became more discriminatory, however. In 1900 a primary law was introduced to regulate the custody of patients. In 1919 another law was approved to facilitate the establishment of public psychiatric hospitals. In 1950 the Mental Hygiene Law was enacted to prohibit home custody. However, these regulations did not assure quality of care or protect service users' rights. Also, after the Second World War, many private psychiatric hospitals were built, but this expansion of the sector was not well thought out or well coordinated. In Japan, the government regulates the private health sector only insofar as it sets standardised fees for treatments and carries out basic quality assurance.

In 1984 a scandal involving the murder of in-patients by nursing staff was reported at a psychiatric hospital. This prompted huge international pressure and the Japanese government passed the Mental Health Law in 1988. In 1995 this law was further revised to include welfare support.

## Service provision

Japan operates a unique medical system in which payment for treatment is met via nationally standardised insurance; service users enjoy free access to the treatment facility of their choice. This financial assurance has sustained high accessibility to care, especially for those who fall under the Services and Supports for Persons with Disabilities Act. In consequence, numerous psychiatric clinics have emerged and in-patient treatment, including an emergency service, is available throughout the country. There are also many mental health and welfare centres, as well as rehabilitative facilities (including day treatment centres, work factories, group homes and community centres). With some variations these services are standardised and available throughout the country.

There has been a steady shift from in-patient to out-patient treatment in psychiatry in Japan. According to the World Health Organization (2005) there are 28.4 psychiatric beds per 10 000 population in Japan. There remains a huge population of elderly patients who have been in hospital for many years, but for newly admitted in-patients the average length of stay is around 2–3 months.

The private sector plays an important role. In 2004, of the total of 1667 psychiatric hospitals, 1370 were private. There has been some discussion regarding the discrepancy between academic psychiatry at universities and practice within private psychiatric hospitals.

The Japanese government has recently undertaken a structural reform of psychiatric services to reduce its expenditure in this area. The Services and Supports for Persons with Disabilities Act seems to be actually causing difficulties in some respects.

Collaboration between psychiatric and medical staff needs to be developed further in Japan. The standard of education of psychiatric nurses is not high. There is not yet a national professional qualification in clinical psychology.

## Service users and stigma

The rights of service users are well protected. The Community Office and the Legal Advisory Board receive complaints from the users of psychiatric facilities and work to support them.

The stigma associated with mental health problems has been lessened through the media and the internet. The media frequently report on the importance of depression, suicide prevention and post-traumatic stress disorder (PTSD), for example. Also, many people are exchanging information and experience through internet 'chat' and 'blogs'. The internet is thereby facilitating a spontaneous anti-stigma movement in the general population.

The royal family in Japan has always been supportive of people with mental health problems. The honorary president of the national Epileptic Society is a member of the royal family and the prince and princess attended the World Congress of Psychiatry in Yokohama. Recently members have spoken rather openly about mental health problems within the royal family.

# Current legislation

Only designated psychiatrists can authorise the involuntary detention or treatment of people with mental health disorders. Under the Mental Health and Welfare Law, the Ministry of Health and Labor designates for such work psychiatrists with more than 5 years' experience and knowledge of the legislative procedures; those who wish to be designated must submit eight case reports, which a board examines to ascertain whether appropriate reference is made to legal procedures and clinical treatment.

According to the law, there are three main types of admission. Voluntary admission is based on consent of the patient. Medical protection admission requires the consent of a responsible relative and the assessment of one designated psychiatrist that the patient needs in-patient treatment. Compulsory admission requires that two independent assessments by designated psychiatrists agree the patient is exhibiting explicit danger of self-harm or harm to others.

A written report should be submitted for medical protection and compulsory admission; regular reports are also required thereafter. The law also regulates the conditions under which seclusion and restraint can be implemented.

The law gives patients the right to meet with a lawyer and to make a claim to the Community Office about treatment under any condition. An officer will visit the facility in response to a claim. Also, there is an annual inspection of psychiatric in-patient facilities.

# Recent developments

## Terminology

The most important recent development has been the substitution of the Japanese term for 'schizophrenia'. The term was previously translated as 'split-of-mind disease'. In 1993 the Japanese Society of Psychiatry and Neurology (JSPN) received a request from a family group to change the translation. After comprehensive discussion, in 2002 the JSPN adopted 'integration dysfunction syndrome' as the official term. This change, which coincided with the World Congress of Psychiatry in Yokohama, launched an active anti-stigma movement (Sato, 2006).

## Specialist qualification

The second significant recent development has been the introduction of a specialist qualification by the JSPN. The project was approved in August 2002 and the first examination was implemented in 2006. For the specialist qualification, candidates are required to attend lectures in a wide range of areas. This system is expected to improve the quality of care provided by Japanese psychiatrists.

## Law on Treatment and Surveillance

The Law on Treatment and Surveillance was implemented in July 2005. It applies to those who are mentally incapacitated and who commit a grave offence. Although there were many disputes in its passing, this law aims to provide a specialised, high-standard, rehabilitative treatment for this population. Under the law, a team composed of a judge, a psychiatrist and a psychiatric social worker decides the need for compulsory out-patient or in-patient treatment.

## Treatment guidelines for schizophrenia and depression

Evidence-based guidelines for the treatment of schizophrenia and depression were developed in Japan in 2004. The American Psychiatric Association's Practice *Guidelines for the Treatment of Psychiatric Disorders* (Compendium 2004) was translated into Japanese and published in 2006. Psychopharmacology algorithms for schizophrenia and depression have been available since 1998.

## Other developments

Other notable recent developments include the introduction of strategic planning to reduce suicides and a project of assertive community treatment.

# Numbers of professionals

Japan has a population of about 128 million, for whom there are around 13 000 psychiatrists, 13 000 clinical psychologists, 3600 psychiatric occupational therapists and 22 000 psychiatric social workers. The number of specialised psychiatric nurses is only 25 (2005 figures).

# Education

Psychiatric training is included in the core undergraduate medical curriculum. The focus is on tutorial teaching and less on lectures. Bedside learning and clinical clerkship are emphasised.

For postgraduate training, there are good psychiatric textbooks available in Japanese. In the past there was no explicit standard for postgraduate training programmes; however, the JSPN now sets a clear standard for the areas to be included in the postgraduate curriculum for specialist qualification.

# Child psychiatry

Relatively few facilities provide effective treatment for children and adolescents. However, several issues affect this population in particular, such as domestic violence, child abuse, withdrawal at home and a lack of motivation to participate in study or work. The government and psychiatrists are trying to develop specialists in this area.

# Psychotherapy

The training for psychotherapy is not yet systematically established. Typically, senior psychiatrists will teach the basics of psychotherapy and the rest will depend on the interest of residents. The JSPN plans to provide standardised psychotherapy training opportunities.

## Research

Numerous high-quality research projects in the mental health field are being conducted in Japan. Especially noteworthy for international colleagues may be studies in neuroimaging, neuropharmacology, neurophysiology and genetics. On the clinical side, social skills training has been rigorously researched. Other clinical projects are investigating cognitive therapy for various populations, the 'Rework Assist Programme' (which seeks to facilitate the rehabilitation of company employees who experience mental health problems), the introduction of electronic patient record systems and clinical paths to improve the quality of care. An active interest in anthropological psychopathology from the German and French traditions has been maintained.

## Professional associations

There are around 85 associations which deal with psychiatric issues. Each usually has an annual meeting, and there are numerous seminars and lectures provided by these associations for both professionals and the general public.

## Conclusion

Access to psychiatric treatments and services is available throughout Japan. Current priorities are the development of community care and the standardisation of professional education and training, as well as treatment. We look forward to exchanging our experiences with international colleagues.

## References

Sato, M. (2006) Renaming schizophrenia: a Japanese perspective. *World Psychiatry*, **5**, 54–56.
World Health Organization (2005) *Mental Health Atlas 2005*. WHO.

# Jordan

## Adnan Takriti

Jordan, one of the most recently established countries in the Middle East, was part of the Ottoman Empire. It was declared a political entity known as Transjordan under the mandate of the British government in 1923, until it gained independence and was declared a Kingdom in 1946. In 1950, Transjordan and the West Bank were united and assumed the current name of the Hashemite Kingdom of Jordan. The next major change for the Kingdom came in 1967, when the occupation of the West Bank and Gaza Strip by Israeli forces caused a massive influx of migrants to the East Bank.

Jordan has a total area of 89 342 km$^2$ and a population of 5 329 000 (2002 statistics). The gross domestic product (GPD) per capita is US$1765. The illiteracy rate (among those aged over 15 years) is 10.3% (5.4% for males and 15.2% for females). Life expectancy at birth is 71.5 years and the infant mortality rate is 22.1 per 1000 births. The unemployment rate is 15.3%.

The Ministry of Health budget is 5.7% of total spending. There is one hospital bed for every 568 citizens and one psychiatric bed for every 9000. There is one physician for 600 citizens and one psychiatrist for every 75 000.

## Evolution of psychiatric services

At the time of the British mandate in Palestine in 1915, all psychiatric services were obtained from Palestine. The only psychiatric hospital (in Bethlehem) was in Palestine. In the late 1950s a visiting psychiatrist from Bethlehem hospital used to attend an out-patient psychiatric clinic once a week. Three separate streams of evolution occurred subsequently, in the armed forces, in the Ministry of Health and in academic psychiatry.

### Psychiatric services in the armed forces

In the early 1960s there was only one psychiatrist, who had been trained at the Maudsley Hospital in London. In 1966 a department of psychiatry was established within the main military psychiatric hospital, in Marka, Amman, the capital city. A graduate training programme was implemented, which was recognised by the British Medico-Psychological Association.

In 1973 the King Hussein Medical Centre was founded and its psychiatric department was established in 1975. However, in 1997 it was transferred to its original place in the Marka hospital; this was considered a setback and a failure on the part of medical administrators to understand the need for a multi-disciplinary approach to psychiatry.

Currently there are 12 qualified psychiatrists who run psychiatric services in the armed forces; most of them were trained in Britain.

## Psychiatric services provided by the Ministry of Health

The need for a psychiatric hospital became apparent after the 1967 war with Israel, when the West Bank fell under occupation. In April 1987 the National Centre for Mental Health was established, with 300 beds. In addition, 150-bed hospitals were established for patients with chronic illness and for rehabilitation. Recently, a centre for the treatment of drug addiction was established, with 46 beds.

There are 30 out-patient clinics throughout the country, which are attended by 33 000 patients annually. There are currently only 8 psychiatrists providing this service, largely because neighbouring Saudi Arabia, which can afford to pay higher salaries, draws many health professionals away from Jordan.

## Academic psychiatry

There are two medical schools in Jordan, at the University of Jordan, in Amman, and at the University of Science and Technology, in the town of Irbid in northern Jordan. Medical students undergo 1 month of training in the government psychiatric hospital in their 5th year. There is no psychiatric department at the University of Jordan, although there are two psychiatrists working at its out-patient clinic. Recently, the University of Science and Technology established a psychiatric unit (with 30 beds) in the newly built university hospital. Undergraduate and graduate programmes are being established.

# Psychiatric journals

The *Arab Journal of Psychiatry* is published biannually under the auspices of the Arab Federation of Psychiatrists. It is published in Jordan although it represents all Arab psychiatrists.

# The private sector

There are 30 private psychiatrists who work exclusively in their own clinics. Psychiatrists in the public sector, described above, are not allowed to work privately. There is one psychiatric hospital, with 70 beds, which serves psychiatrists in the private sector.

## Psychiatric treatments

Trends in psychiatric treatments in Jordan have run parallel to those in Britain, largely because many of the country's psychiatrists have trained in Britain since the early 1960s. Accordingly, tricyclic antidepressants, monoamino oxidase inhibitors and conventional neuroleptics were used. More recently, since the late 1980s, the new generation of antidepressants (e.g. the selective serotonin reuptake inhibitors) and novel antipsychotics have been extensively prescribed. Mood stabilisers, including lithium and various anticonvulsants, are available. Electroconvulsive therapy, abreactive techniques and hypnosis are also used. Psychotherapy is being practised by some psychiatrists who were trained in specialised centres in the UK and USA, generally in the field of cognitive–behavioural therapy; psychodynamic therapies are not practised in Jordan.

Group therapy, occupational therapy and rehabilitation are usually practised for in-patients.

## Educational issues

The universities have their own undergraduate syllabus. Postgraduate teaching is accredited under the auspices of the Jordan Medical Council, which is the medical body that deals with all academic issues. The Council has a psychiatric division that steers the theoretical and clinical aspects of psychiatry. After a 4-year training programme, which covers basic sciences and clinical experience, the candidate sits the psychiatric board examination.

## Professional body

The Jordan Psychiatric Association is a division of the Jordan Medical Syndicate. There are 60 registered psychiatrists.

## Fields allied to psychiatry

Clinical psychologists, social workers and occupational therapists, in addition to psychiatric nurses, are part of the psychiatric teams in the psychiatric hospitals and departments. Generally speaking, there is always a lack of adequate staffing in all these fields, as in psychiatry. There is a Psychological Association run by psychologists, which is licensed by the Ministry of Health. Some members of the Association run clinics in the field of counselling psychology. Unfortunately, there is no collaboration with psychiatrists, at any level.

# The Mental Health Act 2003

The Act provides for the compulsory admission of psychiatric patients, who include those with a drug addiction (to narcotics or psychotropic agents). It states the conditions for the admission and discharge of such patients. The following are notable sections.

## Section 15

A general hospital can allocate a department for psychiatric patients provided that it has on its staff one or more psychiatrists, as well as the required numbers of resident doctors and specialised staff.

## Section 16

Section 16A states that psychiatric patients may be admitted to either a psychiatric hospital or a psychiatric department of a general hospital either voluntarily or compulsorily in the following cases:

- if the patient or the addict needs treatment that is provided only at these facilities
- if the patient is causing harm to him/herself or others, whether this harm is physical or psychological
- if the patient or the addict is causing damage to property
- if a court of law so decides, in accordance with the medical evidence presented.

Section 16B sets out the following conditions for hospital admission (excepting the last, forensic case above):

- an application must be addressed to the hospital manager
- a medical report must be issued by a psychiatrist in support of the application addressed to the hospital manager
- the hospital manager (or whoever is authorised to act on the manager's behalf) gives approval.

## Section 17

In the case of compulsory admissions, the Minister of Health can refer the patient to a psychiatric committee to examine the reasons for admission. Accordingly, the Minister can decide to discharge the patient or to prevent the patient's admission, except where the patient has been admitted as a result of a court hearing.

## Section 18

The attending psychiatrist must discharge the patient after recovery, with the approval of the hospital manager. The patient's family should be notified about the date and time of the discharge. Where the patient was admitted as a result of a court decision, the court should be notified.

# Research and publications

There are limited funds for research. No epidemiological research has been carried out so far in Jordan. Most research work is published locally in one of the two medical journals or in the one psychiatric journal, mainly for the purpose of career progression. The papers mostly address clinical and cultural issues.

# Mental health strategy (1988)

The main goals are:
- the teaching of psychiatry to general practitioners and paramedical staff
- the extension of psychiatric services to all provinces of the country
- the appointment of counselling psychologists and social workers to all schools
- the incorporation of mental health services within primary healthcare.

    A fair portion of this strategy has been implemented. For example:
- by 1995, 100 general practitioners had received training (with notable success), as had 60 paramedical staff
- psychiatrists now cover 36 health centres in Amman, and this programme has been extended to four other muhafazat (governorates)
- psychological counselling centres, staffed by social workers and psychology graduates, have been established in all the main schools in Jordan.

# Cultural issues

Social stigma is quite strong in relation to psychiatric patients and treatments. Consequently, resort is often made to faith healers before or even after visiting a psychiatrist. There is great ignorance about psychiatry in all sectors of society: rich, poor, illiterate and educated. Stigma also affects the status of psychiatry among the other medical specialties. This has restricted progress in the delivery of psychiatric services.

# Sources

Department of Statistics (2002) *Population and Family Health Survey*. Amman: Department of Statistics.

Ministry of Health (1988) *Mental Health Strategy in Jordan*. Report to the World Health Organization. Amman: Ministry of Health.

Shuriquie, N. (2003) Military psychiatry – a Jordanian experience. *Psychiatric Bulletin*, **27**, 386–388.

Website: Jordan Medical Council: www.jmc.gov.jo

# Kuwait

## M. A. Zahid and Adel Al-Zayed

This paper describes the historical background, development and current status of psychiatric services in Kuwait. In addition, present practices and the outlook for further development of services are outlined.

Kuwait is a rich oil-producing country with a gross domestic product (GDP) of US$74.6 billion and an area of 17 820 km². The mid-year population of Kuwait in 2007 was 3 399 637, of whom 30.75% were Kuwaitis, while expatriates, mainly from the Indian subcontinent (39%) and other Arabs (22%), made up the rest (Public Authority for Civil Information, 2007).

The Ministry of Health (MOH) has, over the years, been the principal care provider in the country. Although a number of private hospitals (albeit regulated by the MOH) have taken up some of the load, delivery of psychiatric services is limited to the MOH hospitals. The health services are provided through five general hospitals (one for each health region), nine specialised hospitals, 78 primary healthcare clinics and 38 diabetes clinics, distributed uniformly across the country (Ministry of Health, 2006).

## Prevalent beliefs and practices

Like all Arab communities, Kuwaitis believe in spiritual (jinni) possession, the 'evil eye' and sorcery; these are not uncommonly invoked to explain changes in human behaviour (El-Islam, 1982). For example, obsessional ruminations are invariably attributed to the devil. Faith healers ('sheikhs' or 'masters') are the first source of help chosen by many Kuwaitis. They may recite Koranic verses, tie written verses to the patient's body in the form of amulets or offer the 'washings' of the verses (written on a plate) for drinking. Elaborate anti-sorcery practices by native healers involve the use of 'traces' of material that belong to the victim, to negotiate disengagement by the responsible adverse spirit. Cautery is used to counter painful conditions and also to drive away the jinni, presumed to have overwhelmed the minds of psychotic individuals. Many patients afflicted with mental illness never get to see a psychiatrist and are instead dealt with by faith healers.

# Historical background

The MOH in 1950 first decided to provide psychiatric care for people who are mentally ill. The first asylum was built in Sharq, a district next to Kuwait City. An Egyptian psychiatrist and some Lebanese and Palestinian nurses were entrusted with responsibility for providing custodial care for patients with a mental illness, who were often chained. Shortly after his appointment, the same psychiatrist escorted a patient for treatment to the Al-Asfouria Hospital in Lebanon, one of the modern hospitals at the time. Having witnessed the humane treatment being given to patients there, he decided to introduce similar trends in the management of psychiatric patients in Kuwait. In 1954/55, a barrack-style facility, named the Hospital for Mental and Neurological Diseases, was opened in Sulaibikhat Governorate, to which all psychiatric patients were transferred. Extensions to the hospital over the next decade increased the number of beds from 100 to 400. There were, though, only eight psychiatrists and one assistant registrar to staff the facility.

The psychiatric services remained more or less unchanged during the 1970s. Two major developments took place during the mid-1980s. First, an Amiri Decree (Law No. 74) led to the opening of a 60-bed drug addiction treatment centre. Secondly, the MOH agreed to set up out-patient psychiatric clinics in all the general hospitals.

By the end of 1989, the psychiatric services had begun to look fairly comprehensive. The hospital had more than 400 beds, and provided both an out-patient clinic service 5 days a week and ran a round-the-clock emergency service. Unfortunately, the psychiatric services, like all other institutions of the country, suffered a major setback on 2 August 1990 when Iraqi forces invaded the country. The addiction centre was demolished, all but severely disturbed patients were sent home, the hospital services were restricted to the minimum basic level and the staffing level was reduced to about 10%.

After the liberation of Kuwait on 24 February 1991, the hospital was in moribund state: it had no water supply and no air-conditioning system, and there was severe air pollution resulting from the burning of oil wells by the retreating Iraqis. The country's infrastructure had been ruined. Within 2 months, however, the MOH managed to recruit the necessary staff, and the delivery of the basic medical and psychiatric services was resumed. A specialist centre, the Al-Riggai Centre for Post Traumatic Stress Disorder (PTSD), was established and a Danish group was recruited to identify, evaluate and help patients suffering from PTSD.

In 1993, the main psychiatric hospital was renovated and the addiction centre reopened. Hospital services were regulated by dividing the staff into five units, each responsible for about a fifth of the population of the country. A forensic psychiatry unit was opened. The out-patient clinics in the general hospitals were resumed. A sleep laboratory with an electroencephalogram facility was established. The social services and psychology departments evolved over time, and began making substantial contributions to the delivery of services at all levels.

In 1996, the UK-based Priory Group was hired for 4 years to upgrade services. It was a welcome change. A rehabilitation unit was established. The hospital's policies and procedures were documented. A department of audit and quality assurance was established. The Royal College of Psychiatrists was approached for accreditation of the services, which prompted multiple visits by College delegates.

## The Department of Psychiatry

The Department of Psychiatry, Faculty of Medicine, Kuwait University, established in 1984, is currently staffed by one associate professor, two assistant professors and two technicians. The Department's responsibilities include undergraduate and postgraduate teaching; conducting, supervising and promoting research; and the provision of clinical services in MOH hospitals. It provides block teaching to sixth-year undergraduate medical students, who attend psychiatric rotation in groups of 30–32 for 6-week periods three times a year. Consistent with the curriculum reform programme initiated in the year 2003 by the Faculty of Medicine, the Department has introduced a system of objective structured clinical examination (OSCE) and a clinical problem-based short-essay paper in its teaching programme. The teaching consists of 24 didactic lectures, 25 case conferences in which students are encouraged to present patients and 16 hours weekly of tutor-supervised contact with patients. The assessment procedures include in-course assessments (30%), consisting of a multiple-choice question (MCQ) paper and six OSCE stations, and an annual examination (70%), consisting of an MCQ paper, short-essay questions, eight OSCE stations, and a long case presentation.

The Department, assisted by two senior registrars, eight registrars, one psychologist and a social worker, provides comprehensive psychiatric services to its designated catchment area. Additional hospital-based responsibilities of the Department include organising the programme of continuing medical education (CME) and promoting research.

## Training opportunities

Psychiatry has been the least favoured field for most young local graduates. Nonetheless, the recent improved provision described in the next section seems to have attracted a number of local young graduates. Four graduates, having successfully completed their residency programme abroad, have already returned and joined the MOH. Three more young Kuwaiti undergraduates are undergoing their residency programmes in Canada. Another is currently doing her internship at Harvard Medical School. All of them completed the 1-year internship at the psychiatric hospital before

**137**

proceeding abroad for higher psychiatric training. The recruitment of suitable supervisory senior staff and the documentation of general psychiatry and its subspecialty training posts should lead to the development of a local postgraduate training scheme in the country.

## Current status of services

The psychiatric services took a quantum leap with the completion of a new extension to the hospital in 2005. A new block with 262 beds (bringing the hospital's total to 691) was added and the old drug addiction treatment centre with 100 beds was replaced by a newly built facility with 225 beds. In addition to the existing forensic psychiatry and rehabilitation units, child and family, and old age psychiatry out-patient services were set up. The hospital staff offers advisory, supervisory and consultancy services to the Ministries of Social Affairs, Education and the Interior. The Ministry of Social Affairs has developed institutions for geriatric patients and those with intellectual disability. The Ministry of Education has developed special schools for children with intellectual disability. The Ministry of the Interior has set up a once-weekly out-patient clinic for detainees. All in all, the hospital runs 23 extramural psychiatric clinics organised by the respective ministerial facilities.

## Human resources and adequacy of services

The main psychiatric hospital is staffed by 100 psychiatrists, 61 psychologists, 7 social workers and 451 nurses (Ministry of Health, 2006). There are 20.32 psychiatric and 6.61 substance misuse beds per 10 000 population, and 0.29 psychiatrists, 0.18 psychologists, 0.02 social workers and 1.32 psychiatric nurses per 10 000 population. This is grossly insufficient. Moreover, community psychiatric services are virtually non-existent. The services are restricted to the main psychiatric hospital, albeit with some out-patient clinics in general and specialist hospitals. The provision of services at primary health and community level is absent.

## Psychiatric research in Kuwait

The Department of Psychiatry, together with the hospital staff at the MOH, has largely been responsible for psychiatric research in the country. It has generated more than 50 publications in peer-reviewed international journals during the past 10 years. The research areas have varied with epidemiological, social and biological psychiatry constituting the dominant themes.

## Outlook

The past decade has witnessed substantial development of psychiatric services in Kuwait. The hospital delivers fairly comprehensive psychiatric and substance misuse services and a number of subspecialties have been established. Psychiatry in Kuwait is regarded as a small specialty and there is room for development of allied disciplines, including psychology, social work and occupational therapy. The decentralisation of services to the level of general hospitals, polyclinics and setting up community psychiatric services and the drafting of a mental health act are some of the areas requiring much needed attention. The recruitment of suitably qualified staff to develop the general and the subspecialty services and set up postgraduate training facilities is needed.

# References

El-Islam, F. M. (1982) Arab cultural psychiatry. *TransculturalPsychiatric Research Review*, **19**, 5–24.

Ministry of Health (2006) *Health Kuwait 2006*. Health and Vital Statistics Division, Department of Statistics and Medical Records, Ministry of Health.

Public Authority for Civil Information (PACI) *(2007) Census, 2007*. Ministry of the Interior.

# Laos

## Ken Courtenay and Chantharavady Choulamany

Laos (officially the Lao People's Democratic Republic) is a land-locked country in South East Asia, and one of the three former French colonies of Indochina. Since 1989, when it was opened to foreigners, there has been an influx of non-governmental organisations (NGOs) and tourists. From 1998 tourist numbers have increased every year, and Laos has become the 'must see' destination in a travel industry that craves the exotic. It has an old and rich culture with a diverse population. The climate is tropical, with a cool dry season and a hot wet season, when temperatures reach 38°C.

Laos is bordered by five countries: China, Thailand, Myanmar, Cambodia and Vietnam. It is equal in area to the UK. The country was subjected to heavy bombing during the Vietnam War, which has left a legacy of unexploded ordnance (UXO) in many rural areas. NGOs undertake the decommissioning of UXO. Some 10% of the population emigrated during the Vietnam War.

It is the poorest country in the region and 80% of its population of 5.9 million live in rural areas (World Bank, 2006). Life expectancy is 59 years (UK 78 years) and the child mortality rate is 83 per 1000 (UK 5 per 1000) (World Health Organization, 2006).

Lao people adhere to the principles of Buddhism (60%) and animism (40%). Traditionally, people have gained most social support from their families and Buddhist monks. With economic development, these supports are under threat from the many social changes taking place in the country.

## Economic and social changes

Laos is a one-party, communist state established in 1975. It is one of the 50 poorest nations in the world and is described as one of the 'least developed countries' by the United Nations Conference on Trade and Development (2002). Since 1998 economic and social change has been rapid, especially under the influence of neighbouring Thailand. Inevitably, changes are having an impact on the lives of the people. Telecommunications technology has transformed a society that once cultivated isolation from the outside world. Changes on the land have included deforestation and the creation of dams for hydroelectricity. Migration from rural to urban areas, with the displacement of people, especially the minority ethnic groups, has affected social networks, which in turn has had an effect on the mental health of Lao people (Bertrand & Choulamany, 2002).

## Healthcare in Laos

Health personnel are concentrated in the bigger towns. Access for people in rural areas is difficult because of poor road infrastructure. Consultations with doctors in primary and secondary care are free, as is nursing care. However, patients pay for investigations and medication, as well as the cost of hospital in-patient stays. Medication can be bought without prescription at pharmacies. The government spends 4.6% of its budget on health (UK 16.1%) (World Health Organization, 2006).

## Mental healthcare

Two units in Vientiane (the capital city) are the only facilities in Laos that provide in-patient and out-patient mental healthcare. One is dedicated to the military (103 Hospital) while the other, based in Mahosot Hospital, is in the public healthcare system.

Two senior psychiatrists work at Mahosot Hospital. The professor was educated in Hungary and the second psychiatrist was educated in France. The psychiatric unit opened in 1979 under the guidance of a Soviet psychiatrist. The unit is staffed by these two psychiatrists, a neurologist, ten nurses and four general medical doctors. It has 15 beds. Patients are referred to the unit from the accident and emergency department of Mahosot Hospital and from doctors in other parts of the country; also, families make direct referrals. The duration of stay in the in-patient unit is 21 days, regardless of progress. Patients pay US$1 per day for their care. Family members provide direct care to their relatives while nurses administer drug therapy. After discharge from the hospital out-patient follow-up is available, but it is often not taken up by those who live far from Vientiane. The out-patient department is open every day to review people living in the community.

The general medical doctors in the service have not received formal training in psychiatry. They work in the in-patient unit, providing day-to-day care and advice on drug therapy. They review those who attend the out-patient department and the accident and emergency department of Mahosot Hospital. There are no psychologists in the service. Psychologists from the university academic department advise on the teaching of psychology to medical students but are not actively involved in the clinical work of the mental health unit. In the main, nursing staff provide direct physical healthcare to in-patients and administer drug therapy. They do not undertake psycho-therapeutic programmes. Occupational therapy is not available in the service.

The diagnoses among the in-patients include substance misuse, psychotic disorders, catatonia, delirium, epilepsy and neurotic disorders. The physical conditions on the hospital wards are poor. Air conditioning is not available and so open windows and doors give general ventilation to the wards.

Drug therapy is the mainstay of treatment but the formulary is limited to haloperidol, chlorpromazine, flupentixol, diazepam, carbamazepine and amitriptyline. Private pharmacies sell medication to patients but often families cannot afford to buy it. The adherence to drug regimens is questionable on account of the cost of drugs and erratic out-patient attendance.

## Mental health legislation

Article 18 of the Penal Code relates to the care of people with mental health problems and offending behaviour. There is no legislation on the detention of people who are not suspected of involvement in crime.

## Medical education

Medical undergraduates receive 2 weeks' tuition in psychiatry; however, the course is not popular among students. The academic department is located in Mahosot Hospital but there is a paucity of textbooks, especially ones written in the Thai and Lao languages. The physical conditions of the in-patient unit do not enhance the appeal of working with patients who are mentally ill.

There is no formal postgraduate training for doctors in psychiatry, so doctors must seek it outside Laos. As a result, community doctors, who manage most mental health problems, do not receive training in assessment and treatment. On occasion, they resort to using psychotropic medication.

## Problems and solutions

The economic and social changes of the past decade are affecting the mental health of the people, through the loss of the traditional social systems for supporting and sustaining people with mental illness. The explosion of substance misuse among teenagers and young adults is putting pressure on the psychiatric services and the social cohesion of Lao society. A flexible response to these societal changes is required but is difficult to implement in a country that lacks the infrastructure to support mental health services.

The education of students and postgraduate doctors is poor; further, they have few resources and models of care available to them. The education of staff would help to reduce the stigma attached to mental illness. The four general medical doctors who work in the psychiatric unit in Mahosot Hospital are a resource with great potential because of their interest in working in the service, and yet they have not received training in mental healthcare.

The decrepit state of the in-patient facility reflects the low esteem of mental healthcare in the health service. It contrasts with the state-of-the-art cardiology department in Mahosot Hospital, which has been established by foreign aid. The Ministry of Health needs to invest in mental healthcare to enhance the service that people receive. Improvements in in-patient care are necessary and could happen in conjunction with the development of community care to provide a more robust service for the treatment and after-care of patients. In the absence of established in-patient resources nationwide, there are opportunities to develop local, community-oriented services utilising the health personnel in place to manage mental illness with the support of families and religious leaders. Such innovations would require additional trained personnel at a local level to meet the mental health needs of the people.

Other areas of service need include child mental health, epilepsy, services for people with war-related post-traumatic stress disorder and the development of mental health policy and legislation. The absence of mental health legislation leaves people vulnerable to abuse. The introduction of robust mental health legislation is essential to protect the human rights of patients suffering from mental disorders and prisoners with mental health difficulties.

The problems require investment by the Lao government and foreign aid agencies in health services infrastructure and the education of medical and nursing staff. The current economic and social changes that are taking place in Laos, as it develops economically, provide an opportunity for government to undertake improvements in services that could integrate tradition with modern practice.

# References

Bertrand, D. & Choulamany, C. (2002) Mental health in the Lao PDR. *Juth Pakai*, **5**, 6–10. United Nations Development Programme.

United Nations Conference on Trade and Development (2002) See http://www.unctad.org/

World Bank (2005) See http://web.worldbank.org/

World Bank (2006) World Development Indicators Database, April 2006, at http://devdata.worldbank.org/

World Health Organization (2005) Lao People's Democratic Republic. In *Mental Health Atlas 2005*. See http://globalatlas.who.int/globalatlas/predefinedReports/MentalHealth/Files/LA_Mental_Health_Profile.pdf

World Health Organization (2006) Lao People's Democratic Republic, at http://www.who.int/countries/lao/

# Lebanon

F. Antun, Charles Baddoura and Mounir Khani

Lebanon is a western Asian country with an area of $10\,452$ km$^2$ and a population of around 4 million (excluding the 10 million Lebanese immigrants worldwide). It has approximately 60 psychiatrists, mostly concentrated in the capital, Beirut, although a trend for decentralisation is currently observed. The number of psychiatrists is steadily increasing as postgraduate training centres have been established during the past decade. There are, however, few sub-specialists, owing to a lack of adequate training programmes.

## Training

### Undergraduate training

Six schools of medicine offer medical undergraduate education. The 7-year curriculum includes courses on psychology, psychopathology, psychotherapies and general psychiatry. A typical example would be the undergraduate training programme at the American University of Beirut Medical School, where the Department of Psychiatry offers an undergraduate course to 'Med II' students and a clinical clerkship to 'Med III' students, as well as clinical electives to interns and residents. It also provides training and supervision for psychologists. The course covers:

- *Psychopathology*. A DSM–IV-based course introduces Med II students to normal and abnormal psychological mechanisms as well as the classification and pathophysiology of psychiatric illnesses.
- *Clinical clerkship in psychiatry*. Third-year medical students spend 1 month working on psychiatric cases and attending morning rounds on a psychiatric service. They are supervised by an attending psychiatrist. Students also attend the psychiatry clinic in the out-patient department, where they see new cases and prepare seminars.

The rotation also includes seminars on psychopathology, case presentation and discussions, interview techniques and basic psychotherapy, as well as psychopharmacology. Seminars are held daily and are supervised by the faculty members.

## Postgraduate training

Psychiatrists go through a 4-year postgraduate training programme provided by two universities. This includes a 1-year rotation on medical wards (with a specific focus on neurology) as well as exposure to child, adult and geriatric psychiatry through in-patient psychiatric wards and out-patient facilities. One of these universities (Saint Joseph University, which, since the 1980s, has been affiliated to the Saint Anne Psychiatric University Centre in Paris, France) requires six research subjects, a university diploma in cognitive–behavioural therapy (CBT) and passing a neuropsychiatry examination in order to grant the specialty certificate; the other requires passing the Arab Board of Psychiatry examination (in its three parts).

# Professional bodies and legislation

The Lebanese Psychiatry Association (LPA), founded in the mid-1980s, has a membership of 65 psychiatrists. It holds regular meetings, sponsors psychiatric seminars and closely follows – with the Lebanese Order of Physicians (LOP) – the drafting of legislation. In the absence of national programmes aimed at raising public awareness of psychiatry and mental health, the LPA works with the appropriate authorities to establish a new state strategy that incorporates psychiatry within the core of public health. Such efforts were rewarded in 2000, when, following a study on benzodiazepine use in the Lebanese population (after the war), which found a usage rate of 9.6% and a dependence rate of 50.2% among users (Naja *et al*, 2000), a state law was passed that prohibited selling these drugs without a medical prescription.

# The mental health model in Lebanon

The mental health model in Lebanon has always combined the private and government sectors. Psychiatrists in private practice depend on private general hospitals to admit their patients, some of whom have these costs met by the public sector. Private insurance does not cover mental health, but the cover provided by public sector agencies does (e.g. that provided by social security, the armed forces and civil service unions). There are no governmental mental health institutions as such, and the public sector contracts for beds in private general hospitals.

There are two mental hospitals in Beirut: one that is run by the Order of the Cross, which has a capacity of around 1000 beds, including beds for acute, chronic, child and geriatric patients, as well as facilities for rehabilitation, drug misuse and day care; and the Islamic Mental Hospital, which has a similar capacity, layout and facilities. There is a third such institution in the south of the country – the Fanar Hospital, which is run by a private board. All three hospitals have a relatively high degree of stigmatisation and therefore cater mainly for psychiatric patients with a low degree of social integration.

Recently there has been a vast improvement in public general health services and therefore there is a campaign for a training programme for general practitioners, contracted by the government, in primary care mental health. With this in mind, steps were taken by the Ministry of Health to aid such a programme, taking into consideration the following.

- Research projects are to be funded by agencies and not by the Ministry of Health.
- The majority of health services (including mental health) are private and the government contracts with the private sector for services.
- All 60 or so psychiatrists are in private practice and the majority work with private institutions.
- The mental institutions (which are all private) carry the burden of maintaining a database, of quality assurance and consequently of conducting statistical and epidemiological surveys. They are funded to do so, however, through the Ministry of Health's contracts for in- and out-patient care, and so the data should be available to the Ministry.
- Non-governmental organisations are doing an adequate job in the south but should be further encouraged, since Ministry funds should be reserved for services needed in the whole country.
- Psychologists do not have a professional association, and there are no licensing laws for their practice.
- Awareness and anti-stigma programmes are available through international organisations. Already, anti-stigma programmes for schizophrenia and Alzheimer's disease are under way, with the support of two drug companies.
- Legislation is a very delicate issue as there is no updated Mental Health Act. So far, there have been no problems in consequence, but mental health should have a separate section or department at the Ministry, to handle all policies regarding mental health.
- As part of an ongoing evaluation of services provided by the Ministry, the cost-effectiveness of mental healthcare is being assessed.
- Mental health programmes proposed within the eastern Mediterranean region have been only partially implemented in some countries because of their 'over-ambitious' scope. All eastern Mediterranean countries have a centralised health delivery system except for Lebanon (as it is mostly in private hands). A mental health programme as such would be likely to have a similar fate; instead, improvements to services at different levels and at different times would be much more applicable and beneficial.

These considerations led to a strategy for a primary care mental health programme, with partial incorporation of mental health services into primary care, featuring education programmes in mental health for general practitioners, along the following lines.

- A part-time psychiatrist will be appointed to each primary care centre. The psychiatrist will be paid per weekly visit made. The object of such visits will be consultation on psychiatric patients presented by the general practitioners. Visits can be adjusted according to the needs of each centre. The visits will also feature a form of clinical seminar, where cases are discussed with the general practitioners.

- Psychiatrists will be appointed to the government general hospitals. Their role will be to provide a consultation–liaison service to the hospital and to provide in-patient psychiatric care (the number of beds allocated for the purpose will need to be five to ten or more, depending on the catchment areas of the hospital).
- Therapeutic teams will be created, comprising a psychiatrist, social worker and nurse, and psychologists can be available on demand.
- Ongoing monthly seminars will be given on various mental health topics relevant to general practice.

## Psychogeriatric services

The age profile of the Lebanese population is shifting, as a higher proportion of its population reaches older ages. The existing services will not meet future needs. Although there are private homes that cater for the elderly, there are insufficient beds. A community-based system is needed, spearheaded by the Ministry of Health. This would be more cost-effective than the provision of in-patient beds for the elderly. This programme will be part of the primary care out-patient system, with the addition of a geriatrician and nurses to make domiciliary visits to monitor, and sometimes administer, home care, and also to help families to care for their elderly relatives. Greater public awareness and destigmatisation programmes will also be necessary. In-patient acute care will be in geriatric units in general hospitals. Such a system will minimise the back-log of admissions to homes for the elderly, which will be reserved for advanced cases.

# Research and publications

In the absence of state financial support and because of the multiple wars that have devastated Lebanon, research work is still in its infancy. Nevertheless, some studies have, for example, found similar epidemiological characteristics in the Lebanese psychiatric population to those described in the literature for other countries. Other studies have examined the consequences of the war on psychiatric health, including post-traumatic stress disorder, benzodiazepine misuse and alcoholism. New publications have even appeared in the field of biological psychiatry.

# Conclusion

Psychiatry in Lebanon is moving towards an increase in resources and capacities. The process of health sector reform will undoubtedly give psychiatry its place in the medical community.

# Reference

Naja, W. J., Pelissolo, A., Haddad, R. S., *et al* (2000) A general population survey on patterns of benzodiazepine use and dependence in Lebanon. *Acta Psychiatrica Scandinavica*, **102**, 429–431.

# Malaysia

## M. Parameshvara Deva

Malaysia is a tropical country in the heart of South East Asia, at the crossroads of the ancient east–west sea trade routes. Although independent from British colonial rule only in 1957, it has a recorded history dating back to at least the first century CE, when the region was already the source of valuable mineral and forest produce that found markets in China, India and further west.

Malaysia has an area of over 330000 km², divided between Peninsular Malaysia (formerly known as West Malaysia, south of Thailand) and Sabah and Sarawak (formerly known as East Malaysia, on the island of Borneo, on which are also Brunei and Kalimantan, part of Indonesia). Ethnically, the population comprises 55% Malay and other indigenous people, 33% Chinese and 9% Indians and other groups from South Asia. About 19 million of its 24 million inhabitants live in Peninsular Malaysia, while about 5 million live in the two states in Borneo, which have about three-fifths of the land area. The two eastern states joined independent Malaya in 1963. They are less developed and have fewer social and health services. The widely distributed population centres in these two states are separated by numerous rivers, mountains and few roads, which poses major challenges to the provision of good medical and psychiatric services. On Peninsular Malaysia, however, the long established infrastructure of roads and communications has contributed to better development of health services. Nonetheless, the development of both the east and west has reached a dizzying pace, with huge investments in both infrastructure and social services over the past two decades.

## Development of health and mental health services in Malaysia

There are few records of health services that existed in ancient times but resort to traditional, herbal and religious healing must have started then. They continue to flourish today, despite modern medical and healthcare services being available nationwide. Malay, Chinese, Indian as well as various religious healing practices are available alongside modern medicine.

The modern healthcare system that is in use today was started under British colonial rule largely to cater for the plantation and mine workers in the rubber, palm oil and tin industries, to ensure their productivity, and the expatriate administrators. Indeed, the health service of old was known as the Estates Health Service. This service was expanded gradually to care for others in the country but was almost wholly based in the towns.

The mental health service, similarly, was reportedly started in the late 1700s on the island of Penang to treat colonial sailors. This was later followed by the establishment of a mental hospital in the tin-mining town of Taiping in the 1800s but only in 1911 was a large (4000-bed) purpose-built mental asylum started, in Tanjong Rambutan in Perak, another tin-mining town. This was followed by another mental hospital, of 3000 beds, in Tampoi, Johore, in 1933, a 300-bed mental hospital in Penrissen Road in Kuching, and a smaller, 50-bed mental hospital in Buli Sim Sim in Sandakan, Sabah. There was reported to be only one expatriate psychiatrist in the Central Mental Hospital in Tanjong Rambutan in 1911, and this remained the case for most of the time until independence from British colonial rule in 1957. At independence there were about 1000 medical doctors, of all categories, in the country. There were certainly no local psychiatrists and very few specialists in other fields. Mental healthcare was wholly based on institutions and was custodial in nature.

## Post-independence development of mental health training and services

At independence, Malaysia had no medical school and only a branch campus of the University of Malaya in Singapore. Doctors were trained in Singapore, Sri Lanka, India, Australia or other Commonwealth countries. In 1964, with the setting up of the country's first medical school at the country's first university, the University of Malaya, local training started. Fortunately, the first medical school in the country was blessed with a strong foundation. The Department of Psychological Medicine taught psychiatry in 10 weeks of clerkship. The students were also examined in psychiatry in their final year. This strong presence of psychiatry in the medical curriculum has set the pace for the training of all doctors in the basics of mental health. The model has largely been followed by the seven public medical schools that followed, and contributed in no small way to the general improvement in the detection and treatment by primary care doctors of mental illness in settings other than psychiatric clinics.

In 1973 the first three doctors started training in postgraduate psychiatry in the University of Malaya, to gain their Masters in Psychological Medicine (MPM). This 2-year training programme involved course work, a dissertation and the writing up of six cases treated by the trainee. Since 1988 this has been expanded to a 4-year Masters programme. Today there are three such training programmes in three universities, which together produce some 10–15 psychiatrists per year for the country. The total number of psychiatrists in the country today exceeds 170, of whom about 80 are employed by the Ministry of Health, in all states in the country. Many work in the eight public and four private medical schools. There are about 15–20 trainees in psychiatry entering training every year.

In 1958 the first general hospital psychiatric unit was started in Penang, almost in the very place where the country's first recorded mental hospital was sited about 180 years earlier. This was a major change from the institution-based services for people with a mental illness that was in existence in British times. With major revisions in healthcare that followed independence, and emphasis on community care and rural healthcare, the district or general hospital psychiatric units started to come on stream and efforts at deinstitutionalisation began.

## Service development in mental health

The move to short-stay psychiatric care based in general hospitals was slow because doctors regarded the large mental hospitals as the 'real' treatment agencies for those who were mentally ill. This often kept the units in general hospitals as mere way-stations for patients to be transferred to the two large mental institutions, which were overflowing, with 4000–5000 patients each in 1970. The shortage of psychiatrists – there were only about 17 in 1977 – meant that although there were by then four mental hospitals and about 10 general hospital units, many were not staffed by trained psychiatrists. With the country's economy expanding and shifting from producing primary commodities (whose prices were unpredictable) to producing manufactured goods for export, more resources were available to improve the health services, including mental healthcare. In the late 1980s there was a big push to produce psychiatrists and other specialists. Trainees in psychiatry, who then numbered two or three per year, jumped to 15–20 per year as more training centres were set up. This led to more psychiatrists for services in more parts of the country.

Today there are 32 psychiatric units in general hospitals and district hospitals, with a total of about 1000 beds for acute care. They each have between 20 and 100 beds, one to three psychiatrists, access to occupational therapists, social workers and psychiatric trained nurses, and most have community teams that visit high-risk patients at home. Most (if not all) run their own outreach clinics on a weekly or fortnightly basis in nearby health centres and hospitals that do not have psychiatrists. The two large mental hospitals have managed to bring down their numbers to 1200 and 2000 patients and the two smaller ones have 200 to 300 patients each. These mental hospitals, with just under 4000 beds combined, today treat fewer in-patients and out-patients per year than are treated in the 1000 beds in the general or district hospitals. The acceptance of short-stay psychiatric care in general hospitals by the population represents a major shift, which has largely been achieved not by forcible closure of mental hospitals (as has been the case in several other countries) but by the population's rejection of institutionalism as a mainstay of care.

There are small numbers of child and adolescent psychiatrists, forensic psychiatrists, liaison psychiatrists, rehabilitation psychiatrists, old age psychiatrists and substance misuse specialists, who were trained overseas, but more are being trained every year. As more medical schools come on stream, more academic departments are being set up and more research is being carried out in these departments.

The Ministry of Health's Family Development Division, in cooperation with the psychiatric services, has, since 1997, set up primary care services for people with a mental illness and over 1000 nurses and doctors in primary care help in this care. There are also over 40 day treatment centres for rehabilitation. Rehabilitation itself has changed from work therapy and vegetable farming based at hospital services to social, psychological and occupational therapies and work based on industrial subcontracts. Several of the products made by patients in the sheltered workshops are exported to other countries.

## Mental health of Malaysians

There have been a few recent community surveys, and these have shown that the figures for psychiatric mor¬bidity are generally similar to those of other countries. The usual mix of the severely ill (with schizophrenia, severe depression or mania) in the acute care units is of course different from the case mix seen in primary care clinics or the non-psychiatric wards of hospitals. Around 20% of patients in primary care present with anxiety and depression in Malaysia.

Substance misuse, largely of heroin, is a major problem for which psychiatrists often have to advise treatment and rehabilitation agencies. There is a string of over 30 rehabilitation centres run by government agencies and numerous private and religious agencies that deal with substance misuse. Alcoholism is not as large a problem as it is in some other countries. There are currently no alcohol treatment centres in the country, although Alcoholics Anonymous groups exist in a few places.

Child abuse, violence against women and domestic violence are the focus of attention by several non-governmental organisations and government agencies. The shortage of clinical psychologists, child psychologists, child psychiatrists and other professionals in these fields is a problem that is being addressed.

## Mental health associations

The first mental health association was set up in 1969, in Ipoh Perak. Today there are over a dozen mental health associations covering many of the states. The members are relatives of patients, consumers, mental health professionals and others interested in mental health. Several of these associations also provide rehabilitation services in the community, besides undertaking advocacy and public education and providing advice to the Ministry of Health. The associations come under the umbrella of the Malaysian Mental Health Council and are supported by voluntary donations and fund-raising activities. Several of the mental health associations hold conventions every year, in which lay persons and professionals participate.

## The psychiatric profession in Malaysia

The Malaysian Psychiatric Association (MPA) is the professional association that represents most of the psychiatrists in the country; it was founded in 1977. It has over 120 members (of whom about 20 senior members are also members or fellows of the Royal College of Psychiatrists) and its own *Malaysian Journal of Psychiatry*. The MPA holds national conferences (the Malaysian Conference on Psychological Medicine, now in its 10th session) every year. The MPA was a founder member of the ASEAN Federation for Psychiatry and Mental Health (AFPMH), which was formed in 1981 in Bangkok. It represents psychiatrists in the 10-member Association of South East Asian Nations (ASEAN), which has a population of over 500 million. The AFPMH holds the ASEAN Congress of Psychiatry, now also in its 10th session, every 2 years in rotation in each of the ASEAN countries. Malaysia has hosted the ASEAN Congress of Psychiatry twice, with two of the rotating presidencies being filled by Malaysians. The ASEAN Congresses attract over 500 delegates from the ASEAN countries and the region, as well as Australia and Europe.

## Research

Research in psychiatry in Malaysia is largely university based and usually clinical or psychopharmacological in nature. There are limited resources and expertise in the field.

## Conclusions

For a country that had no university, medical school or local psychiatrists, and which based all its mental healthcare in four mental institutions at independence from Britain in 1957, Malaysia has managed to develop its mental healthcare by moving away from custodial care towards community care. It has started training its own psychiatrists to meet the service and training needs of the country. The time is ripe to establish its own foundation of research, while expanding and consolidating basic and specialised mental healthcare.

## Further reading

Parameshvara Deva, M. (2004) Malaysia: a mental health country profile. *International Review of Psychiatry*, **16**, 167–176.

# Mongolia

## S. Byambasuren and G. Tsetsegdary

Mongolia is a country with an approximate area of 1.5 million km². Its population is 2.5 million, nearly 90% of whom are ethnically Mongolian. Khalkh Mongols form the largest subgroup (approximately 79% of the population); the next largest subgroup is the Kazakhs (5.3%), followed by smaller groups such as Tuvins, Uzbeks, Uighurs, Russian and Chinese. The population is young, with 35.9% under the age of 15 years. The official language is Mongolian. Just under half the population live in rural areas and around a fifth live a nomadic life. About 80% of the land area is suitable for agriculture, mostly for animal husbandry.

According to the statistical data, gross domestic product (GDP) per capita was 500 744 tugriks (approximately US$420) in 2002. In 2000 some 36% of the population were living below the poverty line, and in 2002 the unemployment rate was 3.4%. Education is obligatory for all children aged between 8 and 15 years and the literacy rate is 98% for men and 95% for women.

Life expectancy at birth is 63.5 years (2002). The infant mortality rate is 23.5 per 1000 live births (2003), and the maternal mortality rate is 110 per 100 000 live births (2003). Socio-economic changes such as poverty, unemployment, the destabilisation of family structure, natural and man-made disasters, changes to traditional culture and lifestyle, and urbanisation are major factors affecting mental health. These current social changes result in suicide, street children, acts of violence and substance misuse, especially alcohol-related problems.

## Epidemiological research

According to the results of an epidemiological survey conducted between 1976 and 1984, the prevalence of mental disorders per 1000 population varied widely across the country, from 9.8 in Altai (a mountainous region), to 13.1 in Khangai and Khentii (both also mountainous regions), 18.3 in Dornod (a steppe region), 23.5 in the Gobi (a desert region) and 24.0 in the capital, Ulaanbaatar (Byambasuren, 2000). These figures do not include those people with less severe psychological or psychosocial problems. Epidemiological studies on the prevalence of suicide (Byambasuren *et al*, 2003) and schizophrenia (Khishigsuren *et al*, 2004) have been conducted. According to this research, the number of suicides in Ulaanbaatar increased nearly threefold between 1992 and 2002, to reach 3.0 per 10 000 population. The prevalence of schizophrenia in Ulaanbaatar is 0.97 cases per 1000.

# Mental health legislation and the National Mental Health Programme

Mental health legislation passed in 2000 and the National Mental Health Programme of 2002 have been the key elements of a reform of mental healthcare in Mongolia.

The legislation covers all aspects of mental health, including:

- policy and principles
- the duties of state organisations, business entities and individuals
- mental health promotion
- the structure, management and financing of mental healthcare services
- the rights of people with mental illness
- involuntary admission
- the provision of security and social welfare assistance to people with mental illness.

The aim of the National Mental Health Programme is to reduce the prevalence of mental and behavioural disorders, to create an environment which promotes mental health, and to improve the accessibility of mental healthcare.

# Mental health resources

## Budget

The health budget represents 4.6% of GDP (2003 figures). Of the overall healthcare budget, 5.0% is allocated to mental health. In turn, of the total state mental health budget (to cover treatment, rehabilitation and social care), 90% is spent on hospital care (i.e. the provision of in-patient and out-patient mental healthcare).

## Services

In 1974, the closure of four inter-provincial psycho-narcotics hospitals with 50–75 beds each, located in Khovd, Arkhangai, Darkhan and Dornod provinces, was due to the transition from a centrally planned economy to a market economy.

At present, mental health services for the population are provided through general practice clinics, specialised out-patient clinics and the psychiatric units of general hospitals at the provincial level. There are 5–15 beds in psychiatric units at general hospitals in each of the 21 provinces, giving a total of 194 such beds; there are 23 psychiatrists attached to these units. At the state level, services are provided by the Mental Health and Narcotics Centre (an out-patient facility staffed by 26 psychiatrists), the State Mental Hospital and the Narcotics Hospital (which together have 400 beds and 34 psychiatrists). Thus, nationally there are in total 594 psychiatric beds and 83 psychiatrists. This equates to 2.4 beds per 10 000 population (1.7 psychiatric beds in mental hospitals and 0.7 psychiatric beds in general hospitals) and 3.3 psychiatrists per 100 000 population. There are 4.4 psychiatric nurses, 6.0 psychologists and 3.0 social workers per 100 000 population.

The Mental Health and Narcotics Centre regularly conducts training sessions, and holds meetings on mental health issues and the care of patients for family members, to help integrate patients into family and community life.

## Rehabilitation

Clinics providing psychosocial rehabilitation for people with mental illness have been established in Ulaanbaatar (the Mental Health and Narcotics Centre, the State Mental Hospital and the Narcotics Hospital), Dornogobi, Orkhon, Khovd, Khuvsgul and Bayan-ulgii provinces. These teach music, carpentry, welding, cooking, sewing, herding and farming in order to improve the life skills of patients. For the development of psychosocial rehabilitation, the World Health Organization has provided support by giving 10 gers (Mongolian traditional tents) and a mini-van, and the Geneva Initiative has provided a supply of materials such as sewing machines, musical instruments and games equipment. Also, Open Society and the Soros Foundation supplied four gers. In 2004, the State Mental Hospital built houses for 30 people with mental illness, with support from World Vision.

## Pharmaceuticals

Essential psychotropic drugs are available at all levels of service provision, although supplies are limited by a lack of funds. There is a centrally compiled list of essential drugs, but it is in need of review and update. The antipsychotics on it are chlorpromazine, haloperidol and fluphenazine injections. The chief antidepressant is amitriptyline and the anxiolytic is diazepam. Thus there is a need for the newer drugs.

## Disability benefits for persons with mental disorders

Disability benefits are provided in accordance with the Law on Social Welfare as revised and adopted in 1998.

# Medical education

At present Mongolia has a shortage of mental health specialists. Ninety per cent of medical staff working in the field of mental health were trained during the 1970s and 1980s, and many lack the knowledge, attitude and skills required for community-based mental healthcare. The implementation of the national healthcare reform has led to a need for the reorientation of the medical and nursing curriculum, with a new focus on training in community health, health promotion and prevention.

The Health Law of 1998 includes provisions related to the licensing of medical practitioners and the accreditation of health institutions.

## Undergraduate education

In 2000, the National Medical University substantially revised the undergraduate medical curriculum. The new curriculum consists of 21 'blocks'. Block number 15 is mental healthcare, and is worth 5 credits. The mental healthcare course is run by the departments of anatomy, medical genetics, pharmacology, child psychiatry, psychiatry, medical psychology and general practice. The course time (a total of 200 hours) is divided into lectures, practice and independent practice, and the programme consists of psychiatry (80 hours in total), child psychiatry (36 hours), general practice (28 hours), medical genetics (8 hours), anatomy (12 hours), pharmacology (20 hours) and medical psychology (16 hours).

## Postgraduate education

Postgraduate psychiatric education includes a training course (2–5 months), clinical residency (1–2 years), a Masters degree course (2 years), a refresher training course (2–3 months), PhD (3 years) and a scientific degree (Dr Sc Med).

## International continuing medical education

As part of the Mental Health Project, the World Health Organization's Regional Office for the Western Pacific (WHO/WPRO) conducted a training programme for psychiatrists and family doctors on the integration of mental health into general healthcare and psychosocial rehabilitation. In addition, the WHO has provided support for psychiatrists to receive training abroad on management, community-based mental health and narcotics. The Belgian agency Brothers of Charity sent at its own expense 17 Mongolian doctors and nurses from Ulaanbaatar on a 1-month study tour to visit Belgian mental health facilities for the psychosocial rehabilitation of people with mental illness.

# The mental health information system

A mental health database has been established in the Statistics Department of the Mental Health and Narcotics Centre within the framework of the National Mental Health Programme, which is being implemented jointly with the WHO, for data collection at the national level.

Basic mental health data collected by family doctors are integrated into the national health information system. In 2002–03, the Mental Health and Narcotics Centre conducted a study using existing mental health data in collaboration with other government and non-governmental organisations.

## Mental health promotion and advocacy

Comprehensive mental health promotion and advocacy have been carried out with a view to improving the knowledge and attitudes of the general population with regard to mental health. In 2001, the celebration of World Mental Health Day was later officially included in Government Resolution 224, with the aim of strengthening activities to enhance healthy lifestyles and behaviours.

The Ministry of Health in collaboration with the Ministry of Education, Culture and Science translated and printed the WHO documents Life Skills Education in Schools and Mental Health Programmes in Schools. The secondary school curriculum was revised to introduce elements of life skills, with the consequent preparation and distribution of guidelines and manuals in schools and teaching on this subject. In addition, training courses were held for teachers, school doctors and social workers on the development and implementation of a school mental health programme.

Mental health services for adolescents started with the support of the WHO's project Adolescent Friendly Service. Hope, a telephone counselling service, is present in the two provinces and three districts of Ulaanbaatar. In addition, two private counselling centres have been established in Ulaanbaatar.

Lessons and discussions have been organised for parents on the topic of the common mental and behavioural disorders in children and adolescents. This became an important measure to help parents under¬stand the psychology of their children and to teach them how to assist their children to make the right decisions and overcome difficult issues in their daily life.

New 'relaxation clinics' have been opened in various health facilities across the country.

Training on psychological counselling for the population affected by dzud (wintertime natural disasters) was carried out in the 13 dzud-affected provinces with the assistance of the WHO; this involved around 170 doctors, social welfare workers, Red Cross staff, police and local administrators.

The United Nations Children's Fund (UNICEF), in collaboration with the Mental Health and Narcotics Centre and the National Children's Office, have implemented a project called 'Providing Social and Psychological Support to Children from Areas Affected by Dzud' in the provinces of Khuvsgul, Uvs, Zavkhan and Bayankhongor. Under this project, training was carried out for children from herding families, and promotional materials were disseminated to reduce stress in families and children caused by dzud and to teach the skills required to overcome stress.

## The Mongolian Mental Health Association

The Mongolian Mental Health Association was created in 1999 with the support of the WHO. Its role is to contribute to mental health education and mental health promotion, and to uphold the international norms of rights and social protection of people with mental disorders.

The Association has a membership of psychiatrists, volunteers and representatives of non-governmental organisations. It has carried out a series of public education activities through newsletters and pamphlets which explain the basics of mental health to the public.

## Conclusions

Mongolia is a country which is changing from socialism to a market economy following democratic political reform in 1990. This transition has affected all aspects of Mongolian life: political, economic and social. It has had an effect on the family. Many social problems have emerged as a result of economic decline and inflation, which affect the population generally but vulnerable groups especially.

The national healthcare reform shifted treatment from a specialist to a generalist healthcare delivery system. As a consequence, appropriate training in mental health and psychosocial skills is given to 40% of family doctors. These general practitioners have started to manage patients with mental health problems in their clinics and have included mental health topics in their health education activities in schools and in their home visits, as well as in campaigns promoting healthy lifestyles among the population.

The recent mental health legislation and the National Mental Health Programme have created an environment for the organisation and provision of community-based mental healthcare in Mongolia. Training was carried out not only among health sector personnel (health administrators, doctors at town hospitals, family doctors and mental health professionals) but also among administrators from other sectors, secondary school teachers and patients' relatives. This training facilitated the creation of a supportive environment for mental health problems.

Since 1998, a decrease in the admission and length of hospital stay at the State Mental Hospital has been noted. At the same time, increases in the numbers of patients treated by family doctors as well as those referred have been recorded.

The collaboration and involvement of all key partners is crucial for mental health promotion and prevention. The WHO has played an important role in the introduction of a mental health component in primary healthcare and the development of psychosocial rehabilitation.

**159**

# References and further reading

Byambasuren, S. (1996) *The Indicators of 60 Years' Prevalence of Mental Disorders in Mongolia.* Ulaanbaatar.

Byambasuren, S. (2000) Community-Based Mental Health Service. *Advanced Training Materials for Family Doctors,* **Vol. 3**, p. 291. Ulaanbaatar.

Byambasuren, S., Erdenebayar, L., Tsetsegdary, G., *et al* (2003) Epidemiology of suicides among population in Ulaanbaatar city. *Mongolian Medical Science,* **3**, 40–44.

Erdenebayar, L. & Tsetsegdary, G. (2001) Mental health problems in Mongolia. In *Public Health in the New Millennium, pp. 131–135. Ulaanbaatar.*

Khishigsuren, Z., Gantsetseg, T., Byambasuren, S., *et al* (2004) Epidemiology of schizophrenia in Ulaanbaatar, Mongolia. *Mongolian Medical Science,* **4**, 39–42.

World Health Organization (2001) *Atlas: Country Profiles on Mental Health Resources.* Geneva: WHO.

# Nepal

Pramod M. Shyangwa and Arun Jha

Sandwiched between India and China, Nepal is a small landlocked lower-middle-income country in South Asia. Once a peaceful country, it is striving to overcome the legacy of a 10-year Maoist rebellion, a royal massacre and continuing political chaos. Nepal has been in dispute with neighbouring Bhutan over the repatriation of hundreds of thousands of refugees in several camps in Nepal. In addition, the country experiences frequent natural disasters (floods and landslides) and faces several environmental challenges, including deforestation and a population explosion in southern Nepal.

Slightly bigger than England in size, Nepal is 885 km long and 200 km wide, with an area of 147 181 km$^2$. It has a total population of nearly 28 million, and an annual population growth rate of 2.2%. Life expectancy at birth is 63 years. Almost 90% of the population still live in rural areas and 38% live below the poverty line. Nepal has an annual per capita income of less than US$300 (compared with US$800 in India and over US$1700 in China).

## Health resources and statistics

Healthcare facilities in Nepal are generally poor (Box 1) and beyond the means of the majority. The provision of health services is constrained by low government spending, rugged terrain, lack of health education and poor public expectations. Most hospitals are located in urban areas; rural health facilities often lack adequate funding, trained staff and medicines and have poor infrastructure. In rural areas, patients sometimes have to be carried in a basket through the mountains for 3 or 4 days to reach the nearest primary care centre, which may in any case be devoid of trained medical personnel.

For administrative purposes, Nepal has been divided into five developmental regions, 14 zones and 75 districts. According to the institutional framework of the Department of Health Services, which is one of three departments under the Ministry of Health and Social Welfare, the sub-health posts (SHPs) are the first contact point for basic health services. Each level above the

**Box 1** Health-related facts and figures about Nepal

| | |
|---|---:|
| National health budget for 2007/08 | US$187 million |
| Current per capita health expenditure | US$6.9 |
| Health budget as a proportion of national budget | |
| 2007 | 5% |
| 2009 (projected) | 7% |
| WHO-recommended EHCS (essential healthcare services) package (minimum) | US$35 |
| Number of registered doctors in Nepal | 6719 |
| Number of doctors employed by the government | 1259 |
| Doctor:population ratio | 1:5000 |
| Total number of registered nurses | 11637 |
| Maternal mortality ratio/100000 live births | |
| 1996 | 539 |
| 2009 (projected) | 300 |
| Infant mortality rate/1000 live births | |
| 2001 | 64 |
| 2009 (projected) | 45 |

SHP is a referral point in a network from SHPs to health posts to primary care centres, and to district, zonal and regional hospitals, and finally to the specialist tertiary care centres in Kathmandu. Nepal currently has 10 tertiary care centres, 83 hospitals, 700 health posts and 3158 SHPs. There are a few private non-profit hospitals as well. Almost all the private sector hospitals, including those run by non-governmental organisations, and private, profit-oriented nursing homes are situated in the urban areas.

There are no national epidemiological data on mental health problems in Nepal, but data from other developing countries can help estimate the situation reasonably well. According to the largest international psychiatric epidemiological study so far, by Wang *et al* (2007), unmet needs for mental health treatment are especially worrying in low-income countries. That study, which involved almost 85000 people in 17 countries, revealed that at least two-thirds of people who are mentally ill receive no treatment. One Nepalese study indicated a high point prevalence (35%) of 'conspicuous psychiatric morbidity' (Upadhyaya & Pol, 2003). Common mental illnesses recorded at a recent mental health camp in eastern Nepal included depressive illness, anxiety disorders, schizophrenia, bipolar affective disorder, substance misuse and dementia (Jha, 2007); the camp was also inundated by people with learning disability, epilepsy and complaints of headache. Most people still think that mental illness means becoming crazy or lunatic, being possessed by spirits or losing control of oneself (Regmi *et al*, 2004). Although such perceptions are changing, the majority of the public and even of mental health professionals still believe that mental illness is caused by bad fortune (Shyangwa *et al*, 2003).

The number of psychiatrists has grown from one in 1961 to 40 at present. Although the increase looks dramatic, it is less than one psychiatrist per year. Even in relation to South Asian countries with a comparable cultural and political history, Nepal is under-resourced in terms of mental health staff and services (Box 2). There are fewer than 400 psychiatric beds, only 39 psychiatrists and 48 psychiatric nurses, for a population of some 28 million. There are neither child nor old age psychiatrists, nor any psychiatric social worker in the country. The total number of professionals working in mental health facilities, including the private sector, is only 0.59 per 100 000 population (World Health Organization, 2006).

---

**Box 2** Mental health services and resources in Nepal

| | |
|---|---|
| Population | 28 million |
| Mental health budget as a proportion of the total health budget | 0.8% |
| Number of psychiatrists | 39 |
| Numbers of psychiatric beds | |
| government sector | 94 |
| medical college hospitals | 196 |
| private hospitals/nursing homes | 25 |
| non-governmental organisations | 70 |
| total number of psychiatric beds | 385 |
| Psychiatric bed:population ratio | 1:70 129 |
| Child psychiatrists | 0 |
| Old age psychiatrists | 0 |
| Neurologists | 8 |
| Clinical psychologists | >9 |
| Psychiatric nurses | 48 |
| Psychiatric social workers | 0 |
| Occupational therapists | 1 |
| NGOs in mental health | >8 |

# Mental health policy

The national mental health policy and plan were developed and adopted by the Nepalese Ministry of Health in 1997, but, over 10 years later, they still exist only on paper. The policy nevertheless is meant to ensure the availability and accessibility of mental health services for the entire population, through an integrated mental and general health system, to prepare an adequate mental health workforce, to formulate mental health legislation and to improve mental health awareness among the general public.

On the positive side, there has been some improvement in terms of postgraduate psychiatric training and the introduction of mental health topics in the curriculum of community health workers. Other developments include programmes for traditional healers on orientation and sensitisation to mental disorders and epilepsy.

# Mental health legislation and human rights

There is at present only a draft Mental Health Act in Nepal, and existing practices are based on obsolete laws. The draft Act has created a risk of introducing mental health legislation without the resources necessary to implement it and safeguard human rights. It has a provision for the detention of people who are mentally ill, for assessment and treatment at the only mental hospital, in Kathmandu. Moreover, as happens in some parts of India, treatment and restraint of acutely disturbed unwilling patients are being done in a way which is full of good intentions but which is not technically legal and which is fraught with possibilities of human rights violations (Kala & Kala, 2007).

There are no psychiatric services in any prison and no separate forensic psychiatric service in the country (World Health Organization, 2006).

# Medical education

Medical education started in Nepal in 1978 and the first batch of doctors graduated in 1984. Until 1996, there were only two medical schools; now there are 12 of them (including private schools), which produce over 1000 doctors a year. Several schools run postgraduate medical programmes, but only two have facilities for higher psychiatric training. The quality of these training programmes, including their research components, requires improvement to suit local needs.

In terms of training for primary care staff, only 2% of the training for both medical doctors and nurses is devoted to mental health. One non-governmental organisation is running a community mental health service in seven of the 75 districts of the country. In these seven districts, primary health workers receive regular refresher mental health training (World Health Organization, 2006).

# Mental health services

The World Health Organization (2001) has recorded extremely low levels of mental health service in most developing countries, and Nepal is no exception. A recent assessment of Nepal's current mental health system revealed that the services are not organised in terms of catchment areas (World Health Organization, 2006). There are 18 out-patient facilities, 3 day hospitals and 17 psychiatric in-patient units, in addition to one mental hospital, to serve the entire country.

As the community mental health services are conspicuous by their absence, there is no follow-up care. Community mental health services are limited to a small area in Nepal. The United Mission to Nepal (UMN) initiated community work in 1984 and carried out a series of successful community surveys and training programmes (see, for instance, Wright *et al*, 1989). The development of a national community mental health programme is the most important issue for the Ministry of Health to address. While the importance of psychosocial rehabilitation is recognised, its practice is extremely limited. Similarly, there are no specialist psychiatric services for children or older people, and for those with substance-related disorders the only specialist provision is a de-addiction ward at Tribhuvan university teaching hospital, Kathmandu.

# Challenges and outlook

The near-term future of Nepalese psychiatry does not look bright. If basic mental healthcare is to be brought within reach of the mass of the Nepalese population, this will have to be done through the implementation of the national mental health policy. The World Health Organization (2006), in conjunction with the Nepalese Ministry of Health, has mapped out mental health services and resources for the first time. This is a welcome development and may pave way for future initiatives.

Finally, people affected by the decade-long Maoist civil war, especially women and children, may present with trauma-related psychiatric problems requiring culturally sensitive interventions. Nepal would require international help and support to carry out relevant research to understand and address new and existing mental health challenges.

# References

Jha, A. (2007) Nepalese psychiatrists' struggle for evolution. *Psychiatric Bulletin*, **31**, 348–350.

Kala, K. & Kala, A. K. (2007) Mental health legislation in contemporary India: a critical review. *International Psychiatry*, **4**, 69–71.

Regmi, S. K., Pokhrel, A., Ojha, S. P., *et al* (2004) Nepal mental health country profile. *International Review of Psychiatry*, **16**, 142–149.

Shyangwa, P. M., Singh, S. & Khandelwal, S. K. (2003) Knowledge and attitude about mental illness among nursing staff. *Journal of Nepal Medical Association*, **42**, 27–31.

Upadhyaya, K. D. & Pol, K. (2003) A mental health prevalence survey in two developing towns of western region. *Journal of Nepal Medical Association*, **25**, 328–330.

Wang, P. S., Aguilar-Gaxiola, S., Alonso, J., *et al* (2007) Use of mental health services for anxiety, mood, and substance disorders in 17 countries in the WHO world mental health surveys. *Lancet*, **370**, 841–850.

World Health Organization (2001) *Atlas: Country Profile on Mental Health Resources*. WHO.

World Health Organization (2006) *WHO–AIMS Report on Mental Health System in Nepal*. World Health Organisation & Ministry of Health and Population, Nepal. See http://www.who.int/mental_health/evidence/nepal_who_aims_report.pdf (accessed November 2007).

Wright, C., Nepal, M. K. & Bruce-Jones, W. D. (1989) Mental health patients in primary health care services in Nepal. *Asia Pacific Journal of Public Health*, **3**, 224–230.

# Sultanate of Oman

## Hamed Al-Sinawi and Samir Al-Adawi

The Sultanate of Oman is located in the south-east of the Arabian Peninsula. It has a distinctive history and subcultures. Its seafaring tradition has endowed the country with various ethnic and linguistic groups, with Arabic being a dominant language and Ibadhi being the dominant sect of Islam (Al-Nami, 1971). Oman in the 1970s saw rapid development, triggered by the discovery of oil, which took place under enlightened new political leadership.

## Attitudes to mental illness

As in many traditional communities, modern psychiatric services have yet to play a dominant role in the care of people with psychiatric disorders. Mental illness was largely the preserve of traditional healers, and many people with psychiatric illness are still unlikely to seek psychiatric help until they have reached an advanced stage of irreversible pathology or until 'treatment shopping' from complementary and alternative medicine has failed to provide any benefit (Al-Adawi et al, 2002a).

More positively, however, because an altered mental state is attributed to jinn (and religious teaching affirms the existence of such agents), there is little evidence of pervasive stigma towards people with mental illness in traditional Omani society (Al-Adawi et al, 2002a).

## Common psychiatric illness

Although no formal epidemiological study of psychiatric illness has yet been conducted, anecdotal and impressionistic reports suggest that many types of mental disorders encountered in other countries are common in Oman, although with culturally determined differences in the types of reaction and the incidence (Al-Adawi et al, 1997, 2001, 2002b; Chand et al, 2000).

The Omani population is undergoing a 'demographic transition', with declining death rates complemented by high birth rates. This is likely to be accompanied by an increase in the number of people with psychiatric disorders. There is also an indication that the country is bracing itself for the social and economic consequences of a more youthful population, with far more job-seekers than the labour market can absorb. The traditional passage to adulthood is also changing, as youngsters are expected to marry late and to have children when they are well into their 20s. However, the 'adolescent turmoil' seen in Western societies is not evident in Omani society, which emphasises family obedience.

Some maladjustment indicators of youth are becoming increasingly common. Firstly, the incidence of deliberate self-harm increased from 1.9 cases per 100 000 in 1993 to 12.8 per 100 000 by 1998 among female adolescents (Zaidan *et al*, 2002). Secondly, there has been an increase in the numbers of addicts seeking rehabilitation, drug overdoses and drug-related deaths; there has also been a rise in drug shipments confiscated by law enforcement officers (Al-Harthi & Al-Adawi, 2002). The popular mind-altering substance in Oman appears to be cannabis, although the extent of its use is hard to quantify. Finally, there is evidence that the traditional admiration of a plumpish figure is eroding, and that eating disorders are becoming increasingly common in young Omanis (Al-Adawi *et al*, 1999).

## Psychiatric services

Psychiatry in Oman is generally based on the Anglo-American model. The first steps towards instituting a system in Oman of biomedical care for psychiatric patients were taken in the mid-1970s in a missionary hospital, Al-Rahma Hospital, located in the capital, Muscat, in the northern part of the country. An Indian psychiatrist dispensed out-patient services, which later developed into the provision of custodial care for people with acutely disturbed behaviour. Parallel services evolved in the late 1970s in the southern part of the country.

The first specialised psychiatric hospital, Ibn Sina, was opened in 1983. It started with two wards, one for male and the other for female patients; custodial care was provided for severely disturbed patients and there were also out-patient services. The one hospital catered for the needs of the whole population (then nearly 1.5 million). In the early 1990s, a psychiatric teaching service was initiated within the teaching hospital of Sultan Qaboos University.

There is a universal free mental health service for Omani nationals. Although the majority of patients with a psychiatric illness are likely to 'somatise', individuals whose lives are compromised by psychological disorders are entitled to disability benefits, which are dispensed by the Ministry of Social Affairs.

The World Health Organization (2005) rated the healthcare system of Oman the most efficient in the world. Despite this, as elsewhere, mental health services have been inadequately addressed. There are fewer than 15 registered mental health professionals for a population of nearly 3 million people scattered over 300000 km². Most services are dispensed within general tertiary hospitals, but there are two specialised centres, both in the capital city. Most psychiatrists have been recruited from abroad, although some have been naturalised. Apart from the teaching hospital, the multidisciplinary infrastructures often essential for psychiatric services have remained rudimentary, owing to a lack of suitable staff. There are substandard facilities for occupational therapy and psychiatric rehabilitation remains basic.

The first point of contact for those who seek biomedical care is meant to be the primary care clinics, from where most common psychotropic medications are readily available. However, because of a lack of awareness and of suitable health education, as well as the lack of a close, informed and consistent relationship with professional care providers, there is a tendency for people to seek primary care at tertiary centres. A study has suggested that the majority of these patients present with 'unidentified medical illness' (Al Lawati et al, 2000).

To help non-specialist physicians in primary care clinics to recognise mental disorders, the Ministry of Health, the main provider of healthcare in Oman, has instituted regular training for primary health workers in the recognition of psychiatric disorders, and accompanying manuals are available to help in this endeavour.

## Child psychiatry

Even though Oman's postnatal coverage is the highest among Arab nations (Sulaiman et al, 2001), with the 'baby boom' and a relatively high prevalence of consanguinity the country is also experiencing an upsurge in many childhood disorders (Kenue et al, 1995). Disorders characterised by marked regression in a variety of cognitive, motor and social skills after apparently normal development are also on the rise, with all the consequences for the parents and society of having to care for children with pervasive developmental disorders (Al-Sharbati et al, 2003).

The Ministry of Education coordinates special education and rehabilitation programmes for children with communication disorders, physical disabilities and learning disorders (Ministry of Education, 2002). The government is training school health workers to identify and intervene on behalf of vulnerable children, and some teachers are taking an active part in this campaign. As diverse organisations and professionals provide care for children, there is a need both to standardise taxonomy and to enhance cross-disciplinary communication. To this end, specialised centres for the behavioural and emotional problems of children will be essential.

# Policy and legislation

Mental health policies and legislation have been forthcoming in recent years, with a decree to promulgate a substance misuse policy and a law on the control of narcotics and psychotropic medication. Furthermore, a national mental health programme has been established (World Health Organization, 2005).

# Education

## Undergraduate education

The duration of general medical training in students at Sultan Qaboos University is 7 years (4 years pre-clinical, 3 years clinical). Graduates then spend 1 year on internship, rotating between three out of four specialties (internal medicine, general surgery, child health, obstetrics and gynaecology).

Behavioural science, which encompasses diverse disciplines, including sociology, anthropology and psychology, is taught in the second and third years of the pre-clinical course, in order for Omani trainees to appreciate the social and cultural aspects of illness and well-being. In their sixth year, clinical students spend 8 weeks on a clinical clerkship in psychiatry, which is their first exposure to psychiatry. The 8-week programme includes supplementary lectures on various aspects of clinical psychiatry and allied fields, patient case presentation, case histories and clinical interview.

## Postgraduate education

The psychiatry residency programme was introduced in 1999 under the auspices of the Oman Medical Board, which oversees postgraduate training. The average duration of the training is 4 years, during which the trainee will complete different modules each year before taking the membership examination relevant to his or her specialty.

The psychiatry residency programme did not attract applicants until recently. Five Omani doctors have now completed their residency training in psychiatry (two of whom completed their training in the UK and obtained the MRCPsych). In 2004 two new graduates started their psychiatry residency, followed by three more in 2005. Two more have enrolled in an institution of higher education in the UK, to pursue academic programmes in substance misuse and child and adolescent psychiatry.

# Challenges to psychiatry

Traditional value systems in Oman are collectivist in orientation. In communal society, from birth children are brought up in an environment that ushers them into the collective mind-set; the development of self-hood is generally discouraged, as is expression of emotions. Depending on the level of education, difficulties are attributed to jinn and distress is communicated in psychosomatic rather than psychological ways (Al-Adawi *et al*, 2002*a*). The fact that traditional Omanis attribute ill-health to external agents has two particular implications for psychiatry. When a social impropriety occurs, an individual is likely to attribute his or her difficulty to external forces like jinn, the 'evil eye' or witchcraft. It is not surprising, therefore, that many psychiatric problems are first brought to the attention of traditional healers. The second implication is that distress in Oman is not perceived in psychiatric parlance, as intra-psychic conflict. A psychiatric attempt to heal the 'self' is always going to be difficult in a society where development of the self is not lauded.

A survey of Oman's trainees' interest in psychiatry (Al-Adawi *et al*, 2006) has suggested that the attitudes towards psychiatry and psychiatric services appear to be positive. However, there is little interest in psychiatry as a career. Within the context of increasing mental health problems, this is likely to represent a challenge for the country. At the moment, overseas psychiatrists are filling the gap. However, expatriate health personnel may not be well versed in local traditions and languages.

Unless the profession institutes mechanisms to decode local idioms of distress rather than adhering to biomedical models of mental illness (Littlewood & Lipsedge, 1997), psychiatry is likely to be perceived as medicine for 'crazy people'.

Despite these caveats, within the last two decades, rapid acculturation has occurred in Oman. With modernisation, the social status of Omani individuals has undergone some notable changes. These have been brought about by unprecedented prosperity, expansion of educational opportunities and, most importantly from the point of view of psychiatry, an increased preference for an individualistic rather than the traditional collectivistic mind-set and social behaviour. With these expected changes, psychiatry will have fertile ground on which to flourish.

# References

Al-Adawi, S., Burjorjee, R. N. & Al-Issa, I. (1997) Mu Ghayeb: a culture-specific response to bereavement in Oman. *International Journal of Social Psychiatry*, **43**, 144–151.

Al-Adawi, S., Ghassany, H., Al-Naamani, A., *et al* (1999) Sub-clinical eating disorders: preliminary study of students in Muscat. *Oman Medical Journal*, **15**, 29–29.

Al-Adawi, S., Salmi, A., Martin, R. G., *et al* (2001) Zar: group distress and healing. *Mental Health, Religion and Culture*, **4**, 47–61.

Al-Adawi, S., Dorvlo, A. S. S., Al-Ismaily, S. S., *et al* (2002*a*) Perception of and attitude towards mental illness in Oman. *International Journal of Social Psychiatry*, **48**, 305–317.

Al-Adawi, S., Dorvlo, A. S., Burke, D. T., *et al* (2002*b*) A survey of anorexia nervosa using the Arabic version of the EAT-26 and 'gold standard' interviews among Omani adolescents. *Eating and Weight Disorders*, **7**, 304–311.

Al-Adawi, S., Dorvlo, A. S. S., Bhaya, C., *et al* (2006) Withering before the sowing? A survey of Oman's tomorrow's doctors' interest in psychiatry. *Education for Health* (in press).

Al-Harthi, A. & Al-Adawi, S. (2002) Enemy within? The silent epidemic of substance dependency in GCC countries. *SQU Journal for Scientific Research: Medical Sciences*, **4**, 1–7.

Al Lawati, J., Al Lawati, N., Al Siddiqui, M., *et al* (2000) Psychological morbidity in primary healthcare in Oman: a preliminary study. *Journal for Scientific Research: Medical Sciences*, **2**, 105–110.

Al-Nami, A. K. (1971) *Studies in Ibadhism*. Cambridge: Cambridge University Press.

Al-Sharbati, M. M., Al-Hussaini, A. A. & Antony, S. X. (2003) Profile of child and adolescent psychiatry in Oman. *Saudi Medical Journal*, **24**, 391–395.

Chand, S. P., Al-Hussaini, A. A., Martin, R., *et al* (2000) Dissociative disorders in the Sultanate of Oman. *Acta Psychiatrica Scandinavica*, **102**, 185–187.

Kenue, R. K., Raj, A. K., Harris, P. F., *et al* (1995) Cytogenetic analysis of children suspected of chromosomal abnormalities. *Journal of Tropical Pediatrics*, **41**, 77–80.

Littlewood, R. & Lipsedge, M. (1997) *Aliens and Alienists: Ethnic Minorities and Psychiatry (3rd edn)*. London: Routledge.

Ministry of Education (2002) *Evolution of Educational Statistics in the Sultanate, 1970–2001*. Muscat: Ministry of Education.

Sulaiman, A. J., Al-Riyami, A., Farid, S., *et al* (2001) Oman family health survey 1995. *Journal of Tropical Pediatrics*, **47 (suppl 1.)**, 1–33.

World Health Organization (2005) *Mental Health Atlas*. Geneva: WHO.

Zaidan, Z. A., Burke, D. T., Dorvlo, A. S., *et al* (2002) Deliberate self-poisoning in Oman. *Tropical Medicine and International Health*, **7**, 549–556.

# Pakistan

## Malik Hussain Mubbashar

Pakistan is a country comprising four provinces: Punjab, Sind, Northwest Frontier Province and Baluchistan, in addition to the federally administered tribal areas and the federal capital territory of Islamabad. It is bordered by China, Afghanistan, Iran and India. It has a population of 152 million (excluding an estimated 3–4 million Afghan and Bangladeshi immigrants) and an area of 796 095 km².

The per capita gross national product (GNP) is $483 and the budget of the Ministry of Health is 5% of the national budget, or 0.7% of the GNP (1997 figures). The annual per capita expenditure on health by the Ministry of Health is $3.5, compared with the national expenditure of $31. The ratios of beds, doctors, dentists and nurses to 10 000 population work out at 6.9, 6.0, 0.25 and 4.1, respectively. The mental health budget is 0.4% of the overall health budget.

From a modest beginning in 1947, when there were only three mental hospitals, at Lahore, Hyderabad and Peshawar, and a psychiatric unit at the Military Hospital in Rawalpindi, psychiatric units were gradually established in all the medical colleges of the country, especially during the 1970s.

## Training

At the undergraduate level, behavioural sciences have been incorporated in the curricula of all the medical schools in Pakistan. An indigenous behavioural sciences teaching module has been developed for medical students and a demonstration project of community-oriented medical education with an emphasis on behavioural sciences was established in 1998 in four of the public sector medical colleges in all the provinces of the country.

At the postgraduate level, fellowship (FCSP), MD and diploma courses are available. The College of Physicians and Surgeons Pakistan (CPSP) is the main certifying body for postgraduate training in psychiatry; a four-year training programme leads to a fellowship in psychiatry. This training is carried out at specified institutions under the supervision of certified trainers. The training involves exposure to adult, forensic, child and adolescent, geriatric and liaison psychiatry patients in a graded manner that is monitored by the CPSP through regular reports from the supervisors, trainees and its own inspectors. The trainee has to com-plete a research project and submit a dissertation during this training period, besides attending workshops (organised by the CPSP) on research methods, biostatistics and communication skills. The primary FCPSP examination focuses on basic sciences relevant to psychiatry, while part II forms the summative evaluation at the end of training.

In addition, universities also offer MD and diploma training courses of shorter duration. There are 320 psychiatrists based in major urban centres; of these, 70 are fellows of the CPSP, 50 are members or fellows of the Royal College, and the rest have qualifications from the American Board, European institutions or local universities.

There are two centres at Lahore and Karachi for the training of clinical psychologists; together they train about 30 every year. Currently about 200 clinical psychologists work in the country.

Psychiatric nursing is being offered as a separate subject at all the nursing institutions in the country and a curriculum for psychiatric nursing has been developed. A two-year postgraduate diploma for psychiatric nursing has been initiated in nurse training colleges in the country and so far 52 psychiatric nurses have qualified.

There is no provision for the training of psychiatric social workers at the university departments.

# Epidemiology

Epidemiological studies carried out in Pakistan have shown that 10–66% of the general population suffers from mild to moderate psychiatric illnesses, in addition to the 0.1% suffering from severe mental illnesses (Mumford *et al*, 1996, 1997, 2000; Husain *et al*, 2000).

The prevalence of severe learning disability in children aged three to nine years has been estimated at 16–22/1000 and according to recent (2000) estimates 4 million people misuse substances in Pakistan. The most common substance of misuse is heroin (49.7%) and 71.5% of the abusers are below 35 years of age. There are about 232 facilities for drug detoxification in the country (Sub-committee on Mental Health and Substance Abuse, 2003).

# Development of mental health services

The national programme of mental health was the first such programme to be developed, in 1986, at a multi¬disciplinary workshop; it was incorporated in the 7th–9th five-year national development plan. In the light of the above, it is evident that it will not be possible in the foreseeable future to realise the objective of the programme if reliance is placed exclusively on specialised workers. Instead, the aim is to incorporate mental health services within primary healthcare. This has been initiated in five districts of the country (each of the four provinces, plus Azad Kashmir). The government of Pakistan has now allocated a separate budget of more than Rs22 million for this purpose. This model was initially developed in two sub-districts of Rawalpindi, and is presently being replicated.

The majority of the policy and field-level administrators have been provided, including some from the armed forces. Mental heath training programmes, as part of the ongoing in-service training programmes of the district health development centres, are being initiated in the five target districts. These centres have been set up to build the capacity of primary care personnel to handle common health problems, by organising on-the-job training for them. More than 2000 primary care practitioners have so far been trained in mental health. Similarly, more than 40 000 lady health visitors (LHV), multipurpose health workers (MPHW) and lady health workers (LHW) have received training all over the country, in a decentralised manner, within the district health development centres, using indigenously developed training manuals.

In addition, so far more than 78 junior psychiatrists have been trained in community mental health to act

as resource persons in the development of community mental health programmes in their areas, and to provide the training, referral and evaluation support to facilitate the integration of mental health within primary care. As well as psychiatrists from Pakistan, mental health professionals from Iran, Egypt, Tunisia, Afghanistan, Morocco, Yemen, Sudan, Palestine and Nepal (Mohit et al, 1999) have been trained in community mental health, to act as resource persons in their respective countries.

Another major development has been the incorporation of indicators for mental illnesses as part of the national health management information system.

# Development of a school mental health programme

The school mental health programme works through a series of four phases: familiarisation, training, reinforcement and evaluation (Mubbashar, 1989; Rahman et al, 1998; Saeed et al, 1999).

During the year 2000, a mental health component was included in the teacher training programmes at national level. So far more than 150 education administrators from all provinces have been given orientation training.

Training of master trainers from all provinces (batches of 40 for four months each) started in January 2001. Textbook boards of all provinces are being approached for inclusion of mental health issues in the school curricula being prepared by them.

**175**

## Activities with faith healers

Faith healers and religious leaders are the first port of call for the majority of people with a mental illness. One research project has shown that about 16% of the patients presenting to faith healers in a subdistrict of 0.5 million were given 'medical diagnoses' and referred to the nearest health facility. This marks a significant departure from past practices (Saeed *et al*, 2000).

## Activities with non-governmental organisations

Non-governmental organisations (NGOs) are taking on an increasingly important role in developmental activities. The National Rural Support Programme (NRSP) is an organisation active in the fields of income generation, education, agriculture, forestry, tourism and health; it has direct access to about 20 000 village-level organisations. The NRSP and its sister organisations have agreed to include mental health among all their activities and about 20 000 community activists will be trained each year through this initiative; this highlights the role of mental health in national development activities.

## Research and publications

Lack of indigenous research has been a major hindrance to the rational planning and allocation of resources; however, over the past few years a number of research papers have been published. Major areas of research activity include: mental health policy research, epidemiology (Minhas *et al*, 2001), health systems, economic evaluation of models of mental healthcare delivery (Chisholm *et al*, 2000), the development and validation of research instruments (Saeed *et al*, 2001), the evaluation of intersectoral linkages (Mubbashar *et al*, 2001) and clinical research.

## Legislation

The government of Pakistan has repealed the Mental Health Act of 1912–26. The new mental health law, promulgated on 20 February 2001, embodies the modern concepts of mental illnesses, treatment, rehabilitation, and respect for civil and human rights. The first meeting of the Federal Mental Health Authority to develop an implementation mechanism for mental health ordinance 2001 was held on 29 December 2001. The ordinance provides for the prevention of mental illnesses, and the promotion of mental health through mental health literacy, the establishment of mental health services with stress on community-based services and integration with primary healthcare, the protection of the human rights of people with mental illnesses, and the reduction of stigma and discrimination.

# References

Chisholm, D., James, S., Sekar, K., *et al* (2000) Integration of mental health care into primary care: demonstration cost–outcome study in India and Pakistan. *British Journal of Psychiatry*, **176**, 581–588.

Husain, N., Creed, F. & Tomenson, B. (2000) Depression and social stress in Pakistan. *Psychological Medicine*, **30**, 395–402.

Minhas, F. A., Farooq, S., Rahman, A., *et al* (2001) In-patient psychiatric morbidity in a tertiary care mental health facility: a study based on the case register. *Journal of the College of Physicians and Surgeons of Pakistan*, **11**, 224–229.

Mohit, A., Saeed, K., Shahmohamadi, D., *et al* (1999) Mental health manpower development in Afghanistan: report of a training course for primary health care physicians. *Eastern Mediterranean Health Journal*, **5**, 215–219.

Mubbashar, M. H. (1989) Promotion of mental health through school health programme. *EMR Health Services Journal*, **6**, 14–19.

Mubbashar, S. S., Saeed, K. & Gater, R. (2001) Reaching the unreached: evaluation of training of primary health care physicians. *Journal of the College of Physicians and Surgeons of Pakistan*, **11**, 219–223.

Mumford, D. B., Nazir, M., Jilani, F. U., *et al* (1996) Stress and psychiatric disorder in the Hindu Kush: a community survey of mountain villages in Chitral, Pakistan. *British Journal of Psychiatry*, **168**, 299–307.

Mumford, D. B., Saeed, K., Ahmad, I., *et al* (1997) Stress and psychiatric morbidity in rural Punjab – a community survey. *British Journal of Psychiatry*, **170**, 473–478.

Mumford, D. B., Minhas, F. A., Akhtar, I., *et al* (2000) Stress and psychiatric disorder in urban Rawalpindi: community survey. *British Journal of Psychiatry*, **177**, 557–562.

Rahman, A., Mubbashar, M. H., Gater, R., *et al* (1998) Randomised trial of the impact of school health programme in rural Rawalpindi, Pakistan. *Lancet*, **352**, 1022–1025.

Saeed, K., Wirz, S., Gater, R., *et al* (1999) Detection of disabilities by school children: a pilot study in rural Pakistan. *Tropical Doctor*, **29**, 151–155.

Saeed, K., Gater, R., Hussain, A. & Mubbashar, M. (2000) The prevalence, classification and treatment of mental disorder among attenders of native faith healers in rural Pakistan. *Social Psychiatry and Psychiatric Epidemiology*, **35**, 480–485.

Saeed, K., Mubbashar, S. S., Dogar, I., *et al* (2001) Comparison of self reporting questionnaire and Bradford somatic inventory as screening instruments for psychiatric morbidity in community settings in Pakistan. *Journal of the College of Physicians and Surgeons of Pakistan*, **11**, 229–233.

Subcommittee on Mental Health and Substance Abuse (2003) *Report of the Subcommittee on Mental Health and Substance Abuse. 9th Five Year Plan (1998–2003)*. Islamabad: Planning Commission, Government of Pakistan.

# The Philippines

Udgardo Juan L. Tolentino Jr

The Philippines, known as the Pearl of the Orient, is an archipelago of 7107 islands, bounded on the west by the South China Sea, on the east by the Pacific Ocean, on the south by the Sulu and Celebes Sea, and on the north by the Bashi Channel. The northernmost islands are about 240 km south of Taiwan and the southernmost islands approximately 24 km from Borneo. The country has a total land area of some 300000 km². It is divided into three geographical areas: Luzon, Visayas and Mindanao. It has 17 regions, 79 provinces, 115 cities, 1495 municipalities and 41956 barangays (the smallest geographic and political unit). It has over 100 ethnic groups and a myriad of foreign influences (including Malay, Chinese, Spanish and American).

The last official census (2000) put the population at 76498735. However, the National Statistics Office Population Projections Unit estimated it to be 81081457 in 2003. The annual population growth rate (1995–2000) is 2.36% (a reduction from the 1980s). The population is young: 38% are under 15 years old and only 3.5% over 65 years. Most (83%) of the population is Catholic. The literacy rate is fairly high at 95.1% for males and 94.6% for females, which possibly accounts for the facility with which Filipinos find work abroad. Labour is, in fact, a prime export of the country.

More than half of the Philippine population resides in Luzon. Within that area, the National Capital Region (NCR) has 12.9% of the national population (9906048 inhabitants in 61728 km² of land). It is composed of 13 cities, 4 municipalities and 1693 barangays. Three cities in the NCR have emerged as the most populous: Quezon City, Manila and Caloocan, which have populations of 2.17 million, 1.58 million and 1.18 million, respectively. Among the provinces, Pangasinan is the most populous, with 2.43 million, followed by Cebu, with 2.37 million and Bulacan, with 2.23 million people.

Opportunities brought about by economic development vary from region to region and this has affected internal migration. In 1980, about 37% of the total population resided in urban areas. By 1990, the urban proportion of the population had increased to 49%, with the NCR getting the bulk of this population increase. By the year 1995, more than half of the population

(54%) lived in urban areas and this proportion increased further, to 59%, by the end of 2000.

A 1997 survey conducted by the National Statistical Coordination Board showed a poverty incidence of 31.8%. If this rate is applied to the 2000 population census report, then, for that year, over 24 million Filipinos can be considered poor and therefore likely to be at high risk in terms of health status.

## General healthcare

Health status indicators sourced from the National Statistics Office are shown in Table 1.

The available health resources are not only inadequate but also inequitably distributed. There are 548 government and 1146 private hospitals; the government health workforce comprises 2848 doctors, 4945 nurses, 16 173 midwives and 14 267 staff working in barangay health stations. Based on the population in 1997, the ratio of government health workers to population is as follows: 1 doctor per 9727 people, 1 dentist per 36 481, 1 nurse per 7361, and 1 midwife per 4503. This situation has been aggravated by increasing numbers of health workers gaining employment overseas. A wave of physicians, both general practitioners and specialists, have been shifting to nursing in order to cash in on the great demand for nurses in the USA, the UK and other coun-tries. Already, many hospitals are finding difficulty in keeping experienced nurses and maintaining optimum standards of care as nurses use the hospitals merely to acquire the required minimum clinical experience before seeking employment abroad.

## Mental healthcare: provision and demand

The provision of mental health services is outlined in Table 2. There has been no nationwide study on the prevalence of psychiatric disorders in the

**Table 1** Health status indicators for the Philippines, 2001 and 2002

| Health status indicator | Year 2001 | Year 2002 |
|---|---|---|
| Life expectancy at birth (years) | | |
| Male | 66.63 | 66.93 |
| Female | 71.88 | 72.18 |
| Crude birth rate (per 1000 population) | 26.24 | 25.7 |
| Crude death rate (per 1000 population) | 5.83 | 5.80 |
| Total fertility rate (no. of children per woman) | Not available | 3.23 |

Source: 1995 census-based national, regional and provincial projections, National Statistics Office.

**Table 2** Numbers of psychiatric beds and professionals

| | |
|---|---|
| Total psychiatric beds per 10 000 population | 0.9 |
| Psychiatric beds in mental hospitals per 10 000 population | 0.56 |
| Psychiatric beds in general hospitals per 10 000 population | 0.3 |
| Psychiatric beds in other settings per 10 000 population | 0.03 |
| Number of psychiatrists per 100 000 population | 0.4 |
| Number of neurosurgeons per 100 000 population | 0 |
| Number of psychiatric nurses per 100 000 population | 0.4 |
| Number of neurologists per 100 000 population | 0.2 |
| Number of psychologists per 100 000 population | 0.9 |
| Number of social workers per 100 000 population | 16 |

Source: World Health Organization (2001).

Philippines. However, the World Health Organization (2001) estimates that 1% of the population suffers from severe psychiatric disorders or neurological conditions. In a country where disasters, both natural and manmade, are common, psychosocial problems abound, yet mental health remains a low priority for health agencies.

Some other studies on mental health are listed below.

- Baseline study conducted in a Pampanga municipality by the Department of Health (DOH) Division of Mental Hygiene (1964–67). The prevalence of mental disorders was estimated to be 36 per 1000 adults and children.
- WHO Collaborative Studies for Extending Mental Health Care in General Health Care Services. This was a seven-nation collaborative study conducted in 1980. It found that 17% of adults and 16% of children who consulted at three health centres in Manila had mental disorders. Significant also was the finding that depressive reactions in adults and adaptation reactions in children were frequent.
- University of the Philippines–Philippine General Hospital (UP–PGH) Study in Sapang Palay, Bulacan (1988–89). This found that the prevalence of schizophrenia was 12 per 1000 adults.
- Population Survey for Mental Disorders by the UP–PGH Psychiatrists Foundation, Inc. (1993–94), done in collaboration with the Regional Health Office. This study covered both urban and rural settings in three provinces (Iloilo, Negros Occidental, and Antique). It estimated that the prevalence of mental disorders was 35%. The three most frequent diagnoses among adults were: psychosis (4.3%), anxiety (14.3%) and panic disorder (5.6%). The five most prevalent psychiatric conditions among adolescents and children were: enuresis (9.3%), speech and language disorders (3.9%), learning disabilities (3.7%), adaptation reactions (2.4%) and neurotic disorders (1.1%).

# Current realities of Philippine mental healthcare

## Financing

Only 2–3% of the national budget is allocated to healthcare – a figure way below the World Health Organization's recommendation for developing countries. Of the total health budget, the country spends only 0.02% on mental health. The primary sources of mental health financing, in descending order, are: taxation, out-of-pocket expenditure by the patient or family, and social insurance. Sadly, mental disorders are not covered by most health maintenance organisations, nor by the Philippine health insurance system.

## Policy

The Philippines has as yet no mental health act. The National Health Policy was expressed in the *National Objectives for Health* (1999–2004), which had two key objectives:

- a reduction in morbidity, mortality and disability and complications from mental disorders
- the promotion of mental health through less stressful lifestyles.

The vision enunciated in the National Mental Health Policy is 'better quality of life through total healthcare for all Filipinos'. It provides direction for 'a coherent, rational and unified response to the nation's mental health problems, concerns and efforts through the formulation and implementation of the mental health program strategy'. The goal of the Policy is to achieve 'mental healthcare through the development of efficient and effective structures, systems, and mechanisms that will ensure equitable, accessible, affordable, appropriate, efficient and effective delivery to all its stakeholders by qualified, competent, compassionate, and ethical mental healthcare professionals and service providers'.

Although the National Health Policy was written by the Department of Health, its policies, programmes and guidelines have reached only to the regional level. At the local level (provincial, city and municipal), the Department of Interior and Local Government implements only basic health services, based on available budget, the priorities of local leaders, political will and local realities.

Drug misuse is a major area of concern. It has recently been given a boost with the enactment in 2002 of the Dangerous Drugs Act (Republic Act 9165). With this Act, the Department of Health has been tasked to set standards and monitor the operations of drug testing laboratories, to set standards for the operation of drug treatment and rehabilitation centres, and to accredit physicians who evaluate and treat substance misuse.

Likewise, the Tobacco Regulation Act of 2003 (Republic Act 9211) explicitly assigned to the Department of Health the demand-reduction efforts concerning tobacco dependence and smoking cessation.

**181**

Within the Department of Health, the National Programme for Mental Health is being restructured as the National Programme for Mental Health and Substance Misuse, to reflect the changes imposed upon it by the newly revised drug law.

## Service delivery

The Department of Health's current number of in-patient beds for mental disorders amounts to 5465. Of these beds, 77% (4200) are in the National Centre for Mental Health (NCMH) in the NCR. The rest (23%, or 1265 beds) are distributed across the remaining regions. Only 10 regions have psychiatric in-patient facilities. Mental health units have 25–100 beds; these provide out- and in-patient care, consultation–liaison, and forensic services.

In response to the ill effects of long-term confinement and the advantages of community-based mental health strategies, acute psychiatric units (APUs) were developed. Ten government general hospitals were designated as pilot areas for the development of APUs, which initially provided out-patient services. The objective was to integrate mental health within general healthcare in these centres and to bring mental health services closest to where the need is. This was also part of the process of eventually phasing out the NCMH and distributing patients to psychiatric units in regional medical centres or provincial hospitals. Primary health workers were likewise trained in the identification and management of common psychiatric morbidities in order to prepare the community for the eventual closure of psychiatric institutions.

## Workforce

There are currently 412 psychiatrists in the Philippines. Of these, over half (237 or 58%) practise in the NCR. Similarly, the majority (65%) of the 181 (44%) board-certified specialists practise in the NCR.

All 27 medical schools in the Philippines teach psychiatry in the undergraduate curriculum. There are 12 training centres accredited by the Philippine Psychiatric Association to offer residency training programmes in psychiatry. Of these accredited training centres, eight are in the NCR, 1 in the Cordillera Autonomous Region (Baguio), 1 in Region VI (Iloilo), 1 in Region VII (Cebu) and 1 in Region XI (Davao).

# Challenges to overcome

New mental disorders are emerging, including the behaviour disorders of youth and the mental health consequences of HIV. The absolute and relative numbers of mental and neurological disorders are expected to increase in the years to come. Demographic changes, changed patterns of substance misuse, and the successes of medications (leading to survival of people who would have died from chronic diseases) will contribute to the trend of increasing prevalence of mental health problems.

The rising costs of mental disorders are forcing managed care to the forefront of medical practice in the Philippines. Associated costs arise from: lost employment and productivity, the impact on the productivity and social function of families and carers, and premature death (including suicide). As practised in the USA, a business ethos dictates the practice of medicine.

Thus, there are major challenges to contend with. These include the following:

- the increased incidence and prevalence of mental disorders
- the low priority given to mental health programmes and services
- separation of mental health from general health programmes
- neglect of the psychological needs of people living with chronic diseases
- stigma and discrimination against people with mental illness and substance misuse or dependence, and their families
- limited capacity for research into mental health and evaluation of mental health services
- coping with the effects of social factors negatively affecting mental health (e.g. poverty and the effect of minority status – children, women, ethnic groups – disasters, armed conflict and terrorism)
- weakening of the informal social support given to people in need and of social cohesion in general
- poor community awareness of the nature and determinants of mental health and mental illness
- limited coordination between the Department of Health, the Philippine Psychiatric Association, academia, and other agencies providing prevention, treatment, rehabilitation, disability support and social services, including housing, employment and welfare
- serious shortages of professional workers trained in mental health
- lack of medicines and other resources
- insufficient attention to demand-reduction and harm-reduction strategies for alcohol and substance misuse and dependence.

# Sources

Casimiro-Querubin, M. L. & Castro-Rodriguez, S. (2002) *Beyond the Physical. The State of the Nation's Mental Health: The Philippine Report.* Melbourne: Centre for International Mental Health.

World Health Organization (2001) *Atlas: Country Profiles on Mental Health Resources.* Geneva: WHO.

# Qatar

## Suhaila Ghuloum and Mohammed A. Ibrahim

The State of Qatar is a peninsula overlooking the Arabian Gulf, with an area of 11 400 km$^2$. The Al Thani family has ruled the country since the mid-1800s. The population of just over 860 000 is of a multi-ethnic nature, and predominantly resides in the capital, Doha. Only about 20% of the population is Qatari. Around 73% of the population are between the ages of 15 and 64 years. Life expectancy at birth is 74.8 years for males and 73.8 years for females. The literacy rate is 94.9% for men and 82.3% for women. Arabic is the official language and English is a common second language. The economy is dominated by oil and natural gas, and the country has one of the highest per capita incomes in the world. The per capita government expenditure on health is $574 (international dollars), which is among the highest in the region.

## Historical background

In the Arab world, and Qatar is no exception, the belief in possession by a spirit (jinn), the evil eye and sorcery or witchcraft as the cause of mental disorders was quite strong. The notion continued from pre-Islamic into Islamic periods. These beliefs, and a lack of proper psychiatric care, constituted fertile ground for native and traditional healers (Motawwa) to dominate the scene and become the sole source of care for those who were suffering from emotional and behavioural problems.

The first general hospital (Doha Hospital) in Qatar was built in 1948 and it accepted psychiatric patients. In 1956, another general hospital (Rumailah) was built and there general practitioners looked after psychiatric patients. Before their management in Doha Hospital, people with a psychosis used to be restrained at home or in prison, according to their family's status and resources. Some of them were sent abroad for treatment, especially to Egypt or Lebanon.

Modern psychiatric services were established in 1971, shortly after the country's independence. They were based at Rumailah Hospital. In 1994 the department moved to its current position, at the old Women's Hospital, which is a separate building away from the general hospital that has been specially adapted for the purpose.

## Service provision

The psychiatry department is the main provider of mental health services for the entire population of Qatar. It works with three other psychiatric services, those of the school health system, the armed forces and the police force. The service provides in-patient, out-patient and community care. The emphasis is on general adult psychiatry. However, subspecialties are gradually expanding.

Liaison services are covered on an on-call basis. The psychiatry department is located at a distance from the general hospital, which hinders the development of separate liaison psychiatric services.

Drug dependency is dealt with by the general psychiatric service. There is a plan to establish a purpose-built drug dependency unit for detoxification and rehabilitation. Alcohol dependency is the commonest substance misuse problem and its prevalence is rising.

Child and adolescent psychiatry is provided by the school health system, which has its own child psychiatrists. The psychiatry department functions as a tertiary service, receiving referrals of more difficult cases.

Forensic psychiatry is another independent area, provided by psychiatrists at the medical division of the Ministry of Interior, who work in close collaboration with the department's forensic psychiatrist. Referrals to the department are often for admission, or for the provision of medical reports at the request of the courts, the Attorney-General or the police. The service also provides expert witnesses for relevant authorities. The lack of a medium-secure unit is hampering the delivery of high-quality care for this cohort of patients.

In addition, there are satellite clinics located at other hospitals, namely psychosomatic, dermatology, psycho-oncology and psychogeriatrics.

A recently opened hospital in the north of Qatar has one consultant psychiatrist and a specialist providing the care required.

There is a specialised centre for children and adolescents with learning difficulties and autism. Adults with the same conditions come under general psychiatry.

There is a small private sector, with just four clinics, either stand-alone or within a private hospital setting.

## Community psychiatry

Day care psychiatric services were initiated in 1998, as part of occupational therapy services. Before that, a single nurse was responsible for conducting all home visits and crisis intervention, at an informal level. Community care as a separate entity started in 2001. It includes day care, home visits and crisis intervention. The service has proved invaluable to patients and relatives. The focus is on rehabilitation. Crisis intervention has been introduced more recently, delivered through a multidisciplinary team. Crisis intervention work is currently limited to office hours, although there is an intention to make it a 24-hour service. Several obstacles prevent this service achieving its full potential, stigma being one of the main barriers.

## Resources

The Hamad Medical Corporation, the primary healthcare provider, employs five consultant psychiatrists. This amounts to one consultant psychiatrist per 170 000 population. The total number of non-consultant medical staff is 21. The services are based on a multidisciplinary approach; there are seven psychologists (one based at the oncology hospital), two mental health occupational therapists and three occupational therapy technicians. There is a significant shortage of staff in the social services, with only two social workers for the entire service.

The in-patient bed capacity is currently 56 in total, with separate wards for male and female patients. This is set to increase by 20. The number of out-patient visits per day fluctuates between 70 and 120.

## Training and education

The residency training programme has been focused on the Arab Board examination. It is a 4-year programme, aimed at achieving parts I and II of the Arab Board examination in psychiatry. It started in Qatar in 1994.

Until 2004, there was no medical school in the country. Students were sent abroad on government scholarships, or at their own expense, to study medicine. Weill Cornell Medical College, based at New York, opened its Qatar branch, and the medical programme started in the autumn of 2004. Hamad Medical Corporation became affiliated with the College, and there were subsequent changes in both the undergraduate and the postgraduate training programmes. Although the specialist qualification remains that of the Arab Board, the programme needs to reflect the requirements for the examination and adhere to the College's postgraduate training requirements. This has been rather a challenge. The department will start having a regular influx of medical students on clinical and pre-clinical attachments.

As part of the training programme, regular bedside teaching, weekly case presentations and journal clubs are held, in addition to symposia, often in collaboration with other medical specialties.

## Mental health legislation

The National Mental Health Programme was introduced in 1990. It focuses on raising awareness of mental illness at the levels of legislation, counselling programmes, family involvement and primary healthcare. The

Mental Health Policy and Substance Misuse Policy were both formulated in the 1980s.

However, there is no Mental Health Act as yet. The extended family influence minimises the need for compulsory admission and treatment. It is of great interest to note that even those who are mentally ill respect family authority to a large extent. This system relies on psychiatrists to do their best in working with families in order to admit those who need to stay against their will. There have been serious discussions over the past 2 years to have a Mental Health Act that will be applicable to the six Gulf Cooperation Council countries (Bahrain, Kuwait, Oman, Qatar, Saudi Arabia and the United Arab Emirates).

At present some mentally ill offenders can be kept in the psychiatric in-patient unit for 2–6 weeks, based on a written order from the Attorney-General. Patients with drug dependency problems can also be admitted for treatment by court order.

# Research

The psychiatry department at Rumailah Hospital gives special consideration to research. Epidemiological studies that produce prevalence data are the greatest priority and this is the current focus of research.

# Prospects

Qatar is rapidly growing in terms of its economy, population and infrastructure. There is already a shortage of psychiatric hospital beds and this is expected to rise acutely in the near future. A plan to build a new hospital to reflect this rapid growth is in progress. Attempts are also being made to incorporate psychiatric wards within general hospitals. Fortunately, there has been increasing focus on psychiatry from the Corporation's management. This has resulted in the expansion of the existing structure, as a short-term measure to regulate the services and prevent a bed crisis. Community care has been a focus for improvement, with an ongoing plan to expand services and to build larger facilities to accommodate the growing demand. There is also a plan for a new drug dependency unit.

The Corporation as a whole is working towards accreditation with the Joint Commission on Accreditation of Healthcare Organizations. The process has proved very costly and time and energy consuming, but should ultimately result in medical practice being at an internationally accredited standard.

# Web sources

Further information on Qatar is available at two websites of the World Health Organization:
http://www.emro.who.int/MNH/WHD/CountryProfile-QAT.htm
http://www.who.int/mental_health/evidence/atlas/index.htm

# Singapore

## Siow-Ann Chong

Singapore is a modern city state and the smallest nation (land area of 699 km²) in South East Asia. Its population of over 4 million is multiracial, with the Chinese (76.8%) constituting the majority of the population, followed by the Malays (13.9%) and the Indians (7.9%). The present health system is one that stresses individual responsibility, based on a system of compulsory medical saving accounts and on market mechanisms for the allocation of scarce healthcare resources. There are both public and private healthcare sectors. Since 1985, every public sector hospital has been 'restructured' – to grant some degree of autonomy in operational matters, with the intention of creating competition and financial discipline, although the government still retains 100% ownership of the hospitals.

## Mental health services

Singapore has not engaged in a large move towards deinstitutionalisation, and community care for patients with a mental illness has not received high priority. The Institute of Mental Health (IMH) is the largest mental hospital, with a total bed capacity of 2200, and is the largest provider of mental healthcare. It provides a range of subspecialties, such as child and adolescent psychiatry, geriatric psychiatry, substance misuse, affective disorders, sleep disorders, early psychosis, psychiatric rehabilitation and forensic psychiatry. It provides a range of pharmacological and psychological treatments, as well as psychosocial rehabilitation.

More recently, however, there has been a resurgence in the recognition of the need for community psychiatry, with the establishment of a department of community psychiatry in 2001 within the IMH. The department provides an array of services, including community-based programmes such as the assertive community treatment (ACT) programme, the mobile crisis team (MCT) programme (a rapid-response team for crises in the home) and the community psychiatric nurse (CPN) service (Lim *et al*, 2005).

The IMH is the only statutory institution, in that patients can be admitted, detained and discharged in accordance with the Mental Disorders and

Treatment Act 1985 and the Criminal Procedure Code 1985 of Singapore. The services include assessment of accused persons suspected to be of unsound mind and the psychiatric treatment of offenders who are mentally unwell. Powers to detain persons for treatment exist under the Mental Disorders and Treatment Act. There is currently no community treatment order or other provision to mandate the compulsory treatment of patients in the community.

Three of the restructured general hospitals in the public sector provide a psychiatric service. The numbers of mental health workers and beds in these services are small, however; for example, the number of beds in each ranges from 15 to 26. There are also psychiatric services in the Singapore armed forces, prison services and hospitals in the private sector (there is only one private hospital which solely provides care for people who are mentally ill).

Another important facet of mental healthcare in Singapore is the complementary and supplementary services provided by voluntary welfare organisations (VWOs). The VWOs receive government aid and provide a range of services, from counselling, residential care and day care, to employment and other rehabilitation services, for persons with mental illness.

One characteristic of the present mental health service is the relative lack of involvement of family physicians, especially in relation to patients with chronic mental disorders. The care of such people still very much rests with the specialised services in both the public and private sectors. In the effort to 'right site' the care of those with stable chronic mental disorders to the community, the IMH initiated a programme to induct general practitioners in the care and management of stable patients.

The three major ethnic groups of Singapore contain significant minorities who rely on a mixture of Western and traditional medicines, or who use Western medicine only as a last resort (Somjee, 1995). The practitioners of traditional medicine therefore constitute another important source of help for people who are mentally unwell. Cultural and religious beliefs often prompt patients to turn to spiritual healers (Kua, 2004; Chong *et al*, 2005) but their clinical and socioeconomic impact is unknown.

The emphasis on individual responsibilities demands that the populace is appropriately educated in relation to health matters. This is principally undertaken by a body called the Health Promotion Board. It runs a public education programme called 'Mind Your Mind', initiated in 2001. The programme is spear-headed by the IMH with other partners, including the Ministry of Education, the Ministry of Community Development and Sports, VWOs and other professional bodies. It focuses on raising awareness and the early detection of the major mental disorders, such as depression, anxiety disorders and schizophrenia. It also works towards destigmatising mental disorders and promoting mental well-being (Yeo, 2004).

# Research

In the past 6 years, there has been an emphasis on biomedical research and heavy investments have been made by the Singapore government.

Singapore has the potential to conduct world-class mental health research because of the unique characteristics of the population, the consolidated organisation of psychiatric services and the presence of sophisticated scientific technological platforms like the Genomics Institute of Singapore, which provides cutting-edge technology. There has been a steady growth in research activities, particularly in the areas of psychiatric epidemiology, first-episode psychosis, dementia, pharmacogenetics of tardive dyskinesia, brain imaging and clinical drug trials.

## Workforce issues and training

The quality of mental healthcare depends on the availability and adequacy of the relevant mental health workers: psychiatrists, psychologists, medical social workers, case managers, nurses and occupational therapists.

There are now two medical schools in Singapore, producing between 200 and 250 doctors a year. Psychiatric training, which has been enhanced in the undergraduate curriculum in the past few years, now comprises an 8-week posting in a psychiatry department in a restructured hospital.

Postgraduate training in psychiatry takes a minimum of 6 years. All specialist doctors, including psychiatrists, are certified by a specialist accreditation board appointed by the Ministry of Health. There are only 108 psychiatrists on the specialist register, giving a psychiatrist:population ratio of about 2.6:100 000.

Table 1 shows the number of mental health professionals in Singapore; in each of these categories there is an acute shortage. One reason for this shortage is the absence of local training. For example, there is no doctoral-level programme for clinical psychologists in any of the academic centres in Singapore. Steps are now being taken to address this, for instance with the establishment of a bachelor's degree in nursing at one of the local universities.

## Professional bodies

These include the Chapter of Psychiatrists of the Academy of Medicine, the Singapore Psychiatric Association, the Singapore Psychological Society and the Singapore Association of Counselling.

**Table 1** Numbers of mental health professionals in Singapore

| Mental health professionals | Number | Per 100 000 general population |
| --- | --- | --- |
| Psychiatrists | 108 | 2.6 |
| Clinical psychologists | 30 | 0.7 |
| Registered mental health nurses | 462 | 11.1 |
| Occupational therapists | 22 | 0.5 |

# Mental health policy

The principal problems with the current mental health system include the fragmentation and lack of coordination of services, the rudimentary community mental health services and the shortage of mental health workers. Other challenges facing the country are its ageing population, increasing divorce rates, changing family structures and economic pressures.

The Ministry of Health appointed a National Mental Health Committee in 2005 to draft a national mental health policy and blueprint for Singapore, which aimed to promote mental health in the community, to prevent mental disorders and to allow the early detection, treatment and rehabilitation of persons with mental illness. The Committee has identified four key areas that require the attention of policy-makers and mental healthcare providers over the next 5 years. These are: promotion of mental health and prevention of mental illness; integrated mental healthcare, featuring greater collaboration with general practitioners and the embedding of psychological services into medical teams; the development of the mental health workforce; and mental health research.

# Conclusions

The formulation of the above-mentioned policy and blueprint is a positive step in addressing the gaps in the mental health service. The strategies should include an integrated approach to the mental well-being of children and adolescents, measures to reduce the stigma of mental illness, such as reviewing employment policies and practices to reduce discrimination, establishing support networks for adults to promote positive mental health, and the early detection and treatment of mental illness. The intention is to develop an emotionally resilient and mentally healthy community with access to community-based, comprehensive and cost-effective mental health services.

# Sources

Chong, S. A., Mythily, Lum, A., *et al* (2005) Determinants of duration of untreated psychosis and the pathways to care in Singapore. *International Journal of Social Psychiatry*, **51**, 55–62.

Kua, E. H. (2004) Focus on psychiatry in Singapore. *British Journal of Psychiatry*, **185**, 79–82.

Li, X. (2007) Striking a healthy balance. *Straits Times*, **7 April**, S6.

Lim, C. G., Koh, C. W., Lee, C., *et al* (2005) Community psychiatry in Singapore: a pilot assertive community treatment (ACT) programme. *Annals of the Academy of Medicine*, **34**, 100–104.

Lim, M. K. (2004) Quest for quality care and patient safety: the case of Singapore. *Quality and Safety Health Care*, **13**, 71–75.

Somjee, G. (1995) Public health policy and personnel in two Asian countries. *Journal of Asian and African Studies*, **30**, 90–105.

World Health Organization (2000) *Report 2000 Health Systems: Improving Performance*. WHO.

Yeo, C. (2004) Mind Your Mind: Mental health promotion. In *Case Studies from Countries* (eds S. Saxena & P. J. Garrison). World Federation for Mental Health & WHO.

# South Korea

## Guk-Hee Suh

The Korean peninsula is located between China and Japan. After the Second World War, the Republic of Korea was established in the southern half of the Korean peninsula. South Korea has a total area of 98 480 km² and a population of 48 598 175 (July 2004 estimate). The per capita gross domestic product (GDP), in terms of purchasing power parity, is US$17 700 (2003 estimate) (Central Intelligence Agency, 2004). The illiteracy rate (among those aged over 15 years) is 1.9% (0.7% for males and 3% for females) (2003 estimate). Life expectancy at birth is 75.6 years (72.0 years for males and 79.5 years for females) and the infant mortality rate is 7.2 per 1000 births (2004 estimate). The unemployment rate is 3.4% (2003 estimate). The proportion of the population aged 65 and over is currently 8.7% (2004 estimate) (Korea National Statistics Office, 2003). Over 40% of the total Korean population (i.e. some 20 million) lives in Seoul and its vicinity. South Korea is highly urbanised and modernised. Besides central government, local government is based on seven metropolitan cities and nine provinces.

## Mental health services

There is one hospital bed for every 148 citizens and one psychiatric bed for every 1446. There is one physician for 830 citizens and one psychiatrist for every 19 500 (2002 estimates).

The basic healthcare needs of the Korean population are covered by universal public health insurance, funded by premiums, not taxes. This is compulsory, and there is no private health insurance. None the less, the private sector accounts for approximately 90% of mental health services, as there are too few public facilities. However, the government is responsible for free nationwide healthcare funded by taxes for the poor and aged. Thanks to an active community mental health movement in the public and private sector of psychiatry, since 1995, 242 public health centres nationwide have registered to take care of people with mental illness, including elderly people with dementia or stroke. In 2002, there were 989 specialist mental health facilities in South Korea: 46 community mental health centres, 66 social rehabilitation facilities, 74 mental hospitals, 207 general hospitals with psychiatric out-patient departments, 541 psychiatric clinics and 55 nursing homes.

Table 1 shows the progress in the public mental health project run by the Korean government. Both community and institutional care programmes provide long-term care. Home help services and delivered meals, adult day care, short-stay and respite care and a visiting nursing programme are also available to people with mental illnesses, including elderly people with a mental disability. Table 1 shows that care capacity is being substantially increased. The proportion of the population in need of community care who could be catered for by the maximum community care capacity will increase from 4.7% in 2003 to 72.2% in 2011, and the equivalent proportion of those in need of institutional care from 30.2% in 2003 to 71.0% in 2011 (Table 1).

**Table 1** Projected estimates of the provision for community and institutional mental healthcare in Korea

| Year | 2003 | 2005 | 2007 | 2009 | 2011 |
|---|---|---|---|---|---|
| *Community care* | | | | | |
| Number of home help centres | 120 | 470 | 1020 | 1770 | 2769 |
| Number of day care centres | 166 | 416 | 866 | 1516 | 2561 |
| Number of short-term care centres | 32 | 131 | 356 | 681 | 1079 |
| Total number of community care facilities | 318 | 1017 | 2242 | 3967 | 6409 |
| Maximum community care capacity, n | 15200 | 52700 | 114700 | 200700 | 319930 |
| Number of patients who need community care | 320974 | 353080 | 387528 | 416319 | 442925 |
| Community care capacity rate (%) | 4.7 | 14.9 | 29.6 | 48.2 | 72.2 |
| *Institutional care* | | | | | |
| Number of residential homes (capacity) | 161 (11270) | 245 (17150) | 325 (22750) | 405 (28350) | 488 (34160) |
| Number of nursing homes (capacity) | 120 (8400) | 192 (13440) | 264 (18480) | 355 (24850) | 454 (31780) |
| Number of dementia care hospitals (capacity) | 37 (3852) | 51 (4952) | 65 (6052) | 79 (7152) | 93 (8252) |
| Total number of institutional care facilities | 318 | 488 | 654 | 839 | 1035 |
| Maximum institutional care capacity | 23522 | 35542 | 47282 | 60352 | 74192 |
| Number of patients who need insitutional care | 77836 | 84838 | 92347 | 98624 | 104423 |
| Insitutional care capacity rate (%) | 30.2 | 41.9 | 51.2 | 61.2 | 71.0 |

Source: Ministry of Health and Welfare (2003, personal communication)

To meet the demand for institutional care arising from the increasing numbers of cases of dementia and stroke, special units in nursing homes and dementia care hospitals are being constructed all over South Korea.

A multidisciplinary community-oriented approach has been adopted and close working relationships have been maintained with various professionals caring for people with mental illnesses. In general, each team has a catchment population of about 50 000–200 000, which would include some 3500–14 000 people aged 65 and over. The staff usually comprise one consultant psychiatrist (generally part-time), one community psychiatric nurse, one social worker or psychologist and several volunteers. They draw on a variety of community resources in devising the most effective care pathway for people with mental illnesses and focus on enabling them to stay longer in their own homes. They have responsibility for registration, case management and education. Some of them run day care programmes for schizophrenia, alcohol dependence or dementia. The public sector has been more active in home-visiting outreach activities, while the private sector has been promoting day care rehabilitation. These movements in South Korea have been instrumental in developing infrastructure and providing mental health services.

## Psychiatric treatments

The predominance of the private sector and the relatively generous reimbursement of public health insurance have made Korea a large and early market for novel drugs in psychiatry, although reimbursement for novel drugs has now become subject to much stricter regulation. Atypical antipsychotics and novel antidepressants are much more widely used in South Korea than are traditional antipsychotics and tricyclic antidepressants. Electroconvulsive therapy also has been frequently used; there is no special limitation on its use. Psychoanalysis, psychodynamic psychotherapy, cognitive–behavioural therapy, group therapy and even hypnosis are applied on in-patient wards and out-patient clinics in psychiatry.

## Training

Basic undergraduate training in psychiatry forms part of the curriculum in medical school. Postgraduate training comprises a 4-year residency in psychiatry, in which both the theoretical and the clinical aspects of psychiatry are covered. This leads to the psychiatric board examination. Training programmes are accredited under the auspices of the Korean Neuropsychiatric Association, which is also the medical body that deals with all academic issues.

## Epidemiological issues

There have been several community-based epidemiological studies on the prevalence of mental disorder in South Korea (Cho *et al*, 1998; Suh *et al*,

1999a, 2003; Suh & Shah, 2001). Epidemiological data on the prevalence of mental health problems help to determine the need for care. Dementia and depression are the most common mental disorders and the most severe public health problem, especially in the older population. Korean reports have been comparable to those of Western studies. Suh *et al* (2003) interviewed 1037 people aged 65 and over, and found a prevalence of dementia of 6.6% (Alzheimer's disease 4.2%, vascular dementia 2.4%). A nationwide survey examined the prevalence of depressive symptoms in the Korean population. The prevalence rates using a cut-off score of 16/17 on the CES-D (Center for the Epidemiologic Study of Depression) scale were 23.1% of male adults, 27.4% of female adults and 24.3% of the elderly population (Cho *et al*, 1998; Suh *et al*, 1999a). A community-based survey reported a prevalence of 'the wish to die' within last 2 weeks among elderly respondents of 14.6% (Suh *et al*, 1999b).

A total of 788 000 persons, equivalent to 21% of the South Korean elderly population, were in need of long-term care in 2001. Of these, at least 74 000 needed institutional care, while the remainder required community care. The number of patients with dementia and disturbed instrumental activities of daily living has been estimated at 186 000, and this group will require insti-tutional care at some point (Sunwoo, 2001).

## Problems in mental healthcare in South Korea

There are several problems in mental healthcare in South Korea. First, medical, psychiatric and social welfare services are separate, which means that integrated care is not available. This separation originated from an artificial distinction between 'treatment' and 'care'. Second, sub-acute care facilities are too scanty: there are generally only acute care and chronic care facilities. Differentiation of function in facilities is necessary, for example 'hostel' for mild cases and 'nursing home' for severe cases. Third, public care facilities are too few (less than 10% of the overall mental healthcare provision). Most facilities are private and this leads to frequent conflict between consumers, government and suppliers. However, the Korean government has substantially increased its expenditure on healthcare and social welfare to meet the unmet need. It is also actively considering the adoption of a long-term care insurance system, similar to those that have been adopted in Germany and Japan.

## Conclusion

The private sector provides approximately 90% of mental health services in South Korea. These services are in short supply for the population, despite the relatively high number of psychiatrists. Thanks to an active community mental health movement in the public and private sectors of psychiatry and the long-term care plan being implemented by the Ministry of Health and Welfare, better care provision is expected. Although services have actively been trying to move away from institutionalisation to community-based care, the inadequate number of fully qualified community mental health professionals, prejudice towards mental illnesses among the general population and less active participation of board-certified psychiatrists make this move difficult. However, a large investment in infrastructure, the development of programmes for community care, upgraded training and active research will lead to a more modern, community-based, multidisciplinary approach to healthcare in South Korea.

# References

Central Intelligence Agency (2004) *World Factbook*. Available at www.cia.gov/cia/publications/factbook/geos/ks.html. Last accessed 22 November 2004.

Cho, M. J., Nam, J. J. & Suh, G. H. (1998) Prevalence of symptoms of depression in a nationwide sample of Korean adults. *Psychiatry Research*, **81**, 341–352.

Korea National Statistics Office (2003) *Statistical Annual 2002*. Daejeon: Korea National Statistics Office.

Suh, G. H. & Shah, A. (2001) A review of the epidemiological transition in dementia – cross-national comparisons of the indices related to Alzheimer's disease and vascular dementia. *Acta Psychiatrica Scandinavica*, **104**, 4–11.

Suh, G. H., Cho, D. Y., Rhoo, I. K., *et al* (1999a) Prevalence and risk factors of depressive symptomatology among the Korean elderly. *Journal of the Korean Geriatrics Society*, **2**, 49–60.

Suh, G. H., Kim, J. K., Jung, Y. J., *et al* (1999b) Wish to die and associated factors in the rural elderly. *Journal of Korean Geriatric Psychiatry*, **3**, 70–77.

Suh, G. H., Kim, J. K. & Cho, M. J. (2003) Community study of dementia in the older Korean rural population. *Australia and New Zealand Journal of Psychiatry*, **37**, 606–612.

Sunwoo, D. (2001) *Survey of the Long-Term Care Service Need of Old Persons and Policy Direction*. Seoul: Korean Institute for Health and Social Affairs.

# Sri Lanka

Nalaka Mendis

Relative to its economic indicators, Sri Lanka has a high health status. The life expectancy in the year 2001 was 70.7 years for males and 75.4 years for females. Maternal and infant mortality rates have shown a downward trend over the past half century and now are around 2.3 per 10 000 live births and 16 per 1000 live births, respectively. These trends are mainly due to the high literacy rate and comparatively large investments made in health and social welfare.

The situation regarding mental healthcare services is very different. As in many developing countries, negative attitudes to mental illness, social stigma and a lack of appreciation of the suffering and disability caused by mental illness have resulted in low priority being given to mental healthcare services in Sri Lanka. This situation is, however, beginning to change.

## Overview

Major psychiatric illnesses form the bulk of the clinical load of psychiatrists in Sri Lanka. The suicide rate, though declining, is still higher than global average rates (De Silva & Jayasinghe, 2003), and alcohol-related problems are rising (World Health Organization, 1999). Drug misuse, which appears to be less of a problem than alcohol misuse, is mainly confined to heroin and cannabis (Ratnayake & Senanayake, 2002).

Long-term mental illness has a considerable social, economic and health burden (De Mel, 2001). The fast-growing elderly population, which will amount to 21% of the overall population by 2020, is likely to pose enormous mental health problems. Thirty years of civil disturbances coupled with ethnic violence have resulted not only in trauma but also a range of other problems, including loss of life, refugees, displacement, the disruption of the physical and social infrastructure as well as the poor economic performance of the entire country. The inevitable mental and psychosocial distress associated with the above problems, especially in the north and the east, compounds the existing mental health burden.

In the absence of a formal referral system, patients have the liberty to consult any mental health professional – or any other type of healer – in any part of the country. In view of the concentration of services in urban areas and also because of the perception that services in urban areas are of better quality, many patients gravitate towards these centres.

Increasingly, the majority of acutely disturbed patients tend to seek psychiatric help early; however, others, especially those with somatic manifestations, tend to seek psychiatric help when the initial treatment by a range of healers, including those in the general healthcare services, fails.

Most psychiatrists working for the government or for a university additionally engage in private practice after their contracted working hours. Almost all patients prefer to seek private services at least initially and resort to public services only when they are pressed financially to do so.

Mentally ill offenders and those coming under the Mental Health Act are directly referred to mental hospital for admission and care. Police and social care agencies are generally reluctant to force the involuntary admission of patients living in the community.

Responsibility for the development of mental health services belongs to the Director of Mental Health Services, who works with the Advisory Council on Mental Health. Because all health services are organised in a very complex and bureaucratic manner, taking decisions and implementing them is a tedious process. However, attempts are being made to implement, in stages, both the recommendations of a presidential taskforce set up 1998 and the National Plan to strengthen mental health services, which was prepared by a consultant from the World Health Organization (Ministry of Health, 2001).

The present public mental health services are organised around hospitals, which have no direct formal responsibility to a catchment area or a community.

## In-patient services

The two large mental hospitals located in the suburbs of Colombo provide nearly 2500 in-patient beds. Long-stay patients occupy more than half of these. In addition to voluntary patients from all over the country, those referred by the courts, other units and involuntary patients reside in these institutions. The mental hospitals at present operate with severe staff constraints, as many positions are vacant. It is inevitable that, under these circumstances, the quality of patient care often has to be severely compromised. Although the need to develop provincial mental health services while phasing out the mental hospital facilities in Colombo is accepted by all stakeholders, practical steps towards realising this have not been taken.

The teaching hospitals and provincial general hospitals have a total of about 500 mental health beds in open wards. The average duration of an in-patient stay in a general hospital unit is around one to two weeks.

## Out-patient services

Most major hospitals and some small hospitals offer out-patient clinics and day facilities. Basic psychotropic drugs and facilities for electroconvulsive therapy are available in most of these, while almost the whole range of drugs is available at the teaching hospital units, including newer drugs, which are also available in the private sector.

Non-medical mental health professionals carry out mainly psychological interventions. However, except in a few academic departments there are no clinical psychologists working in the publicly funded mental health services.

## Rehabilitation services

With the assistance of the Nations for Mental Health programme, a project has begun to settle long-stay patients from the mental hospitals in the community. Recently, the Ministry of Health initiated a programme to develop intermediate-stay units at provincial level. Already about five such units are functioning. A few non-governmental organisations conduct residential rehabilitation programmes in the community.

An organisation called Sahanaya has been conducting a community-based rehabilitation programme since the early 1980s through its community mental health centre in Colombo. In addition, a number of innovative community-based programmes are being conducted in the central, north and eastern provinces at the initiative of psychiatrists and other mental health professionals.

The general health services provide detoxification and support for those with alcohol- or drug-related problems. In addition, a few state and non-governmental facilities provide residential care.

## Specialised mental health services

Two child psychiatrists provide a specialised service in the children's hospital in Colombo, while a general psychiatrist with training in forensic psychiatry provides a forensic service at one of the mental hospitals. Residential facilities run by the social services tend to house children with severe learning difficulties and behaviour problems.

During the past two decades there has been a steady growth of counselling centres in the country, mostly in the non-governmental and private sector. There has been a phenomenal growth of counselling programmes conducted by foreign organisations in the north and the eastern provinces, many of which are directed at war-related issues.

## Promotion, prevention and social care

Health programmes – school health, maternal and child care and adolescent programmes – have been successful in incorporating aspects of mental health.

**199**

The Ministry of Social Services has been increasingly active in supporting the social needs of those with mental illness, especially those with a long-term illness.

# The Mental Health Act and mental health budget

The Mental Health Act, amended in 1956, focuses on involuntary treatment and it mandates a mental hospital to house all patients coming under the Act. The inability of the present Act to meet the needs of those with mental illness was recognised as far back as 1971 and since then a number of committees have produced drafts at various times.

At national level, the budget for mental healthcare, which amounts to about 1% of the overall health budget, is wholly allocated to the mental hospitals. However, individual general hospitals meet their own mental healthcare expenses.

# Training

The academic departments of psychiatry in all six medical schools have undergraduate training programmes, which feature one to two months of clinical attachments as well as classroom teaching. The five-year postgraduate training programme in psychiatry initiated in 1981 at the Postgraduate Institute of Medicine, University of Colombo, has so far produced more than 70 psychiatrists, but Sri Lankan mental health services have been able to retain less than half this number.

The requirement of a research thesis as a part of the postgraduate programme in psychiatry has resulted in trainees being introduced to research. The numbers of research presentations by psychiatrists at scientific meetings and publications in local and international journals have increased over the past 10 years. Suicide, trauma, epidemiology, alcohol and long-term mental illness are some of the areas focused on.

In order to take psychiatry to the secondary care level, Sahanaya, with the support of the Ministry of Health, initiated a three-year training programme for doctors in 1999. At present, nearly 40 medical officers in mental health serve at secondary care hospitals, thus complementing services rendered by psychiatrists. In 2001, at the request of the Ministry of Health, a one-year diploma programme was initiated and already 10 people have graduated. They are to be posted to secondary care hospitals to develop new hospital and community services.

The general nursing programme includes training in psychiatry for two months at a mental hospital. A postgraduate training programme established in 1965 unfortunately continued only for two years; however, a similar training programme was initiated in 2001.

# Professional bodies

The Professional Association of Psychiatrists (which is to be renamed the College of Psychiatrists), established in the 1970s, has become more active in the recent past. There are a number of civil society or non-governmental organisations working in the area of mental health, the National Council for Mental Health being the oldest and most active. Most non-governmental organisations are engaged in providing a range of services, but advocacy and activism in mental health receive minimal attention.

# Future challenges

During the past few decades there have been significant developments in the field of mental health. Most of these have been on the initiative of local groups in universities, non-governmental organisations or in the private sector.

There is an urgent need to provide accessible basic services of good quality to meet the emerging needs of people living in the community. In order to realise this objective, there is a requirement for a coordinated development strategy at national level, with political leadership and the support of an effective mental health planning and implementation unit.

The challenge for the Ministry of Health is to strengthen its leadership role in the development of mental health at a national level and to work towards a common goal in partnership with other government agencies, non-governmental agencies, universities, other groups and international agencies.

# References

De Mel, N. (2001) Summary of findings. In *Caring for Long Term Mentally Ill: Impacts, Needs and Options* (eds S. Jayasinghe, N. de Mel & V. Basnayale), pp. 44–45. Colombo: Smart Media.

De Silva, D. & Jayasinghe, S. (2003) Suicide in Sri Lanka. In *Suicide Prevention: Meeting the Challenges Together* (ed. L. Vijayakumar), pp. 179–182. Hyderabad: Orient Longman.

Ministry of Health (2001) *National Mental Health Plan, Strategy to Strengthen Mental Health Care in Sri Lanka*. Colombo: Ministry of Health.

Ratnayake, Y. & Senanayake, B. (eds) (2002) *Handbook of Drug Abuse Information*, pp. 10–12. Colombo: Research and Publication Unit, National Dangerous Drugs Control Board.

World Health Organization (1999) *Global Status Report on Alcohol (331 WHO/SAB/99.11)*. Geneva: WHO.

# Syrian Arab Republic

Iyas Assalman, Mazen Alkhalil and Martin Curtice

The following view was espoused in a 1903 *Lancet* editorial describing psychiatric services in the East: 'The treatment of lunatics in the East has not yet fully emerged from the clouds of ignorance and barbarism which have surrounded it for ages.' One of the first reformers was 'Mr. Theophilus Waldmeier, a gentleman resident in Syria, who commenced in the spring of 1896 the work of helping and providing for the numerous sufferers from mental disease in Syria and Palestine.' He attempted to introduce the methods of humanity and science in this field. In 1939 Bernstein described his visit to the Maristan Arghoum, a psychiatric hospital, in the city of Aleppo. He observed the complete lack of medical supervision, 'bad' patients being chained and the despotic rule of the 'keeper' of the hospital.

## Demographics

The Syrian Arab Republic has a total area of 185 180 km², of which approximately 80 000 km² is cultivable land; the remainder is desert and rocky mountains. The country's population in 2006 was estimated at 18.717 million. The population growth rate was 2.45%; 39.4% of the population were below 15 years of age and 3.3% above 65 years. In 2006, the crude death rate was estimated to be 4 per 1000 population per annum and the crude birth rate 30 per 1000 per annum. In the same year, life expectancy at birth was estimated at 72 years.

The socio-demographic correlates of psychiatric morbidity among low-income women in Aleppo, Syria, were studied by Maziak *et al* (2002), who concluded that the prevalence of 'psychiatric distress' was 55.6%, but there was no categorisation of these psychiatric disorders. The study used a special questionnaire based on items not relating to psychosis from the 20-item Self-Reporting Questionnaire (SRQ–20), as well as questions about background information considered relevant to the mental health of women in the population studied. (The SRQ–20 was developed primarily as a psychiatric screening tool to suit primary care settings in low- and middle-income countries.) 'Psychiatric distress' was related to a number of factors, including women's illiteracy, polygamy and physical abuse, most of which are amenable to intervention. It is the authors' opinion that women's education is a very important factor for the mental health of this population. In 2006, mental illnesses contributed 0.2% of the total mortality, according to the Ministry of Health (no further details were given).

# General health services

In 2005 the health expenditure per capita was US$58. This is very low in comparison with the UK (where the health expenditure per capita was US$2900 in 2005). The Ministry of Health budget was 1.4% of the government budget in 2005.

With respect to human resources, in 2006 there were 78196 physicians, 27636 dentists and 54855 qualified nurses and midwives. The overall provision per 10000 population of physicians, dentists and nursing and midwifery personnel was 14.8, 7.4 and 18.8, respectively.

The health system is based on primary care and is delivered at three levels: village, district and provincial.

# Mental health services

Currently there are 65 psychiatrists and 40 psychiatric residents in the whole country.

## Public sector

General adult psychiatry is the main specialty in Syria. Three different government ministries – Health, Defence and Higher Education (Damascus University) – provide this service.

The Ministry of Health runs the two main psychiatric hospitals:

- There are 800 beds at Ibn Sina Hospital, in Damascus, distributed over 18 wards, of which 600 are for male patients and 200 for female patients. Approximately 100 of these patients are under legal confinement.
- Ibn Khaldoun Hospital, in Aleppo, has 400 beds, 250 of which are for male patients and 150 for female patients.

In addition, there is a 30-bed addiction treatment centre in Damascus, with three psychiatrists, three psychotherapists and two social workers, who provide the service and supervise trainees. The Ministry of Health also runs community psychiatric out-patient clinics, which operate in nearly every big city in Syria; there are four such clinics in Damascus. They are run by trained psychiatrists and offer consultations and medical interventions but no psychological input.

The Ministry of Defence service includes two military general hospitals that have mental health departments. The biggest is Tishreen Hospital, with a 40-bed department.

The Ministry of Higher Education runs Damascus University Hospital (Al-Moassat Hospital), which has a psychiatric ward with 12 beds for the purpose of undergraduate and postgraduate training.

### Specialist services

There are special foundations attached to the Ministry of Work and Social Affairs that provide treatment and rehabilitation for patients with intellectual disability. Child and adolescent psychiatric services are provided through non-governmental organisations and the above foundations. They deal with patients suffering from intellectual disability, autistic spectrum and other behavioural disorders. These foundations have clinical freedom and a lot of government support. They offer treatment and support to patients and their families under supervision of licensed psychiatrists and psychologists.

## The private sector

While there is a private health system, there is currently limited private health insurance and so most patients who choose to be treated privately pay for their healthcare out of their own funds.

### Private hospitals

There are only two private hospitals and both are in Damascus. They offer acute admission, as well as long-stay and out-patient clinics. Medical treatment and some psychotherapy are available. The larger is Al-Basheer Hospital, with 50 beds; the other is a recently established day hospital for adults, which also incorporates a special centre for autistic children.

A hot-line has been set up with the help of the private sector to offer free consultations and advice to people with mental health issues.

### Private clinics

There are 65 private clinics in Syria; most (45 clinics) are in Damascus, and 10 are in Aleppo; the other 10 clinics are located in the other big cities, for instance Homs. The main specialty of these clinics is general adult psychiatry. There are only two child and adolescent psychiatrists in Syria.

# Mental health policies and legislation

The rules governing mental health and psychiatric treatment in the Syrian Arab Republic are derived from the health legislation issued in 1981 by the Ministry of Health. Currently, a draft Mental Health Act is under discussion.

In 2001 the Ministry of Health established a Psychiatric Directorate to improve and develop services.

Admitting a patient to a psychiatric hospital is done either informally or under a court order. A responsible psychiatrist or a family member can raise concern about a patient's mental state. Following a referral, a committee of three psychiatrists will decide whether an informal admission is appropriate. After the patient has been in hospital for 1 week, another assessment by the same committee is done to validate the decision and the management plan.

If a patient refuses informal admission, she or he must be assessed by a psychiatrist in the community, who will then submit a report to a court. The judge may order an assessment by a general forensic doctor (there are no forensic psychiatrists in Syria). If the doctor decides to admit the patient, the committee of three psychiatrists decides the management plan.

If a patient commits an offence, a court may order an assessment by a special committee and if the patient is found to be mentally ill she or he will be detained in a high-security unit.

# Professional bodies

Most of the 65 Syrian psychiatrists are members of the Syrian Psychiatric Association, which was established in 1996. Psychiatric residents can have honorary membership. The Association has an important role in medical education and training, by arranging conferences and lectures.

# Training

## Undergraduate training

Medical students have formal training in psychiatry as part of the syllabus for internal medicine. It includes lectures and clinical training during the fourth and fifth year (4 weeks each).

## Psychiatrists

There are three different training schemes attached to the three ministries that provide the services (see above), with a total of 40 psychiatric residents.

Each scheme is a 4-year programme and at the end of it the doctor is granted either a masters degree in general adult psychiatry (Damascus University scheme) or a certificate to practise general adult psychiatry. The curriculum includes general adult psychiatry, addiction treatment and a compulsory 6 months in neurology.

There is a proposal for a temporary, instead of permanent, licence for psychiatrists, to be renewed every year, to ensure that high standards are maintained in clinical practice.

## Psychiatric nurses

There are no psychiatric nurses in Syria, but instead general nurses with psychiatric experience. The Ministry of Health has acknowledged this problem and now psychiatric nursing is part of the nursing curriculum.

## Psychology and psychotherapy

The Faculty of Education and Psychology in Damascus University is currently running 4-year courses to train students in social and psychological specialties. Students obtain a diploma in social counselling or a diploma in psychological counselling. Students can take a higher degree in clinical psychology and get a masters degree in cognitive–behavioural therapy.

Syria has very few psychodynamic psychotherapists; most of those there are have trained abroad. Other forms of psychotherapy (solution focus therapy, cognitive–behavioural therapy, behavioural therapy, art therapy, music therapy and so on) are not practised.

# Research in psychiatry

Despite the existence of a few research projects, it is very rare for any of the results to be published. Every masters student in psychiatry is expected to conduct and produce a research thesis.

# The future

The government is trying to develop modern psychiatric care by encouraging the establishment of more community-based services and smaller centres, and in addition involving the private sector more in the delivery of services. Syria is opening its market to some private insurance companies, and this may have a beneficial effect on service development.

# Acknowledgement

We thank staff of the Queen Elizabeth Psychiatric Hospital Library for their assistance in the preparation of this paper.

# References and sources

Bernstein, E. L. (1939) American Journal of Psychiatry, 95, 1415–1419.

*Lancet* (1903) 17 January, p. 189.

Maziak, W., Asfar, T., Mzayek, F., *et al* (2002) Socio-demographic correlates of psychiatric morbidity among low-income women in Aleppo, Syria. *Social Science and Medicine*, **54**, 1419–1427.

Ministry of Health (2006) See http://www.moh.gov.sy

World Bank (2005) See http://www.worldbank.org

World Health Organization (2005) Syrian Arab Republic. In *Mental Health Atlas 2005*. See http://www.who.int/mental_health/evidence/atlas

# Tajikistan

Alisher Latypov, Vladimir Magkoev, Mutabara Vohidova and Zulfia Nisanbaeva

Tajikistan, in Central Asia, gained its independence in 1991, with the break-up of the Soviet Union. There followed a period of civil war, 1992–97. In 2003, 64% of Tajikistan's population was poor, which was defined as living on less than US$2.15 per day at purchasing power parity by the UN *Appeal for Tajikistan* (2006). The Tajik healthcare budget appropriations decreased from 4.5% of gross domestic product in 1991 to 1.3% in 2005. The average annual rate of population growth is 2.19%. The estimated 7 320 815 population of the country is mainly rural (73.5%) and about 38% of the country's population is under the age of 14. Life expectancy at birth is 62 years for males and 68 years for females. The infant mortality rate is 106.49 deaths per 1000 live births.

Tajikistan has a state-regulated system of healthcare which increasingly depends on unofficial private payments for medical services (70% of total spending in recent years). In 2005, Tajikistan presented its draft National Development Strategy with three fundamental priorities: public administration reform, private sector development, and development of human potential. The main priorities for development of the healthcare system in Tajikistan are:

- reform of the healthcare system, including development of the private sector and attraction of investment
- improvement of maternal and child health
- a significant slow-down in the spread of HIV/AIDS, a reduction in infectious diseases and the eradication of certain infections that can be controlled by vaccination
- improved availability, quality and effectiveness of medical services (National Development Strategy, 2006).

## Mental health policy and legislation

The legal framework for public health-related activities is the Law of the Republic of Tajikistan 'On Protection of Health of the Population', of 15 May 1997. It contains, *inter alia*, some provisions dealing with mental health. According to article 53 of this law, people with mental illnesses are categorised as those who 'pose a threat to surrounding people', along with people with tuberculosis, sexually transmitted diseases, leprosy, AIDS and other infections.

Activities in the field of mental healthcare provision have not been specifically regulated up to 2002 from the legal point of view. At present, these are governed by the Law of the Republic of Tajikistan 'On Psychiatric Care', adopted on 2 December 2002. Furthermore, there is a Decree of the Ministry of Health of Tajikistan, 'On Measures for Further Improvement of Psychiatric Care', of 9 February 2001, which approved 17 regulations on the provision of psychiatric care.

The only document which has an element of strategy on mental health in Tajikistan is the *Strategy of the Republic of Tajikistan on Protection of Health of the Population for the Period to 2010*. Task 6 of this strategy is entitled 'Improvement of Mental Health' and is aimed at improving significantly, by 2010, psychosocial support for the general population and people with mental disorders and ensuring improvement in the psychosocial status of people. This envisages:

- implementation of comprehensive measures on reduction of prevalence of mental disorders, and improvement of people's capacities to cope with life stressors
- establishment of comprehensive care services for people with mental disorders.

In 2005, at the Ministerial Conference in Helsinki, the Tajik Minister of Health signed the *European Declaration and Action Plan on Mental Health*.

# History of psychiatry in Tajikistan

By the 1990s, a network of psychiatric institutions, including dispensaries, hospitals and mental health offices, had been established in Tajikistan. In-patient care was by far the predominant form of psychiatric service available, and hospital stay tended to be long. In the process of treatment of mental disorders, preference was given to biomedical interventions, such as psychopharmacotherapy or shock therapy.

The condition of post-Soviet mental health services in Tajikistan can be defined as critical, based on many indicators: availability of the qualified staff; provision of food; the state of the wards, facilities and utilities at the mental health institutions; and the availability of effective therapies. In 1996, in psychiatric hospitals of Lakkon and Leninsky districts, 311 of about 700 patients died mainly because of lack of food. The physical infrastructure of the mental health services was dilapidated. In many psychiatric care facilities there were no decent windows or doors; in-patients slept on beds with no mattresses, while dressed. There was little regard for basic hygiene (Médecins Sans Frontières, 2003).

Since 2005, first in-patient and then out-patient psychosocial rehabilitation programmes have been introduced by the Global Initiative on Psychiatry.

# Incidence and prevalence of mental disorders

The Tajik Ministry of Health has provided the quantitative data on mental disorder shown in Table 1.

# Mental health service delivery

According to the Pharmaciens Sans Frontieres Comite International (PSFCI) report on the assessment of psychiatric institutions in the Republic of Tajikistan released in 2006:

> there were 17 psychiatric institutions in the Republic of Tajikistan, divided in four groups of medical institutions with bed capacity i.e. psychiatric hospitals, psychoneurological dispensaries, psychoneurological centres and psychoneurological departments. Psychiatric departments within central

**Table 1** Prevalence and incidence of mental and behavioural disorders in the Republic of Tajikistan as registered by the psychiatric services, 2001–05

| Mental and behavioural disorders | ICD–10 block | 2001 | 2002 | 2003 | 2004 | 2005 |
|---|---|---|---|---|---|---|
| *Prevalence* | | | | | | |
| Total | F00–F09, F20–F99 | 39634 | 41300 | 40998 | 40951 | 41177 |
| Schizophrenia, schizotypal and delusional disorders | F20–F29 | 10654 | 10805 | 10938 | 11069 | 11219 |
| Mood disorders | F30–F39 | 656 | 685 | 673 | 673 | 688 |
| Neurotic, stress-related and somatoform disorders | F40–F48 | 1681 | 1668 | 1688 | 1782 | 1699 |
| Behavioural syndromes associated with physiological disturbances and physical factors; and disorders of adult personality and behaviour | F50–F69 | 1192 | 1198 | 1202 | 1210 | 1227 |
| Mental retardation | F70–F79 | 19390 | 20341 | 20015 | 20230 | 20408 |
| *Incidence* | | | | | | |
| Total | F00–F09, F20–F99 | 1402 | 1388 | 1370 | 1338 | 1406 |
| Schizophrenia, schizotypal and delusional disorders | F20–F29 | 351 | 386 | 418 | 450 | 491 |
| Mood disorders | F30–F39 | 37 | 23 | 16 | 26 | 28 |
| Neurotic, stress-related and somatoform disorders | F40–F48 | 38 | 43 | 49 | 48 | 36 |
| Behavioural syndromes associated with physiological disturbances and physical factors; and disorders of adult personality and behaviour | F50–F69 | 24 | 25 | 25 | 35 | 46 |
| Mental retardation | F70–F79 | 629 | 691 | 569 | 543 | 563 |

Source: Tajik Ministry of Health.

district hospitals substitute for psychoneurological hospitals in districts with small populations. Therefore, there are in total 2 hospitals, 2 departments, 2 psychoneurological centres and 11 psychoneurological dispensaries in Tajikistan. PSFCI found that 69% of the hospitals' budget needs were not covered. Allocated State budget resources (1,561,166.00 Somoni or about 520,390.00 USD in 2005) were mainly intended to cover wages, food and medicines expenses. (PSFCI, 2006)

# Mental health workforce

Institutionally, mental healthcare services in Tajikistan are provided within the public health and social sectors. According to the most recent (end of 2005) assessment of psychiatric institutions in Tajikistan, the evaluated structures were employing 102 doctors. Of those, 75 were psychiatrists and 27 were experts in narcology.

Table 2 provides Ministry of Health statistics on mental health professionals, including drug treatment specialists, by region in 2003 and 2004.

# Education and training

Undergraduate and graduate medical and pharmaceutical education and training in Tajikistan are provided by the Tajik State Medical University named after Avicena. The overall duration of education and training of a medical doctor is between 7 and 8 years: basic medical education (bachelor's level) takes 5 years, and graduate (master's level) education is another 2–3 years.

Graduate training in psychiatry lasts 2 years. According to the syllabus, psychiatry-related courses take 882 hours per year or 1764 hours altogether over the 2 years of postgraduate training. The educational programme of other medical students also devotes some hours to psychiatry. This includes 1764 hours for drug treatment specialists, 60 hours for neurologists and 36 hours for general practitioners.

**Table 2** Total number of psychiatrists and narcologists in Tajikistan in 2003 and 2004, by region

| Region | 2003 | 2004 |
|---|---|---|
| Dushanbe City | 72 | 70 |
| Regions of Republican Subordinations | 29 | 25 |
| Sogd Region | 58 | 54 |
| Khatlon Region | 26 | 25 |
| Gorno-Badakhshan Autonomous Region | 5 | 5 |
| Total | 190 | 179 |

Source: Tajik Ministry of Health.

Medical education is multidisciplinary and the curriculum is developed in compliance with the state standard for graduate education in Tajikistan, approved by Resolution No. 95 of the Government of Tajikistan of 23 February 1996.

Postgraduate training of medical and pharmaceutical professionals is conducted by the Tajik Institute for Postgraduate Training of Medical Professionals, which was established in 1993. Such postgraduate 'upgrade' courses are to be undertaken by medical professionals every 5 years on a mandatory basis.

Training and education of nurses are provided by medical colleges and vocational schools.

## Substance misuse

In 2002 the United Nations Office on Drugs and Crime (UNODC) estimated the number of drug users in Tajikistan at 45 000–55 000 (UNODC, 2002).

Specialised medical drug treatment in Tajikistan is provided exclusively by the narcological centres established in Soviet times. In 2005, 1040 individuals received in-patient treatment at such centres, of whom 96.4% were diagnosed with heroin addiction (F11.2 according to ICD–10). In 2001–05, the narcological facilities treated 4818 in-patients in total.

## Mental health and human rights

According to a report from the Tajikistan Bureau on Human Rights, on access to psychiatric care in Tajikistan (Sanginov & Romanov, 2006), violations of fundamental human rights are common in psychiatric institutions. In particular, the following are often not met: the right to information, notably regarding patients' rights; the right to equal reward for equal labour; the right to an adequate environment; the right to the best available treatment; economic and social rights.

Patient's participation in discussion of the treatment plan and the giving of informed consent for treatment are not in place, and patients play only a passive role. They are almost never informed of their diagnosis and their health condition (they are often told simply that they have developed a psychiatric illness).

Drinking water is often unavailable. There is a shortage of electricity, especially in winter. Daily schedules are repetitive; most patients have nothing to do but to sit and stare at the walls around them. Wards lack furniture except for metal beds. The freedom of movement of patients is very limited, even within the institutions.

Psychiatric patients do not have an opportunity to ask for alternative psychiatric examination. There is no institute of independent psychiatric expertise in Tajikistan (Sanginov & Romanov, 2006).

# Conclusion

Tajik psychiatry 'flourished' during Soviet times, when the biomedical approach to treatment was paramount. The collapse of that system and the subsequent civil war in Tajikistan led to a major emergency in psychiatry in terms of migration of qualified staff, dilapidation of buildings and disintegration of services. As Tajik society recovered from deep social and economic crisis, the provision of mental health services gradually stabilised. While the financial capacity of the government is still very limited, the Central Asian region as a whole, and Tajikistan in particular, are the focus of many international donors and non-governmental agencies. As some of them prioritise the social sector and in a few cases mental health, new psychosocial rehabilitation services are being developed and opportunities exist for further improvement of mental healthcare in Tajikistan.

# Sources and references

Central Intelligence Agency. *The World Fact Book, Tajikistan*. See https://www.cia.gov/cia/publications/factbook/geos/ti.html (last accessed 23 April 2007).

Médecins Sans Frontières (2003) *'Will You Remember Me?' A Question from the Patients of Psychiatric Institutions in Tajikistan. Report of Médecins Sans Frontières on the Situation in Psychiatric Institutions in the Republic of Tajikistan*. Médecins Sans Frontières, Dushanbe, Tajikistan.

*National Development Strategy of the Republic of Tajikistan for the Period to 2015*, draft, 2006. See http://www.untj.org (last accessed 23 April 2007).

PSFCI (2006) *Report on the Assessment of Psychiatric Institutions in the Republic of Tajikistan*. PSFCI.

Sanginov, K. & Romanov, S. (2006) *Access to Psychiatric Care in Tajikistan*. Tajikistan Bureau on Human Rights.

*UN Appeal for Tajikistan* (2006) See http://www.untj.org (last accessed 23 April 2007).

UNODC (2002) *Regional Conference on Drug Abuse in Central Asia: Situation Assessment and Responses*. Conference Report. UNODC.

# Thailand

Pichet Udomratn

Thailand is located in Southeast Asia and covers an area of 513 115 km². In 2006 its population was approximately 64 million. The major nationality is Thai. About 80% of the total population live in rural areas. The country is composed of 76 provinces, divided into a total of 94 districts and 7159 sub-districts.

## Prevalence of mental illnesses

The latest data concerning the prevalence of mental disorders in Thailand were obtained from a national survey conducted in 2003. The survey was a two-step cross-sectional community survey using AUDIT (Alcohol Use Disorders Identification Test) and MINI (Mini-International Neuropsychiatric Interview). There were 11 700 participants, aged 15–59 years, selected by stratified two-stage cluster sampling. The top three problems found (1-month prevalence) were alcohol use disorders (28.5%), major depressive disorder (3.2%) and generalised anxiety disorder (1.9%) (Siriwanarangsan et al, 2004).

## Mental health policy and legislation

The current mental health policy was formulated in 1995. Its main components are advocacy, promotion, treatment and rehabilitation, but it also includes sections on administration and technical development. The policy plan is to promote mental health and prevent mental health problems, to expand and develop treatment and rehabilitation services, to develop a management system to reform all aspects of mental health services, and to develop modern psychosocial and other technical knowledge in order to apply them fruitfully to Thailand's mental health situation (World Health Organization, 2001).

There is at present no mental health legislation, although a Mental Health Bill, which was drafted by the Department of Mental Health and then revised according to suggestions from service providers, carers and ex-patients during a public hearing process, has been submitted to parliament. However, parliament was dissolved in February 2006 following an army coup and we must now wait until we get a new parliament to approve the Bill. The Mental Health Bill is, in essence, similar to the legislation enacted in other countries, in that all persons in need of psychiatric treatment either will be able to access it voluntarily or will be compulsorily brought to a hospital for evaluation and to receive treatment.

# The healthcare system

The system was originally set up (before 2001) so that those with a medical problem were expected to consult first in the primary care setting; then, if necessary, they would be referred to secondary and if necessary tertiary care. (These services are described below.) However, in reality, patients could go directly to any level they chose. Many were first seen at secondary or tertiary settings, including university hospitals. Except for those with a psychosis, referral of patients from primary to secondary care seldom happened – patients were referred directly to a tertiary service or a psychiatric hospital.

Since the last government introduced the policy of universal coverage under its '30 baht healthcare scheme' in 2001 (30 baht is approximately 0.60 euros), referral systems have been strengthened. Under this scheme, people who have no health insurance must register with a nearby hospital. If they are ill, they can go to that hospital and pay the hospital only 30 baht per visit. This covers all kinds of treatment, from medication to open-heart surgery. If doctors at the registered hospital cannot treat that patient for any reason, they will refer the patient to a larger hospital, which will in turn send the bill for reimbursement back to the first hospital.

The government allocates a yearly budget to each hospital according to its number of registered patients. The hospitals received 1202 baht per registered patient per year in 2003, which increased to 1308 baht in 2004, 1396 baht in 2005 and to 1659 baht for 2006. This budget is meant to cover all expenses, including salaries, equipment and materials. Under this scheme, patients now are unable to visit a doctor in a secondary or tertiary care setting without a referral letter from the registered hospital, unless they are prepared to pay all of the expenses out of their own pocket (Udomratn, 2006). In October 2006, the new interim government scrapped payment of 30 baht per visit but the system remains the same.

## Primary care services

These cover all areas of the country and fall under the administration of the Ministry of Public Health, except in Bangkok, which is under the Bangkok Metropolitan Administration. The services located nearest the local communities are the sub-district health centres, each of which is run by three or four health workers. Their main function is the prevention of illness, although they also provide treatment for simple illnesses or problems. If the problem is beyond their ability they refer the patient to the district (community) hospital. There are about 8800 sub-district health centres covering the whole country.

The second level of primary care service is the district hospital, which typically has one or two physicians, between five and seven nurses and 10–30 beds. The largest district hospital has 120 beds. Out-patient services are the main provision. Currently there are approximately 695 district hospitals in Thailand.

## Secondary care services

These are the responsibility of the general hospitals, which typically have 100–120 beds and are located in each of the 76 provinces. A few provinces have two general hospitals. Typically, five specialised services (medicine, paediatrics, surgery, obstetrics and gynaecology, and orthopaedics) are provided by the general hospitals. There may be a psychiatric unit in the general hospital, but this will usually be supervised by a non-psychiatrist physician and a psychiatric nurse: only about a third of the general hospitals have a psychiatrist as the head of the psychiatric unit.

## Tertiary care services

There are about 20 tertiary care hospitals, with 150–200 beds or more, located in the larger provinces. Patients with complications are referred from primary and secondary care. More specialists are available in these hospitals and some have psychiatric staff.

Medical school hospitals also provide tertiary care. There are eight medical schools in seven universities in Thailand. One is under the control of the Ministry of Defence and one is run by a private organisation.

# Mental health services

Before 1964, all mental health activities were located in mental health or psychiatric hospitals. Psychiatrists and their colleagues acted as the sole providers of services. During the First to Third Five-Year National Health Plans (1962–76), mental health activities were extended to community health services.

Nowadays psychiatric care is provided in the government, private and non-governmental sectors. The public sector, mainly supported by the government budget, includes the Ministry of Public Health, the Ministry of Education, the Interior Ministry, the Ministry of Defence and the Office of the National Police. The Ministry of Public Health includes the Department of Mental Health, the Office of the Permanent Secretary and the Medical Department, which oversees many psychiatric units and psychiatrists.

All government hospitals face the problems of too many patients, lack of staff and under-financing. Most hospitals have additional income from fees and donations, but even so their total expenses are almost always higher than their total income.

At the moment there are about 400 psychiatrists working in Thailand. Most are public sector employees who also have a private practice outside their official hours. Not only is the number of psychiatrists insufficient but there is also a lack of other mental health personnel (Table 1), especially occupational therapists, of whom there are only 49 nationally (ratio 1:1 271 610). Moreover, the distribution is also skewed, with more than half the total number of psychiatrists working in Bangkok (Table 1) and most of the rest working in the other big cities.

Most specialised care is offered by the psychiatric hospitals. In 2001, there were nine of these, with a total capacity of 8893 beds (Boonyawongvirot, 2003). They provide in-patient services, out-patient clinics, emergency services, rehabilitation services, education and training, and mental health promotion and prevention services. There are also two mental health centres, which provide out-patient services and which emphasise mental health promotion and prevention. There are also two subspecialty psychiatric hospitals, the Forensic Psychiatric Hospital and the Institute of Mental Health for Children and Family.

## Problems of the mental healthcare system

The main problems to be found in the mental healthcare system in Thailand can be summarised as follows:

- The number of mental health workers is insufficient (Table 1).
- General physicians and general practitioners are not confident in the assessment and management of psychiatric patients. Some psychiatric disorders, especially depression, are under-diagnosed, whereas other diagnoses are made too often, such as anxiety disorders. Many patients receive anxiolytic or antidepressant medication in sub-therapeutic doses. (Patients with a psychosis are an exception, as most are directly referred to psychiatric hospital.)

**Table 1** Mental health personnel and proportion to the whole population, by region[1]

| Region | Psychiatrists | | Psychiatric nurses | | Psychologists | | Social workers | |
|---|---|---|---|---|---|---|---|---|
| | n | Ratio[2] | n | Ratio[2] | n | Ratio[2] | n | Ratio[2] |
| Bangkok | 218 | 1:26 267 | 173 | 1:33 099 | 42 | 1:136 338 | 117 | 1:48 942 |
| Central | 75 | 1:195 374 | 481 | 1:30 464 | 44 | 1:333 023 | 78 | 1:187 859 |
| North | 31 | 1:391 111 | 308 | 1:39 365 | 45 | 1:269 432 | 84 | 1:144 338 |
| North-East | 39 | 1:551 120 | 551 | 1:39 009 | 48 | 1:447 785 | 61 | 1:352 356 |
| South | 24 | 1:346 315 | 222 | 1:37 439 | 17 | 1:488 916 | 33 | 1:251 866 |
| Total | 387 | 1:161 005 | 1735 | 1:35 913 | 196 | 1:317 902 | 373 | 1:167 048 |

1. Data from the Department of Mental Health, Ministry of Public Health, 2003.
2. Ratio: ratio of staff to regional/national population.

- The primary and secondary care services have little opportunity to care for psychiatric patients during the continuation and maintenance phases of their illness because of limited supplies of medications. District hospitals usually have only haloperidol for schizophrenia and amitriptyline or imipramine for depression. Although the Ministry of Public Health added fluoxetine (generic) to the list of essential hospital drugs a few years ago, only the central hospital and a few general hospitals are able to supply this. Atypical antipsychotics have only just been supplied to psychiatric hospitals, university hospitals and some central hospitals, but they are not covered by health insurance unless the medical committee of the hospital decides, on a case-by-case basis, that they are necessary. The shortage of psychiatric drugs at local hospitals, the long distances that patients have to travel to get treatment, and the high cost of travel (because of increasing fuel prices) are also problems for continuation of treatment.
- Patients and their families have a poor understanding of psychiatric disorders. In the case of psychoses, most have some knowledge about the symptoms but tend to believe that they were caused by stress, worry or supernatural influences. This may result in patients discontinuing their treatment early.
- During the continuation and maintenance phases of treatment, even though some mental health teams in general hospitals can monitor symptoms, adjust the doses of drugs and provide psychosocial intervention, often the patients and their families still prefer to see a psychiatrist, and this overloads many psychiatrists in tertiary care.

## Role of carers

In January 1995, the PRELAPSE (Preventing Relapse in Schizophrenia) programme was introduced in Thailand. This was implemented in five psychiatric hospitals under the Department of Mental Health. Preliminary results showed that for patients with schizophrenia whose families joined this programme, the readmission rate decreased by 44% and the length of hospital stay decreased for 50% of patients (Udomratn, 1999). After evaluating these preliminary results, the Department transformed this programme into the 'Technology for Caring Relatives of Schizophrenic Patients' programme and some hospitals integrated it into their routine services. Many relatives who joined in the educational activities later agreed to meet regularly and formed clubs at various psychiatric hospitals throughout the country. These clubs went on to form the Association for the Mentally Ill (AMI), in 2003. The AMI now receives funding from the Thai Health Promotion Foundation, the Health Systems Research Institute of Thailand and other agencies. The AMI has contributed to many activities related to mental health promotion and prevention, and to increasing awareness of mental health problems in Thailand.

# Conclusions

Psychiatric services in Thailand, as in many low- and middle-income countries, still face shortages of mental health workers. Mental health problems are not well recognised by general practitioners. Patients' poor understanding of psychiatric disorders causes a delay in seeking help and frequently early discontinuation of drug treatment.

Many strategic plans have been initiated by the Thai Department of Mental Health, with the aim of increasing human resources and providing a better quality of care in both general and psychiatric hospitals. Destigmatisation campaigns have been run. We expect a brighter future for Thai psychiatric patients and their families within the next decade.

# References

Boonyawongvirot, P. (ed.) *(2003) Mental Health in Thailand, 2002–2003.* ETO Press.

Siriwanarangsan, P., Kongsuk, T., Arunpongpaisan, S., *et al* (2004) Prevalence of mental disorders in Thailand: a national survey, 2003. *Journal of Mental Health of Thailand,* **12,** 177–188.

Udomratn, P. (1999) The progress of the PRELAPSE program in Thailand. *Journal of the Psychiatric Association of Thailand,* **44,** 171–179.

Udomratn, P. (2006) Psychiatry in Thailand. In *Textbook of Psychiatry in Asia* (eds E. Chiu, H. Chiu, E. H. Kua, *et al*). Peking University Medical Press.

World Health Organization (2001) *Atlas: Country Profiles 2001.* Available at http://w3.whosea.org/LinkFiles/Health_and_Behaviour_tha.pdf. Last accessed 23 October 2006.

# Timor-Leste

Zoe Hawkins

The Democratic Republic of Timor-Leste (East Timor) occupies the eastern half of the island of Timor, which lies north-west of Australia and within the eastern Indonesia archipelago. The population is approximately one million, of whom 45% are below the age of 15. Average life expectancy is 59.5 years and 50% of the population live below the national poverty line of US$0.88 per day. The official languages are Tetun and Portuguese, with Indonesian also used. The majority of the population are Catholic but also hold traditional animist beliefs.

Timor-Leste, a Portuguese colony for over 400 years, was invaded by Indonesia in 1975 following Portugal's rapid decolonisation. During the following 24 years of occupation, anti-insurgent and terror campaigns were carried out by the Indonesian military, with mass internal displacements of people and war-induced famines. Following a majority vote for independence in a 1999 referendum, a violent backlash from pro-Indonesia groups caused further deaths and mass destruction of buildings and infrastructure. Intervention by Australian-led peacekeeping forces restored stability, and the territory was administered by a United Nations mission until full independence was gained in 2002.

## History of mental health services

During the years of Indonesian administration there were no mental health services in East Timor. In 1999, Psychosocial Recovery and Development in East Timor (PRADET) was founded by a partnership of mental health practitioners from Australia. Sixteen Timorese health workers underwent basic mental health training in Australia and returned to form the core staff of PRADET (Zwi & Silove, 2002). In addition to providing assessment, diagnosis and treatment for people with mental illness, the staff of PRADET trained district health nurses in their follow-up care.

In 2002, the government established the East Timor National Mental Health Project (ETNMHP) as its mental health service, with technical support and training provided by a team of Australian mental health workers. PRADET continued as a local non-governmental organisation (NGO) to complement government services by providing psychosocial support, counselling and community education. In 2008, the ETNMHP became the Department of Mental Health within the Ministry of Health.

## Psychiatric morbidity

An epidemiological study conducted in 2004 reported a point prevalence of psychosis (meeting DSM–IV criteria) of 1.35% and post-traumatic stress disorder of 1.47% (Silove *et al*, 2008). Since January 2008, the mental health service has seen a total of 3881 clients, of whom 1026 (26%) have had a primary diagnosis of epilepsy. There are no data on the prevalence of different mental disorders within the remaining case-load. However, mental health workers report that psychotic disorders form the majority of cases, followed by depressive disorder.

## Mental health policy and legislation

The government has a national mental health strategy (Ministry of Health Timor-Leste, 2005), which emphasises both a primary care approach to mental health services and partnerships with non-government service providers. There is currently no mental health legislation.

## Infrastructure

The 260-bed National Hospital (Hospital Nacional Guido Valadares) is located in Dili, the capital, and provides secondary and tertiary healthcare services. There are also five regional referral hospitals in the districts. The National Hospital acts as the national referral centre and is the principal clinical training centre for health personnel studying in Timor-Leste. At present there is no mental health bed allocation and no psychiatric hospital.

Each of the 13 districts in Timor-Leste has a district health office, where clinical services for the area are coordinated and supervised.

Sixty-five community health centres (CHCs) – approximately one per subdistrict – provide primary healthcare services, including out-patient clinics, simple laboratory testing, health promotion and preventive health services such as immunisations. Eight CHCs have in-patient facilities.

There are 193 health posts located across Timor-Leste, which are smaller health centres staffed by midwives and nurses. Basic drugs are available but there are no laboratory or in-patient services. In addition, a programme called Integrated Community Health Services (Servisu Integradu da Saúde Communitária, SISCa) provides monthly community-based health services within each village, including health promotion, and interventions in areas such as nutrition, maternal and child health, infectious disease prevention and environmental health.

# Mental health services

All basic health services, including mental health and medication, are provided free of charge to Timorese people. Two internationally recruited psychiatrists (from Cuba and Papua New Guinea) work in Timor-Leste. Both are based in Dili, although one makes brief visits to the districts. Essentially, there are 1.14 psychiatrists per 100 000 population in Dili, and 0 in the rest of the country.

Each district has an allocated mental health worker with basic training in mental health and a background in nursing or public health. In addition, 25% of CHCs have a general nurse who has also received basic training in mental health. These nurses form the primary service for people presenting with mental illness, with more difficult cases referred to the mental health worker for case management. Referrals for initial assessment can also be made directly to counsellors working in PRADET. District case-loads range between 100 and 200 clients, with referrals coming from the police, families, the church and village chiefs. There are no social workers or psychologists working in the government or NGO services.

## Pharmaceutical interventions

Psychotropic medication is ordered by the district health office from the central medical stores in Dili (Serviço Autónomo de Medicamentos e Equipamentos de Saúde, SAMES), based upon calculations of monthly use from each CHC. The medication is delivered by truck to each district every 3 months and distributed to CHCs. Clients or family members must then collect the prescription from the CHC themselves. Basic psychotherapeutic drugs are available and can be prescribed by the two psychiatrists, the district mental health workers and more senior general nurses.

# Health workforce training

## Pre-service training

The Ministry of Health, through the Institute of Health Sciences (Instituto de Ciências da Saúde, ICS), provides pre-service training to health workers in the country. This includes upgrading nurses and midwives to diploma 3 level, and providing courses in laboratory technology, pharmacy technology, anaesthetics nursing, eye-care nursing and radiography at diploma 1 level.

Currently, two out of every three doctors in the country (162 out of 243) are from Cuba. This is a result of a joint initiative between the governments of Cuba and Timor-Leste known as the Cuban Medical Brigade, which provides primary care physicians and other health staff from Cuba to fill vacant posts within Timor-Leste.

The Ministry of Health collaborates with the Cuban Medical Brigade and the National University of Timor-Lorosae (Universidade Nacional

Timor-Lorosae, UNTL) in providing pre-service courses in medicine (currently 150 students), nursing (50 students per year) and midwifery (50 students per year). Two private universities provide undergraduate training in public health.

In addition, through assistance from the Cuban government, a pre-service medical training programme for nearly 700 Timorese students is provided in Cuba. Psychiatry is taught in a 10-week block during the fifth year. A small number of Timorese students have donor-funded scholarships to attend medical schools in other countries.

## Postgraduate training

There is no formal postgraduate training of health personnel in Timor-Leste. However, there are more than 100 scholarship holders pursuing postgraduate training courses in Indonesia, Fiji, Malaysia and Papua New Guinea. There is currently one Timorese doctor completing postgraduate training in psychiatry in Papua New Guinea.

# Traditional healers and religious beliefs

There are strong animist beliefs in Timorese culture. People with mental illness (*bulak*) and their families may feel they are being punished by an ancestral spirit for causing offence, perhaps by walking across a sacred area or swimming in a sacred river. The spirit takes the form of a tree or stone in the village. People who suffer from epilepsy (*bibi maten*, literally 'dying goat') are sometimes thought to have an angry ancestor spirit within them. Traditional healers use herbal treatments, which may include berries from the 'spirit' tree. An animal might be sacrificed and its blood poured over the stone or tree. The healers use trances, smoke, chanting and beating the person with a mental illness to remove the angry spirit. These actions are used in parallel with Catholic practices, with the family praying for forgiveness at the graveyards of the ancestors, and attending church to pray for healing.

# The way ahead

Conflict, violence, large-scale human rights abuses and civil unrest are all elements of Timor-Leste's recent history, and have been shown to be associated with poor mental health (Mollica *et al*, 2005). In the context of this history, and as a young, low-income country, Timor-Leste is addressing significant challenges in the areas of infrastructure, human resources, financial constraints (short- and long-term prioritisation of resources) and poverty.

The mental health system can begin to address these challenges by improving access to mental healthcare, strengthening and expanding the mental health workforce, and prioritising long-term funding for mental health.

Mental health education and promotion activities must be maintained and further developed to reduce stigma and discrimination. The implementation of appropriate and comprehensive mental health legislation is necessary to protect the human rights and dignity of Timorese people with mental disorders.

# References

Ministry of Health Timor-Leste (2005) *National Mental Health Strategy for a Mentally Healthy Timor-Leste*. Ministry of Health, Democratic Republic of Timor-Leste.

Mollica, R. F., Cardozo, B., Osofsky, H., *et al* (2005) Mental health in complex emergencies. *Lancet*, **364**, 2058–2067.

Silove, D., Bateman, C. R., Brooks, R. T., *et al* (2008) Estimating clinically relevant mental disorders in a rural and an urban setting in postconflict Timor Leste. *Archives of General Psychiatry*, **65**, 1205–1212.

Zwi, A. & Silove, D. (2002) Hearing the voices: mental health services in East Timor. *Lancet*, **360**, s45–s46.

# Turkey

Bulent Coskun

The Republic of Turkey has a population of 67.4 million (year 2000) and covers 783 563 km²; administratively it is divided into 81 provinces. A few national statistics from 2000 are: infant death rate 41.9/1000; life expectancy at birth 68 years; unemployment rate 6.6%; gross national product (GNP) per capita US$2965; and adult literacy rate 87.32% (females 80.64%; males 93.86%) (State Statistics Institute, 2003).

Turkey is going through a period of continuous transition. Geographically, the country is a bridge between Asia and Europe (for this reason it has historically been a path for invasions and cultural exchanges) and therefore between the Western world and the Middle East. It is a secular republic but a large majority of the population is Islamic, and it is the only country with these features in NATO and Europe.

Even physically the land is in continuous transition – it is not stable and suffers great damage from earthquakes almost every four or five years, the largest in recent times being on 17 August 1999 in the Marmara region. The state of change is reflected in daily life as well. For example, the traditional, extended family structure is transforming into the more nuclear type. Some traditional national characteristics are being challenged. 'Turning the corner' has been the motto of many people, as the values and preferences of individuals, families and even institutions keep changing. The effects of the long-term high inflation rate, serious financial limitations and separatist activities (with armed conflict in the eastern part of the country) have all played a crucial role. Many people living in the villages have migrated to the peripheries of some of the larger cities or have left the country to work abroad, typically in Germany, France, The Netherlands or Belgium. The specific mental health problems of these migrants have been the subject of comparative studies (Gilleard, 1983; Van der Stuyft et al, 1993; Diefenbacher & Heim, 1994; Yazar & Littlewood, 2001).

Another characteristic feature of Turkey is the series of contrasts seen in almost all aspects of life, which inevitably is reflected in mental health issues, in terms of both psychosocial structure and psychiatric treatment.

None the less, there is stability in many respects, and this has an impact on psychosocial well-being. Solidarity often extends beyond family bonds, to members of the same village or even region. In almost every city there are areas where people from the same region of the country live together and offer each other social support.

Another important factor to be considered is the strong interpersonal links among the people. Traditionally people tend to talk about their difficulties and to share their feelings. Although sometimes such social support may be undermined by intrusive and prescriptive attitudes, it is still possible to say that solidarity among people in general helps them to adapt to and overcome difficulties. This was observed after the devastating earthquake in August 1999 in Marmara. While therapeutic help was made available, most of the inhabitants of the tent cities served as 'patient listeners' to each other all through the long, empty days after the earthquake (Aydin, 2001).

# Forty years of mental health policy development

The psychiatry practised in ancient Anatolia and even the relatively well developed psychiatric services during the period of the Ottoman empire are beyond the scope of this paper, which focuses on current psychiatry in Turkey. But to understand today and the vision for tomorrow, a brief overview of the recent development of mental health policy is necessary.

In the 1960s, improvements to the curative and rehabilitative services through their vertical organisation was the goal. Mental health dispensaries in Istanbul and Ankara served as extensions of the mental hospitals and so had only a limited remit regarding prevention and mental health promotion. At that time, a stand was taken against use of the Turkish equivalent of 'lunatic' and for its replacement by a term equivalent to 'mentally ill patient'. Efforts were made by the Ministry of Health to prepare a mental health policy, although only a few meeting notes remained when the next attempt at the same Ministry was made in the 1980s (Bayülkem, 1998).

At the time of the second attempt to draw up a policy on mental health, in the 1980s, I was in charge of the mental health department at the Ministry of Health. The goal then was the integration of mental health into primary healthcare (i.e. a horizontal approach) with promotion and prevention activities in addition to the improvement of curative services. For inter-sectoral and interdisciplinary coordination there were efforts to get the involvement of different ministries, universities and non-governmental organisations, with the support of the World Health Organization (WHO). Five regions were established, each with one of the country's five mental hospitals at the centre. Regulations were put in place regarding referral to those centres and the follow-up of patients after discharge. The role of provincial mental health divisions was detailed, with emphasis on local mental health coordination councils (Coskun, 1987, 1988). Although most of the plans were prepared in close collaboration with regional and local staff, their implementation was limited and not much could be achieved in terms of a permanent outcome.

Through the early 1990s, there were health reform studies at the Ministry, where mental health issues were discussed once more. Most important in that decade was the epidemiological study of mental health (Erol *et al*, 1998). After the Marmara earthquake in 1999, the need for an overall policy with local action plans was once more realised at ministry level. A more organised process has been planned, with the financial support of the World Bank; a permanent but flexible structure is now being worked on, with contributions from different sectors and disciplines (Ulug, 2003).

## Provision of psychiatric services

Most psychiatric services are provided by hospitals attached to the Ministry of Health. The private sector accounts for only 150 of the total of 6146 beds. At the five mental hospitals run by the Ministry of Health there are 5570 beds in total, while the two hospitals attached to the Ministry of Social Security have 426 beds (Ministry of Health, 2002). A considerable portion of these beds are still occupied by long-stay patients, which limits the number of beds available for other patients, many of whom are therefore repeatedly re-admitted shortly after being discharged too soon. The programme on referral procedure mentioned above, with special guidelines for patient follow-up at a local health centre after discharge, was planned to decrease the number of repeat admissions, but the new procedure has not been universally adopted.

The number of psychiatric beds in general hospitals is not detailed in the current statistics, but the number of psychiatrists working at general hospitals gives an idea of the scale of those institutions' provision of psychiatric services: of the 398 psychiatrists working at hospitals attached to the Ministry of Health, 238 work in general hospitals and 138 at the five specialist psychiatric hospitals. The tendency to set up psychiatry divisions at general hospitals has increased the provision of local help for people with psychiatric problems. Psychiatrists mainly work in large cities and in the western parts of the country. According to the figures of the Psychiatric Association of Turkey, 760 psychiatrists out of 1149 (i.e. around two-thirds) are located in Istanbul, Ankara and Izmir.

This uneven distribution also pertains to psychologists. Six psychology departments provide master and doctorate education. Legally (as set out in a statute dating from 1930) clinical psychologists must work under the supervision of psychiatrists. But especially in large cities there are many private clinics run by psychologists, a few of whom are without proper clinical psychology training. On the other hand, most clinical psychologists are well trained, but they need their legal status to be looked at urgently. Similar to psychiatrists, 149 of 266 psychologists working within the Ministry of Health are at general hospitals, compared with 34 working in specialist psychiatric hospitals.

There are few psychiatric social workers and psychiatric nurses; most of the latter work within higher nurse education. None the less, there are many highly experienced nurses working in psychiatric clinics, although they are not entitled to call themselves psychiatric nurses.

## Consumers of mental health services

An epidemiological study was carried out by the Ministry of Health on the mental health status of the Turkish population (Erol *et al*, 1998). Among the representative sample of 7479 people the prevalence of psychiatric disorders in the past 12 months according to ICD–10 criteria was 17.2%. The three most common psychiatric illnesses were pain disorder (8.4%), major depression (4%) and a specific phobia (2.7%). The professional first contacted for psychological problems was: a psychiatrist (39%), another specialist (e.g. an internist or neurologist) (33%), a general practitioner (21%) or a religious healer (3.6%). The three disorders with the highest rates for any contact were: panic disorder, obsessive–compulsive disorder and somatisation disorder.

The same report revealed that antidepressants were the most commonly used psychotropic medication. Five per cent of the general population interviewed were using psychotropic agents (antidepressants were used by 66% of these, sedatives by 23%, antipsychotics by 7% and anti-epileptics by 2%). Fifty-one per cent had received medication from 'other' specialists, 22% from psychiatrists, 18% from general practitioners and 5% from pharmacists, while 4% had taken them without making a professional consultation (Erol *et al*, 1998).

Other than the above-mentioned disorders, conversion disorder and dissociative disorders are commonly observed and draw scientific attention (Tutkun *et al*, 1998; Sar *et al*, 2000; Kuloglu *et al*, 2003).

There are some newly founded associations that focus on the rights and welfare of psychiatric patients and their relatives, most of which are currently led by professionals who wish to promote 'consumer-led' services (Ankara University Psychiatry Department, 2000). This support for patients' rights follows on from more general discussions of human and consumer rights in the country.

## Education and research

Mental health education and education in the behavioural sciences are overlapping areas in the formal training of different disciplines. At medical schools, in addition to behavioural sciences in the first year, theoretical and practical psychiatry is provided in later years, and there is a four-week practical course in the final year.

It is often argued that six years of medical training is not sufficient to equip the practitioner with the necessary knowledge and skills to handle psychiatric evaluation and care, so that in-service training is needed to provide better integrated care at primary healthcare level. Sometimes there are discussions regarding the motivation for those in-service training programmes – there is a view that some programmes are too closely associated with the pharmaceutical industry and attempt to encourage the use of medication by specialists other than psychiatrists and by local primary care practitioners.

Psychiatric training is provided at 36 university psychiatry departments and 12 training hospitals, most of which are attached to the Ministry of Health. Child and adolescent psychiatry has been a separate specialty since 1995.

An increasing number of multi-centre research projects are being carried out, some with international collaboration (Ustun & Sartorius, 1995). The psychiatry department at Hacettepe University is a collaborating centre of the WHO.

Some other topics for research include: the pathways to psychiatric care, the use and effectiveness of psychotropic drugs, the effects of disasters, consultation–liaison psychiatry, attitudes and behaviour towards people with a mental illness, and the epidemiology of some psychiatric disorders.

## Law and ethics

Ethical rules for psychiatric practice were established in June 2002 by the Psychiatric Association of Turkey; the rights and responsibilities of psychiatrists were underlined with reference to patients' rights, and recommendations were set out on ethical issues regarding research and publication procedures.

Some mental health issues are covered in articles of the Turkish constitution, such as the duty of the state to provide for the physical and mental health of individuals, and the rights to live freely and to develop physical and mental well-being; limitations to these rights can be defined only by law, and there is a prohibition against torture and the undermining of human dignity.

The civil law was renewed in January 2002. It now details the civil rights of citizens and the conditions for the limitations of those rights; it also covers the marriage and divorce of mentally ill people.

The criminal law stipulates special conditions for the treatment of mentally ill offenders.

Lack of an overall mental health law continues to be a concern for the mental health profession. The Psychiatric Association of Turkey has chosen to begin work on a draft law for the protection of the rights of psychiatric patients, rather than a 'mental health law'. In this draft there are items on principles relating to, for example, the rights of patients, including issues on privacy, consent to treatment and involuntary hospitalisation, as well as the roles of psychiatrists and judges. Currently the congruency of this draft and implementations of the new civil law are being studied. The next step will be to send the revised draft to the Ministry of Justice for amendment, before it is submitted to parliament.

# Conclusions

In Turkey at present, the main concerns for psychiatry are:
- the development of a mental health policy
- improved education and training in psychiatry
- better psychiatric care
- increasing the amount of collaborative research
- work against stigmatisation
- collaboration with the consumers of mental health services and their relatives
- the integration of a mental health component into primary healthcare and general healthcare
- mental health promotion and illness prevention.

The rapid changes in socio-economic conditions, the effects of the media, the unstable socio-political situation, the high percentage of young people in the population, unemployment and people not being able to get higher education are other, more general areas of concern.

The national decision makers do not seem to be aware of the effects of psychosocial realities beyond referring to these issues in their public speeches. Mental health specialists should spare more time and energy to collaborate with decision makers at local and national level, bearing in mind that the improvement of mental health and psychosocial well-being is far beyond the capacity of (mental) health specialists to deal with by themselves.

# References

Ankara University Psychiatry Department (2000) *Associations and Foundations Acting on Mental Health Issues in Turkey* [in Turkish], pp. 3–48. Ankara: 36th National Psychiatry Congress Press.

Aydin, M. (2001) *Relationship Between Perception of Trauma and Attribution of Meaning and the Development of PTSD among Individuals Who Experienced the Marmara Earthquake* [in Turkish], pp. 81–84. Dissertation thesis, Kocaeli University.

Bayülkem, F. (1998) *Historical Development of Neurology, Neurosurgery and Psychiatry in Turkey* [in Turkish], pp. 155–165. Istanbul: Arbas.

Coskun, B. (1987) Resources, difficulties and solutions regarding mental health services in Turkey [in Turkish]. *Toplum ve Hekim*, **44**, 11–15.

Coskun, B. (1988) Activities of the Department of Mental Health [in Turkish]. *Mental Health Bulletin*, **1**, 7.

Diefenbacher, A. & Heim, G. (1994) Somatic symptoms in Turkish and German depressed patients. *Psychosomatic Medicine*, **56**, 551–556.

Erol, N., Kilic, C., Ulusoy, M., *et al* (1998) *Report on the Mental Health Profile of Turkey* [in Turkish], pp. 95–100. Ankara: Eksen Tanitim.

Gilleard, E. (1983) A cross-cultural investigation of Foulds' hierarchy model of psychiatric illness. *British Journal of Psychiatry*, **142**, 518–523.

Kuloglu, M., Atmaca, M., Tezcan, E., *et al* (2003) Sociodemographic and clinical characteristics of patients with conversion disorder in eastern Turkey. *Social Psychiatry and Psychiatric Epidemiology*, **38**, 88–93.

Ministry of Health (2002) *Statistics of the General Directorate of Curative Services*. Available on CD-ROM. Istanbul: Ministry of Health.

Sar, V., Tutkun, H., Alyanak, B., *et al* (2000) Frequency of dissociative disorders among psychiatric outpatients in Turkey. *Comprehensive Psychiatry*, **41**, 216–222.

State Statistics Institute (2003) *Turkey with Statistics 2002*, pp. 1–4. Ankara: State Statistics Institute Press.

Tutkun, H., Sar, V., Yargic, L. I., *et al* (1998) Frequency of dissociative disorders among psychiatric inpatients in a Turkish university clinic. *American Journal of Psychiatry*, **155**, 800–805.

Ulug, B. (2003) National Mental Health Policy Conference convened in Ankara [in Turkish]. *Bulletin of the Psychiatric Association of Turkey*, **3**, 6.

Ustun, B. & Sartorius, N. (1995) Background and rationale of the WHO collaborative study on 'Psychological Problems in General Health Care'. In *Mental Illness in General Health Care: An International Study* (eds T. B. Ustun & N. Sartorius), pp. 1–18. New York: Wiley.

Van der Stuyft, P., Woodward, M., Armstrong, J., *et al* (1993) Uptake of preventive health care among Mediterranean migrants in Belgium. *Journal of Epidemiology and Community Health*, **47**, 10–13.

Yazar, J. & Littlewood, R. (2001) Against over-interpretation: the understanding of pain amongst Turkish and Kurdish speakers in London. *International Journal of Social Psychiatry*, **47**, 20–33.

# United Arab Emirates

Valsamma Eapen and Omer El-Rufaie

This paper will focus on the current state of mental health services in the United Arab Emirates (UAE) and reflect on the various public health, socio-economic and psychosocial factors that have a major impact on the mental health needs of the population. It is to be borne in mind that the services described in this paper are in a state of rapid change, as the country is witnessing one of the fastest rates of development in the world.

## Society and culture

Situated in the Arabian Gulf, the UAE has an approximate area of 84000 km2 and a population of 4.1 million (UAE Census, 2005). Males constitute 67.6% of the population and females 32.4%; 20% are under the age of 15 years and only 1.8% are aged over 60 years (UAE Census, 2005). The literacy rate is 75.6% for men and 80.7% for women. Only 21.9% of the residents of the country are Emiratis (UAE citizens), while the remainder comprise expatriates from nearly 120 countries who have come to work in this oil-rich country. The largest ethnic group among the resident population is Asian, with the majority from the Indian subcontinent. The official language is Arabic and the official religion is Islam.

The UAE federation, formed in 1972, consists of seven emirates (Abu Dhabi, Dubai, Sharjah, Ajman, Um Al Qaiwan, Fujairah and Ras Al Khaima). The UAE is a high-income country, itself rich in oil reserves and also lying in a strategic location along the transit route of the world's crude oil. The proportion of gross domestic product (GDP) spent on health is 3.5%. Life expectancy at birth is 71.3 years for males and 75.1 years for females (World Health Organization, 2004).

### Sociocultural and traditional influences

In the UAE, tradition and religion are paramount. Mental health, reflected in good behaviour and conduct, is expected, as outlined by the Muslim religion. This also leads to the notion that supernatural forces can cause mental health problems. Consequently, self-blame and guilt resulting from the belief that mental health symptoms are a punishment for sins are not uncommon among people with mental disorders.

The usual first stop on the help-seeking route for mental illness is the traditional healer. In a study of the help-seeking preference for mental health problems in children, Eapen & Ghubash (2004) found that only 37% preferred to consult a mental health specialist. Alternative remedies are also much sought after, including Ayurvedic, homeopathic and herbal medicines.

The effects on mental health of social change associated with the rapid pace of development and Western influences have been the subject of several studies (e.g. Ghubash *et al*, 1994). While education, employment and social opportunities have started to improve perceptions of and attitudes to mental illness, the stigma associated with mental disorder is still a major factor that prevents individuals from seeking appropriate treatment.

# Mental health policy and legislation

Since the formation of the country 36 years ago, significant progress has been made in the area of health, with most infectious diseases being eradicated. Vaccines as well as state-of-the-art treatments are available for most diseases. However, mental health is lagging behind in terms of policies, facilities and staff.

As yet there is no mental health policy at national level, although efforts have been initiated. A newly commissioned national committee is expected to develop proposals for a national mental health programme. A previous committee, established in 1991, made proposals for the universal provision of mental health and substance misuse services through primary healthcare, but this has not been satisfactorily implemented.

Federal Law 28, enacted in 1981, contains sections on the definition of 'mental disorders', 'next of kin' and 'specialist'. There is also a section on the role of authorities and police in relation to psychosis and the detention of involuntary patients. The question of criminal responsibility is addressed by Sharia Islamic law and the courts rely on psychiatric reports for addressing the issue of insanity. Attempted suicide is a crime and homicide may result in the death penalty.

# Mental health services

The psychiatric services, like physical health services, are primarily delivered through a public health system administered by the Ministry of Health. The recent formation of separate health authorities and the introduction of health insurance cover for all employees as stipulated by the government are rapidly changing this scenario, particularly in the emirate of Abu Dhabi and to some extent in Dubai. As a result, both private sector establishments and private–public partnerships are coming into existence. For example, in the emirate of Abu Dhabi, partnerships exist between the Health Authority of Abu Dhabi and leading international healthcare providers such as the Johns Hopkins International, the Cleveland Clinic, the Medical University of Vienna and Bumrungrad International Limited. The government of Dubai, in collaboration with Harvard Medical International, is developing the Dubai Healthcare City as the world's first 'healthcare free zone'; this is a self-regulated environment providing a platform for regional and international medical institutions to set up their own facilities in Dubai.

Psychiatric services are delivered primarily through out-patient clinics in general hospitals and polyclinics, as psychotropic medication requires prescription by a specialist. Primary care facilities play a limited role, while community psychiatric services are nonexistent. In-patient facilities are available in the emirates of Abu Dhabi (Abu Dhabi Psychiatric Hospital, with 163 beds, and Al Ain Hospital, with 30 beds), Dubai (Al Amal Hospital, with 80 beds at present and a plan for considerable expansion; as well as a small unit at Rashid Hospital) and Ras Al Khaima (which has a hospital with 10 beds). Individuals needing in-patient treatment in other emirates are referred to one of the nearest general hospitals with psychiatric staff (e.g. Sharjah). The purpose-built Abu Dhabi Psychiatric Hospital also has a dedicated unit for child psychiatry, a day care facility, a secure forensic psychiatry facility (30 beds) and a unit for addiction disorders. Police and prison services are integral to the substance misuse programmes, although treatment is offered on a voluntary basis for those who comply with the regulations of the treatment unit.

The delivery of psychiatric services through primary care is best developed in the city of Al Ain, which hosts the only academic psychiatry department in the country. This initiative was launched in 1991, and is accompanied by ongoing efforts to train primary care physicians and carry out psychiatric research (El-Rufaie & Absood, 1993). A similar initiative was started in 1995 for mental health problems in children at the primary care level through the school health services. This was followed by the launch of a school mental health screening programme (Eapen, 1999).

# Psychiatric training

The Academic Department of Psychiatry at the Faculty of Medicine and Health Sciences, UAE University, was started in 1990 with the primary mission to contribute to the undergraduate educational programme in psychiatry and behavioural sciences, which is oriented to the needs of the UAE community. The psychiatry clerkship is an 8-week programme, and every effort is made to meet the highest international standards of quality in training, to enable its graduates to compete for advanced training at top centres around the world.

The graduate training programme currently offered is a structured multi-centre 4-year residency programme. The clinical training is complemented by an academic component organised by the university department, Al Ain, and the residents take the Arab Board Examination in Psychiatry.

## Psychiatric subspecialties and allied professions

The Academic Department of Psychiatry in Al Ain was instrumental in establishing child psychiatry services in the Al Ain Medical District. The Department is solely responsible for providing these services, which include out-patient, in-patient and consultation–liaison services at the two teaching hospitals in Al Ain, and receives referrals from other emirates. In the absence of the subspecialty for intellectual disability, provision of services in the area of developmental psychiatry is also undertaken. At the community level, the Department has pioneered the introduction of a comprehensive school mental health screening programme initially in Al Ain, and then at national level, utilising the structure and resources of the school health services.

## Main areas of research

The Academic Department of Psychiatry in Al Ain is the centre for psychiatric research. The main areas of activity are:
- epidemiological studies (e.g. Abou-Saleh *et al*, 2001; Eapen *et al*, 2003)
- diagnosis and classification of disorders (e.g. Hamdi *et al*, 1997)
- translation, development and validation of psychiatric instruments (e.g. Daradkeh *et al*, 2005)
- personality and psychosocial aspects of physical illness (e.g. Eapen *et al*, 2006)
- transcultural psychiatry (e.g. Salem, 2006)
- biological and genetic research (e.g. Bayoumi *et al*, 2006)
- mental health and special populations (e.g. Swadi & Eapen, 2000).

## Workforce issues and resources

In general, psychiatric services are limited, with an estimated 1.4 psychiatric beds per 10 000 population. The services are considerably understaffed when compared with other high-income countries, with only 2 psychiatrists, 1 psychologist, 1.2 social workers and 11 psychiatric nurses per 100 000 population. Proficiency in Arabic is considered desirable, which poses a considerable challenge to recruitment.

## Outlook

Since the formation of UAE as a federation of seven emirates 36 years ago, the country has made phenomenal progress in all areas, including health, but mental health has not received the attention it deserves. In this regard, development of a national mental health policy and a comprehensive review and implementation of legislation should take priority.

Programmes are needed for special populations, such as children and the elderly. Currently, psychiatric services are primarily hospital based, but there should be a broader vision in service delivery, with initiation of community outreach services, strengthening of clinical services, and integration of mental health with primary care services. The staff shortage is significant and urgent attention should be given to improving training opportunities. Significant research data exist regarding the nature and occurrence of mental disorder, as well as on some of the culture-specific risk factors and unique clinical presentations. These data could form the basis for the planning and development of a comprehensive mental health service in the country.

# References

Abou-Saleh, M., Ghubash, R. & Daradkeh, T. (2001) Al Ain Community Psychiatric Survey. I. Prevalence and socio-demographic correlates. *Social Psychiatry and Psychiatric Epidemiology*, **36**, 20–28.

Bayoumi, R., Eapen, V., Al-Yahyaee, S., *et al* (2006) The genetics of primary nocturnal enuresis: a UAE study. *Journal of Psychosomatic Research*, **61**, 321–326.

Daradkeh, T. K., Eapen, V. & Ghubash, R. (2005) Mental morbidity in primary care in Al Ain (UAE): application of the Arabic translation of the PRIMEMD (PHQ) Version. *German Journal of Psychiatry*, **8**, 32–35.

Eapen, V. (1999) School mental health screening: a model for developing countries. *Journal of Tropical Paediatrics*, **45**, 192–193.

Eapen, V. & Ghubash, R. (2004) Mental health problems in children and help seeking patterns in the UAE. *Psychological Reports*, **94**, 663–667.

Eapen, V., Jakka, M. E. & Abou-Saleh, M. T. (2003) Children with psychiatric disorders: the Al Ain Community Psychiatric Survey. *Canadian Journal of Psychiatry*, **48**, 402–407.

Eapen, V., Mabrouk, A., Sabri, S., *et al* (2006) A controlled study of psychosocial factors in young people with diabetes in the United Arab Emirates. *Annals of the New York Academy of Sciences*, **1084**, 325–329.

El-Rufaie, O. E. F. & Absood, G. H. (1993) Minor psychiatric morbidity in primary health care: prevalence, nature and severity. *International Journal of Social Psychiatry*, **39**, 159–166.

Ghubash, R., Hamdi, E. & Bebbington, P. (1994) The Dubai Community Psychiatric Survey: acculturation and the prevalence of psychiatric disorder. *Psychological Medicine*, **24**, 121–131.

Hamdi, E., Yousreya, A. & Abou-Saleh, M. T. (1997) Problems in validating endogenous depression in the Arab culture by contemporary diagnostic criteria. *Journal of Affective Disorders*, **44**, 131–143.

Salem, M. O. (2006) Religion, spirituality and psychiatry. *Royal College of Psychiatrists SIG Newsletter*, **21**, 1–15.

Swadi, H. & Eapen, V. (2000) A controlled study of psychiatric morbidity among developmentally disabled children in the United Arab Emirates. *Journal of Tropical Pediatrics*, **46**, 278–281.

*UAE Census* (2005) See http://www.zu.ac.ae/library/html/UAEinfo/UAEstats.htm.

World Health Organization (2004) *Country profile UAE*. In Mental Health Atlas. WHO.

# Yemen

## Maan A. Bari Qasem Saleh and Ahmed Mohamed Makki

The Republic of Yemen, on the south-western coast of the Arabian Peninsula, was formed in 1990 when North and South Yemen united. Yemen covers 527 970 km². The capital is Sana'a. The country is divided into 20 governorates and one municipality. It has an elected president, an elected House of Representatives, and an appointed Shura Council. The president is head of state, and the prime minister is head of government. Suffrage is universal for people aged 18 and older. The population of Yemen according to the 2004 census is about 20 million, but recent years have seen the arrival of many refugees.

Mental health in Yemen has been fortunate to receive government support, albeit modest, and benefits from human resource development projects. These projects have enabled Yemeni students to study psychiatry, psychology, psychiatric nursing and social work abroad. Mental health in Yemen has developed within a context of social development against wars, internal struggles, poverty, high rates of reproduction and illiteracy. Mental health disorders are closely connected to myth, superstition, witchcraft and jinns. There continues to be stigma associated with mental health and, by extension, with psychology and psychiatry.

## Human resources

A survey conducted by the Yemeni Mental Health Association (YMHA) in 2006 gave a figure of 3580 professionals with at least a BA in psychology. These include 139 people working in higher academic institutions. There are 198 psychiatric nurses and 45 psychiatrists and neurologists, giving one psychiatrist or neurologist per 500 000 population. There are only three child psychiatrists in the country and they work between hospitals and universities.

## Educational and training institutions

Two types of institution provide education and training. First, within the undergraduate programme, four departments of psychiatry, housed in university faculties of medicine, serve the national educational and accreditation professional development needs. The training programme in general medicine lasts 6 years. Medical students spend one semester in psychiatry and two in the behavioural sciences or medical psychology. Activities in psychiatry departments are limited to teaching, lecturing and examination, and do not include research or service activities to the community. Reasons for this include scarce resources and consequent limitations and loss of motivation, social stigma associated with mental health issues, newness of the discipline, and a critical shortage of experienced specialists.

Second, since 2003 the Yemeni Council for Medical Specialisation under the Ministry of Health has run local academic qualification programmes in psychiatry and clinical psychology. The qualification for this specialisation is dependent on the Arab Board System (a 4-year course). Unfortunately, there is little interest in psychiatry and to date there have been only three graduates of the diploma programme.

In 2003, a national academic qualification programme was established that provides 1 year of post-baccalaureate training in clinical psychology. By 2007, 30 individuals from the Sana'a and Aden governorates had graduated.

# Mental health services

## Psychiatric hospitals

There are only four psychiatric hospitals treating mental illness in Yemen; the one in Aden, built in 1966, is the oldest on the Arabian peninsula. The total number of beds in the country is nearly 850 (YMHA, 2006) and these are available in only four governorates. These hospitals are for adults and have no special sections for children. Patients who have a mental illness wander the streets of cities and towns. Others, in their thousands, are detained in family homes in oppressive conditions, which is especially difficult for women, for whom the oppression is twofold.

## Psychiatric clinics in general hospitals

In response to the World Health Organization's direction concerning the provision of mental health services in governorate hospitals, a number of mental health out-patient clinics have been developed at public hospitals, to which psychiatrists are appointed. However, these services are not provided by all public hospitals, and are subject to suspension or termination due to staff shortages and budget constraints.

## Psychiatric clinics in prisons

Patients who are mentally ill and who have a criminal record can be detained in correctional facilities. The second National Conference for Mental Health held in Sana'a in 2004, organised with the International Committee of the Red Cross, recommended that patients with a mental illness be separated from prisoners and placed in mental health hospitals.

## Private nursing homes

There are estimated to be only five private nursing clinics, in four governorates, with a capacity of approximately 100 beds (YMHA, 2006). Some have no beds and function as out-patient clinics.

## Private clinics

There are about 45 private mental health clinics in Yemen run by psychiatrists (YMHA, 2006). Psychologists work in some of these clinics, supervised by psychiatrists. Drugs and electroconvulsive therapy (ECT) are typical treatments in these settings. Some work within a collective therapeutic team model. There are no designated clinics for children.

## Patient management and treatment

Successfully treating mental illness often involves using drugs prescribed by psychiatrists and, in rural areas, by psychologists. Although effective, medication is of limited use, as drugs are unaffordable for most. The use of ECT remains widespread. Few evidence-based treatment programmes are considered appropriate for this culture. There are individual settings where institutional or individual initiatives have led to the establishment of models that demonstrate the potential and effectiveness of mental health services in the Yemeni context.

## Psychiatric hospital data in Yemen

Statistical data obtained from Yemeni psychiatric hospitals gave a patient population of 29 519 (YMHA, 2006). Paranoia with schizophrenia was the most common diagnosis, followed by emotional disturbances (depression and anxiety), while epilepsy, still classed as a mental illness, was in third place.

## Epidemiology of suicide

Suicide is a problem of great sensitivity, and much stigma and shame are connected to the act. According to available official data, suicides in Yemen totalled 243 in 2006 (YMHA, 2006), with the use of a firearm being the most common means.

# National Mental Health Programme

The National Mental Health Programme was established in the late 1980s with help from the World Health Organization and the Ministries of Health from North and South Yemeni governments of the time. The project concentrated on treatment in mental hospitals and care of patients with a mental illness by qualified psychiatrists. The National Mental Health Programme responded to recommendations put forward by the first National Workshop on Mental Health in Yemen, in October 2002, organised with the International Committee of the Red Cross. The Mental Health Programme was established by ministerial resolution and administered within the primary care division of the Ministry of Health.

The Programme is still being developed and requires support in both human and material resources as well as the development of a database of resources, statistics and epidemiological information.

## Non-governmental organisations

In Yemen, non-governmental organisations (NGOs) focusing on mental health have increased in quantity and quality since the Associations Law of 2001 permitted the formation of professional organisations. By 2006, there were seven associations in the country, with a membership of 1280 (Saleh, 2008).

The Yemeni Psychiatric and Neurological Association (YPNA) was established in 1989, while the YMHA was established in 1998. In general, most associations are new and struggling but continue to advocate for and provide services. These associations play influential roles in campaigning against physical, mental and sexual violence towards women and children. They organise celebrations for International Mental Health Day, conferences, workshops, seminars, publishing endeavours, radio and television programmes, and contributions to journals and magazines in mental health. Finally, they advocate for the establishment of a formal code of ethics and a Mental Health Act, often at great personal and emotional expense, which is rarely acknowledged.

## Publications

There are two bi-annual journals published by the Yemen Psychological Association (YPA) (20 volumes), another by the Doctor and Clinical Psychologists' Association (DCPA) (3 volumes) and two newsletters published periodically by both the YMHA (30 volumes) and the Aden Central Psychiatric Hospital (10 volumes) (YMHA, 2006). The main obstacles are a lack of financial resources and technical facilities for printing and dissemination.

## Research

Research in mental health is not well developed, because of a lack of capacity and the absence of research institutions. Graduate (PhD and

MA) students and teaching faculty conduct most mental health research in universities. The YPA and the YMHA take an active role in launching research initiatives and community surveys related to a variety of mental health issues, including violence against women and children, qat addiction, female genital mutilation and suicide. A lack of sustainable funding remains the biggest obstacle to research.

# Mental health and leadership

In November 1989, the President of the YPNA, Dr A. Khleadi, also became President of the Arab Psychiatric Association. In 1997 and in 2001, two professors from the Department of Behavioural Sciences, Faculty of Medicine Aden University, became vice presidents of the World Federation of Mental Health for the Middle East Region (Dr Hassen Khan and Dr Maan Saleh). In 2002, Dr Ahmed Makki became a member of the Shura Consultative Council and reporter for its Health Committee. In 2003, Dr Dugysh, from the Aden governorate, became the first neuropsychiatrist to be elected as a Yemeni member of parliament.

# Future challenges and goals

Until Yemen develops its own research base, addressing the population's mental health needs will require creativity and commitment. Developing short- and long-term programmes requires adapting research knowledge and both regional and international experiences appropriately to the Yemeni landscape while accelerating Yemeni progress in the field.

Goals for the future include:

- fostering qualitative and quantitative improvements in graduate and postgraduate higher education and training in mental health (doing so will enable Yemen to train specialists with culturally appropriate skills who can respond to the needs of society)
- offering annual scholarships abroad, for at least 5 years, across the different fields of mental health, with sensitivity to issues of gender
- broadening the faculty role so that university professors can engage in research while being supported by a clear administrative and legislative mandate
- increasing the number of educational campaigns to reduce the stigma of mental illness
- mandating a political and national strategy for mental health that includes the participation of the Ministry of Health, Yemeni universities (faculties of medicine) and related mental health NGOs
- improving and developing services in all the governorates
- getting the Ministry of Health, specialised associations, and concerned scientific departments of Yemeni universities to prepare laws to protect those who are mentally ill and to promote and develop the field as a priority

- strengthening communications with regional and international institutions with respect to mental health and its financing
- joining efforts to establish an accurate database that is methodical and up to date, and that uses contemporary techniques in data collection and manipulation.

# Sources

Ministry of Planning (2000) *Human Resource Development Report.* Ministry of Planning.

Ministry of Planning (2004) *Annual Statistics Book.* Ministry of Planning.

Ministry of Health (2007) *Report on The National Program of Mental Health: The Present Situation of Mental Health (unpublished).* Ministry of Health.

Saleh, M. A. (2008) Experience of Mental Health Association in Yemen. *Journal of Social Science, Aden University,* 22, 55–62.

YMHA (Yemeni Mental Health Association) (2006) [Survey] *Al-Seha-Al-Aqilia,* No. 29–30.

# Australasia

# Australia

Alan Rosen

Australia, a vast continent of 7 700 000 km² (including the island state of Tasmania), is roughly the size of Western Europe or mainland USA, but with a population of only 20.2 million (2004 estimate), mainly concentrated in coastal areas.

Australia's official language is English and its largest religion is Christianity (76.4%). Of the current population 92% are Caucasian, 7% Asian and 1% 'other' in origin, including 350 000 who claim Aboriginal descent. Australia's population growth once relied largely on migration from Britain, and to a lesser extent Ireland, but after the Second World War it was broadened by refu-gees and others from many other parts of Europe. Since the 1970s there has been more substantial migration from Asia. While refugees continue to be taken in and supported, Australia takes a tough stance on unauthorised arrivals, including prolonged detention, which is beginning to be softened due to growing public concern.

The Commonwealth (national) government is responsible for general policy directions in health, disability, education, employment and so on. The state governments retain responsibility for organising all their own health services and facilities, including mental health services. Consequently, such provision is diverse. Further, Australia has developed a substantial private medical sector, now funded nationally by taxpayers through the Health Insurance Commission, as well as via private health insurance schemes.

## Epidemiology

A national cross-sectional community survey of mental health and well-being (Andrews *et al*, 1999; Jablensky *et al*, 1999) was conducted via lay surveyors from the Australian Bureau of Statistics. It revealed that 17.7% of adult Australians met criteria for the common anxiety, affective and/or substance use disorders. More than 20% were likely to have a diagnosable and treatable mental disorder when psychotic, cognitive and personality disorders were included. Only 38% of individuals with a mental disorder (more women than men) sought professional help, which is concerning, and in most cases this was from a general practitioner rather than from a specialist mental health professional. Half as many Australians have a long-term mental disorder as have a long-term physical disorder, with physical disability being more common in the elderly and mental disability being more prevalent in young adults.

Psychotic disorder was found to be associated with a higher prevalence of severe physical illnesses and a much lower access to appropriate medical and surgical interventions (Lawrence *et al*, 2001).

The funding for a new national community survey, which may well have a longitudinal component, was announced by the federal government in July 2005.

## Policy developments and shift in service provision

A National Mental Health Policy was first endorsed by all Australian health ministers and published in 1992. It has been elaborated upon in two further National Mental Plans. These will be the subject of a forthcoming paper in International Psychiatry. Together they have sought to promote mental health, increase the quality and responsiveness of services, and to forge a consistent approach to mental health service system reform among Australian states and territories. They also represent a shift over more than a decade to community reprovision from former reliance on psychiatric hospitals. This has occurred with a slight growth in the number of acute beds, mainly in general hospitals, and a 63% decrease in long-stay hospital beds, and partial compensation in the growth of supervised community residential placements, crisis and assertive community treatment teams.

## Mental health legislation

Although each state and territory has its own Mental Health Act, a template model Mental Health Act upholding the rights and responsibilities of people with mental illness was developed centrally in the early 1990s (as part of the First National Mental Health Strategy). A Rights Analysis Instrument was subsequently developed by the Federal Attorney-General's Department, which is now used to calibrate all state and territory mental health legislation with the United Nations Principles for the Protection of Persons with Mental Illness and the Improvement of Mental Health Care (United Nations, 1991; Whiteford & Buckingham, 2005).

## Workforce and training

Australian public mental health services are largely staffed by interdisciplinary teams of at least five fully professional disciplines: psychiatry; psychiatric nursing; psychology (particularly clinical psychology); occupational therapy; and social work. Variably, depending on location, teams may also include rehabilitation or vocational counsellors or instructors, and indigenous and transcultural mental health workers. Increasingly, paid consumer and carer advocates, consultants or teams are being employed in such services. Case management is generally shared between nursing and allied health professions, as Australian standards and guidelines do not support the development of a generic case manager role, either by merging professions or on a non-professional basis (Rosen *et al*, 1995; Gianfrancesco *et al*, 1996; Rosen & Teesson, 2001; National Mental Health Strategy, 2003; Rosen, 2005).

Following a medical course of 4 years (graduate) to 5 or 6 years (undergraduate) and 2–3 years of rotating hospital resident posts, trainee psychiatrists undergo a 5-year (or more) training period that combines apprenticeship and coursework. This now includes advanced training in a subspecialty over the last 2 years, which may be child and adolescent psychiatry, adult psychiatry, aged-care psychiatry, consultation–liaison psychiatry, psychotherapy and so on, and which results in the trainee becoming a Fellow of the Royal Australian and New Zealand College of Psychiatrists (RANZCP – on which see Boyce & Crossland in this issue).

Nurses are trained on university general nursing courses for 3 years and then may attain postgraduate certificates while working in their chosen specialty (e.g. mental health nursing).

Allied professionals usually have a bachelor degree in their chosen profession, often taking 4 years, but they are being increasingly encouraged to proceed to masters or doctorate level, particularly in psychology.

There are over 2000 psychiatrists; although only around 20% were in public practice (Henderson, 2000), this proportion is growing (it grew by 37% over the decade to 2002) and the number of psychiatrists in private practice has been shrinking by 2–3% per year since 1997 (Whiteford & Buckingham, 2005). Boyce & Crossland in this issue indicate that 40% of Australian psychiatrists now work in the public sector and 60% in the private sector. The apparent difference is explained by the probable increasing proportion of Australian psychiatrists now doing a combination of public and private practice. The RANZCP Workforce Study 2005 revealed that 23% of Australian psychiatrists work solely in public practice, 41% solely in private practice and 36% in both. Comparison with an earlier survey (Australian Medical Workforce Advisory Committee, 1999) indicates a slow decrease in the number of psychiatrists working predominantly in private practice and a slow increase in the numbers of psychiatrists working predominantly in public practice.

There were an average of 87.5/100000 full-time equivalent professional staff employed in specialist mental health services by 2001–02, including 9.7/100000 medical, 57.1/100000 nursing and 20.7/100000 allied health workers (Department of Health and Ageing, 2004). The clinical staffing levels in public mental health services (Department of Health and Ageing, 2004) totalled nearly 18 000 by 2002, having grown by 25% since 1992–93, and consisted of 62% nursing, 22% allied health, 10% medical professionals and 6% others. There is currently a shortage in psychiatry of registrars and nurses, as in other Australian health specialties.

## Resourcing

In 1999 more than 20% of the health burden in Australia was attributable to mental disorders, yet only 5% of the national health budget was spent on mental health (Andrews *et al*, 1999). This proportion of expenditure grew only marginally, to 6.5%, in 2001–02 as derived from World Health Reports (Rosen *et al*, 2004). Total expenditure on mental health services in 2001–02 was A\$3.09 billion, of which 58.2% was spent by the states on the public mental health system, 37.1% was spent by the commonwealth government mainly on pharmaceutical subsidies, general practitioner and private psychiatrist rebates, and 4.7% by private health funds, mainly for private hospital services (Department of Health and Family Services, 2004).

## Research

Particular, sometimes outstanding contributions have been and are being made by Australians to psychiatric research in many areas, as listed by Henderson (2000): the phenomenology and treatment of both the depress¬ive and the anxiety disorders; abnormal illness behaviour and somatisation disorder; illness prevention and health promotion; the epidemiology of mental disorders and the social environment; the epidemiology of mental disorders in late life; the neurobiology of schizophrenia; early intervention in the psychoses; mental health service system research; the mental health of indigenous peoples; alcohol and drug misuse; post-traumatic stress disorder; and psychiatry and ethics. To these I would add research in: mental health literacy, stigma and mental health first aid; telepsychiatry and related strategies for rural/ remote areas; classification, phenomenology and treatment of depression; consultation–liaison psychiatry; the psychological health of asylum seekers in detention, of refugees and of traumatised populations; medico-legal provision; psychosocial (including family) interventions; crisis and assertive community case management and residential alternatives to in-patient care; interdisciplinary roles, teams and leadership; outcome measurement; and consumer and carer participation in services.

## Conferences and forums

Each mental health professional grouping runs its own annual congress or conference, and there are many national and international special interest meetings.

There is a strong independent movement, the Mental Health Services Conference of Australia and New Zealand (www.themhs.org) (Andrews,

2005), which is co-owned by all mental health professions, managers and consumer/carer networks, which promotes joint conferences, binational debates and forums, and mental health service achievement awards for local integrated services, early intervention, comorbidities, rural and remote services, indigenous and transcultural mental health services, consumer and carer service initiatives, mass media representations of mental illness and services (print and electronic). The MHS conference begins with separate indigenous, consumer, carer leadership and provider training forums, with all these constituencies coming together for the last 3 days.

## Conclusion

Mental health reforms in Australia have resulted in considerable achievements (see forthcoming paper in International Psychiatry). However, after 5 years of real growth of integrated community and local hospital mental health services from 1992 to 1997, many community-based psychiatric services are now being increasingly starved of resources, and others were never adequately developed. This plus increasing presentations involving severe comorbidity with substance misuse, particularly in males, has put severe pressure on emergency departments, acute in-patient units and consultation–liaison teams. Private sector resources are not rationally distributed and public health administrations siphon mental health budgets continually. Australia still compares poorly with other Western countries in terms of the proportion of its gross domestic product and health budgets spent on mental health (Rosen *et al*, 2004). So although on paper the Australian National Mental Health Policy has been world class, its implementation has proven patchy and fragile. We now need to lift our game, and call for a consistent indepen¬dent umpire, a National Mental Health Commission or equivalent.

## Acknowledgements

Thanks are due to Sylvia Hands for assistance with the manuscript, and to BBC News Country Profiles – Australia (2004) (http://www.bbc.co.uk/1/hi/world) and Infoplease Country Profiles, Commonwealth of Australia, High Beam Research (2004) (http://www.infoplease.com/ipa/AD107296.htm) – for demographic details.

## References

Andrews, G. (2005) Editorial. The crisis in mental health: the chariot needs one horseman. *Medical Journal of Australia*, **182**, 372–373.
Andrews, G., Hall, W., Teesson, M., *et al* (1999) *The Mental Health of Australians. National Survey of Mental Health and Wellbeing, National Mental Health Strategy.* Canberra: Commonwealth Department of Health and Aged Care.

Australian Medical Workforce Advisory Committee (1999) *The Specialist Psychiatry Workforce in Australia. AMWAC Report 1999.7*. Sydney.

Department of Health and Ageing (2004) *National Mental Health Report for 2000–2002*. Canberra: Commonwealth of Australia.

Gianfrancesco, P., Miller, V., Rauch, A., *et al* (1996) *National Standards for Mental Health Services*. Canberra: Australian Health Ministers National Mental Health Working Group.

Henderson, S. (2000) Focus on psychiatry in Australia. *British Journal of Psychiatry*, **176**, 97–101.

Jablensky, A. V., McGrath, J., Herrman, H., *et al* (1999) *People Living with Psychotic Illness: An Australian Study 1997–98: National Survey of Mental Health and Wellbeing, National Mental Health Strategy*. Canberra: Commonwealth Department of Health and Aged Care.

Lawrence, D., Holman, C. D. J. & Jablensky, A. V. (2001) *Duty to Care: Preventable Physical Illness in People with Mental Illness*. Perth: University of Western Australia. See http://www.populationhealth.uwa.edu.au/welcome/research/chsr/chsr/consumer_info/duty_to_care. Last accessed 26 August 2005.

National Mental Health Strategy (2003) *National Practice Standards for the Mental Health Workforce*. Canberra: Commonwealth of Australia, Department of Health and Ageing.

Rosen, A. (2005) The Australian experience of deinstitutionalization: the effect of Australian culture on the development and reform of its mental health services. *Acta Scandinavia Psychiatrica Supplementum*, in press.

Rosen, A. & Teesson, M. (2001) Does case management work? The evidence and the abuse of evidence-based medicine. *Australian and New Zealand Journal of Psychiatry*, **33**, 731–746.

Rosen, A., Miller, V. & Parker, G. (1995) *Area-Integrated Mental Health Service (AIMHS) Standards*. Sydney: Royal North Shore Hospital and Community Mental Health Services.

Rosen, A., McGorry, P., Groom, G., *et al* (2004) Australia needs a mental health commission. *Australasian Psychiatry*, **12**, 213–219.

United Nations (1991) *The United Nations Resolution 46/119 on the Rights of People with Mental Illness and the Improvement of Mental Health Care*. New York: United Nations.

Whiteford, H. & Buckingham, W. J. (2005) Ten years of mental health service reform in Australia: are we getting it right? *Medical Journal of Australia*, **182**, 396–400.

# New Zealand

A. P. McGeorge

New Zealand's healthcare system has undergone significant changes in recent times, among them being the establishment in 1993 of a purchaser/provider split and the specific attention given to the development of mental health services. Funding for mental health services (Fig. 1) increased from NZ$270 million in 1993/94 to NZ$866.6 million per annum in 2004/05, a real increase (adjusted for inflation) of 154% (Mental Health Commission, 2006). The bi-partisan political commitment sustaining this funding has had a major impact on the development of recovery-based and culturally specific models of care unrivalled by few countries in the world. However, recent reports (Mental Health Commission, 2006) indicate that, particularly with regard to access, much still remains to be done to address the mental health needs of New Zealanders.

New Zealand is a Pacific country of 4.15 million people. At the last census (2001), with three responses allowed per person, 80% identified themselves as being European, 15% as being indigenous Maori, 6.5% Pacific Island and 6.6% Asian, with other ethnicities accounting for less than 1% of the population. These categories are very broad and only partially describe the

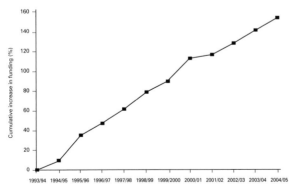

**Fig. 1** Real cumulative percentage increase in public funding for mental health services in New Zealand, 1993/94 (NZ$270 million baseline) to 2004/05. Source: Mental Health Commission (2006).

situation that exists in New Zealand. For example, while 91% identified with one ethnicity, 44% of Maori identified with multiple ethnicities (Ministry of Social Development, 2006).

The median age of the population is 36 years. The overall male/female gender ratio is 0.99. The unemployment rate currently stands at around 4%.

## Healthcare structure

While there is a substantial private sector in medicine and particularly in surgery, the public and not-for-profit sectors dominate over the private sector in the delivery of mental health services. For example, less than 10% of psychiatrists in New Zealand work in the private sector.

The Ministry of Health oversees the development and delivery of health services. It implements government policy and is responsible for the regulation and statutory oversight of the Mental Health Act 1992.

Health services are funded by the Ministry via 21 district health boards, which are responsible for the health of defined populations and catchment areas. Each district health board, guided by the objectives of the Ministry of Health's 2000 *New Zealand Health Strategy* and 2001 *New Zealand Disability Strategy*, has a board comprising appointed and elected members that reports to the Minister of Health through the Ministry of Health. Specialist public services, non-governmental organisations (NGOs) and primary healthcare organisations are funded by the district health boards to provide a range of in-patient and community mental health services.

## Epidemiology

The recently published *New Zealand Mental Health Survey* (Ministry of Health, 2006) indicated that mental disorder is common: 46.6% of the population were predicted to meet criteria for any mental disorder with the exception of psychoses (because the Composite International Diagnostic Interview – 3 instrument used does not generate diagnoses for such disorders) at some time in their lives, with 39.5% having already done so and 20.7% having a disorder in the past 12 months.

The prevalence of disorder in any period is higher for Maori and Pacific people than for other ethnic groups. For instance, the prevalence of disorder in the past 12 months is 29.5% for Maori, 24.4% for Pacific people and 19.3% for others. Much of this burden appears to be associated with the youthfulness of the Maori and Pacific populations and their relative socio-economic disadvantage.

Psychotic disorders have an estimated prevalence of approximately 0.3% of the population; however, in a study of in-patient units in Auckland, New Zealand's largest city, they accounted for around half of all acute psychiatric admissions, with schizophrenia being the most common diagnosis (Wheeler *et al*, 2005).

# Workforce

Recent reports show that major improvements in the workforce have taken place over the past 10 years. There are still, however, significant workforce deficits in mental health services in New Zealand (Ministry of Health, 2005a). For example, although most positions in urban districts are now filled, overall the psychiatric workforce remains depleted compared with international benchmarks. New Zealand has 288 psychiatrists (albeit 528 medical officers overall – Table 1), including 59 child psychiatrists, representing overall ratios of approximately 1 general psychiatrist per 18000 people and 1 child and adolescent psychiatrist for 70000 people, compared with recommendations from the World Health Organization of 1/10000 and 1/50000, respectively (Andrews, 1991). Major deficits in the workforce remain in child and adolescent mental health services, Maori and Pacific Island clinicians and in-patient care (Table 1).

# Legislation

The main pieces of legislation relating to persons with mental health disorders are the Mental Health (Assessment and Compulsory Treatment)

**Table 1** Selected mental health and addiction occupational group workforce

| Occupational group | Total number | Proportion of workforce who are Maori (%) | Proportion of workforce who are Pacific Islanders (%) |
| --- | --- | --- | --- |
| Addiction practitioners[a] | 950 | 22 | 4 |
| Nurses | 3052 | 13.2 | 2.7 |
| Support workers[b] | 1423 | 33 | 8.2 |
| Psychiatrists and other medical practitioners[c] | 528 | 3 | 0.4 |
| Psychologists[d] | 1404 | 4.3 | 0.2 |
| Social workers | 311 | | |

[a] There are approximately 850 alcohol and drug workers and 100 problem gambling practitioners.

[b] This is the number of graduates of the National Certificate in Mental Health Support Work. Note that not all mental health support workers have completed the National Certificate, and not everyone who has completed it is working in mental health.

[c] Includes specialists (288), medical officers special scale (65), registrars (166) and 'other' (5). Although the survey recorded no Pacific doctors working in psychiatry, this table includes two Pacific practitioners because there is at least one psychiatrist and one training in psychiatry who would identify themselves as Pacific.

[d] Of the current surveyed registered psychologists (907), a total of 788 work in the fields of clinical psychology, rehabilitation, psychotherapy and counselling. The ethnicity percentages are from those surveyed.

Source: Ministry of Health (2005a).

Act 1992, the Protection of Personal and Property Rights Act 1998, the Human Rights Act 1993, the Privacy Act 1993 and the Health and Disability Commission Act 1994. Other legislation relevant to mental health includes the Criminal Procedure (Mentally Impaired Persons) Act 2003, which gives the court powers to order individuals with mental impairment who have been charged with or convicted of an imprisonable offence to accept compulsory care and rehabilitation under the Mental Health Act if mentally ill, or, in the case of people with intellectual disabilities, the Intellectual Disability (Compulsory Care and Rehabilitation) Act 2003.

The Mental Health Act seeks to protect the rights of the individual, including treatment in the 'least restrictive' circumstances, and to promote community care. It set a high threshold in terms of determining disorder by specifying that disorders must be severe and pose a serious risk to the patients themselves or others.

## Planning and development

The process of deinstitutionalisation began in New Zealand in the 1970s and resulted in the closure of most of the psychiatric hospitals during the 1980s. It was not, however, until the 1990s that the process was comprehensively planned, implemented and realistically funded.

Three key documents from the Ministry of Health now form the National Mental Health and Addiction Strategy. These include:

- *Looking Forward: Strategic Directions for Mental Health Services* (1994)
- *Moving Forward: The National Mental Health Plan for More and Better Services* (1997)
- *Te Tahuhu – Improving Mental Health 2005–2015: The Second New Zealand Mental Health and Addiction Plan* (2005).

*Looking Forward* confirmed the strategic commitment to the shift from institution-based to community-based delivery of services, backed up by sufficient in-patient services for acute care. The two main goals of the strategy were:

- to decrease the prevalence of mental illness and mental health problems within the community
- to increase the health status of (and reduce the impact of mental disorders on) consumers, their families, carers and the general community.

In 1996, a nationwide review of mental health services was undertaken by Judge Ken Mason. Recommendations from the resulting report (Ministry of Health, 1996) included a major increase in funding for mental health services, and the establishment of a three-member Mental Health Commission with a remit:

- to monitor the implementation of the National Mental Health and Addiction Strategy
- to reduce discrimination against people with mental illness
- to ensure the mental health workforce was strengthened.

Several factors have been responsible for the progress made in the development of mental health services in New Zealand. However, the Mental Health Commission's (1998) 'blueprint' for mental health services has proven to be one of the most important initiatives spurring change. The blueprint specified costed configurations of mental health services for populations of 100 000 people. It aimed to deliver services, when fully implemented, to the 3% of the population most severely affected by mental illnesses, including age-related services for adults, children and youths, and the elderly. It has been augmented by a series of national strategies covering mental health promotion and prevention, workforce development, Maori, Pacific Island and Asian mental health, primary healthcare, activity and outcomes measurement. Maori mental health in particular has received attention through the development of culturally specific services run 'by Maori for Maori'.

More recently, a second *Mental Health and Addictions Plan, Te Tahuhu – Improving Mental Health*, has been developed by the Ministry of Health (2005*b*). Covering the period 2005–15 it encompasses:

- promotion and prevention
- building mental health services
- responsiveness
- workforce and culture for recovery
- Maori mental health
- primary mental healthcare
- addiction
- funding mechanisms for recovery
- transparency and trust
- working together.

## Progress

Figure 2 indicates how resource development in mental health services has increased relative to the blueprint guidelines over the period 1998–2003. Although relatively static since 1993, the configuration of in-patient and community residential beds had changed dramatically before that time, with reductions in in-patient beds and increases in community NGO beds. Since 1993, significant increases in both community clinical and non-clinical staff have taken place, in line with the blueprint. Community services now account for 69% of mental health services, whereas in the late 1980s the reverse was the case.

The Mental Health Commission (2007) has estimated that, at best, 1.9% of the population are now accessing public mental health services. This result falls below expectations – the target was 3% – but needs to be seen in the context of the increasing range and quality of services. It is also anticipated that, as primary healthcare initiatives unfold, access to services for people with low-prevalence disorders and specialist services for those who are more seriously mentally ill will increase.

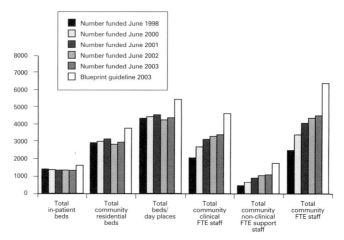

**Fig. 2** Overall trends in beds and community staff funded from June 1998 to June 2003. (FTE, full-time equivalent.) Source: Mental Health Commission (2006).

# References

Andrews, G. (1991) *The Tolkein Report: A Description of a Model Mental Health Service*. University of New South Wales at St Vincent's Hospital.

Mental Health Commission (1998) *Blueprint for Mental Health Services in New Zealand*. Mental Health Commission.

Mental Health Commission (2006) *Report on Progress 2004/2005*. Mental Health Commission.

Mental Health Commission (2007) *Te Haererenga mo te Whakaoranga The Journey of Recovery for the New Zealand Mental Health Sector*. Mental Health Commission.

Ministry of Health (1996) *Inquiry Under Section 47 of the Health and Disability Services Act 1993 in Respect of Certain Mental Health Services (also known as the Mason report)*. Ministry of Health.

Ministry of Health (2005a) *Tauawhitia te Wero – Embracing the Challenge: National Mental Health and Addiction Workforce Development Plan 2006–2009*. Ministry of Health.

Ministry of Health (2005b) *Te Tahuhu – Improving Mental Health 2005–2015. The Second New Zealand Mental Health and Addiction Plan*. Ministry of Health.

Ministry of Health (2006) *Te Rau Hinengaro: The New Zealand Mental Health Survey*. Ministry of Health.

Ministry of Social Development (2006) *The Social Report 2006*. Ministry of Social Development.

Wheeler, E., Robinson, E. & Robinson, G. (2005) Admissions to acute psychiatric inpatient services in Auckland, New Zealand: a demographic and diagnostic review. *New Zealand Medical Journal*, **118**, U1752.

# Papua New Guinea

## Florence Muga

Papua New Guinea is an independent commonwealth in the South Pacific, lying just north of Australia and sharing its western border with Indonesia. The population of Papua New Guinea is 5.2 million, of whom 87% live in rural areas (2000 census) (National Statistics Office, 2003). The country has a very rich culture; for example, there are over 800 distinct language groups (although Papua New Guinea has less than 0.1% of the world's population, it is home to over 10% of the world's languages).

Administratively, Papua New Guinea is divided into four regions, which are further divided into a total of 20 provinces. The capital city is Port Moresby. Travel between the capital city and the provinces is generally by air, since Papua New Guinea's limited road network does not connect all the provinces to one another.

The gross national income is US$580 per capita and the government spends 7% of its total budget on health (UNICEF, 2006). Only 0.7% of the total health budget is spent on mental health (World Health Organization, 2005).

## Health indicators

The average national infant mortality rate is 82.2/1000 live births for males and 72.2/1000 for females, while the maternal mortality ratio is a horrific 370/100000 live births (National Statistics Office, 2003). There are, however, wide provincial variations. Life expectancy at birth is 56 years (UNICEF, 2006). The doctor:population ratio is currently about 1:11000, but disproportionately more doctors work in the urban areas than in the rural areas. The nurse:population ratio is 1:400.

## Mental health resources and services

Public psychiatric services fall under the Social Change and Mental Health section of the Division of Curative Services within the National Department of Health. The resources in terms of facilities and workforce at the different care levels are summarised in Table 1. There are only five psychiatrists practising in the country, giving a national ratio of 1 per 1 000 000, but since all the psychiatrists are in the capital city, the true ratio is 1 psychiatrist for every 70 000 people in the city and zero for the rest of the country. The number of psychiatric nurses per 100 000 population is 0.09 and the number of social workers per 100 000 population is 0.04 (World Health Organization, 2005). The number of psychiatric beds per 10 000 population is 0.24, of which 0.17 per 10 000 are in the sole mental hospital and 0.07 per 10 000 are in the general hospitals (World Health Organization, 2005).

The commonest psychiatric conditions treated at out-patient level are depression and anxiety disorders. The commonest causes of admission are psychotic illnesses, mostly schizophrenia, bipolar disorder and cannabis-induced psychosis. Nearly all patients admitted with cannabis-induced psychosis are men under the age of 30 years. Papua New Guinea does not (at least as yet) have a problem with hard drugs such as heroin.

There are at present no private psychiatrists, no private psychiatric hospitals and no clinical psychologists in the country. Neither are there any neurologists, although there is one neurosurgeon.

There are no community-based services for people who are mentally ill. Patients in the community are looked after by their families.

Apart from clinical services, mental health services available to the public include mental health talks to schools as part of the 'healthy schools programme', radio broadcasts on mental health issues and a weekly mental health column in one of the daily newspapers. World Mental Health Day is celebrated publicly every year in several provinces; in addition to this, the mental health services are represented at the annual 'Health Expo' in the capital city. Posters and leaflets explaining mental health issues are distributed to the public free of charge at such venues. The public's response to these services has always been very encouraging.

## Mental health policy

The goal of the mental health programme is to improve access to mental health services at provincial and district levels and to improve the capacity at community level to support and maintain patient care and rehabilitation (Ministry of Health, 2000). This is to be achieved by 2010 through the following strategies (Ministry of Health, 2000):

- psychiatric patient care and treatment shall be free of charge
- Laloki Psychiatric Hospital shall remain the national referral centre
- four referral and supervising units shall be established at regional level
- psychiatric units shall be established at all provincial public hospitals
- all physicians caring for adult patients in public hospitals shall be responsible for hospital-based psychiatric units in the absence of psychiatrists

**Table 1** Mental health facilities at different healthcare levels in Papua New Guinea

| Level | Facilities | Staffing | Services offered |
|---|---|---|---|
| Tertiary (capital city) | 60-bed Laloki Psychiatric Hospital | 2 psychiatrists[a]<br>12 psychiatric nurses<br>29 other general clinical health workers | Long-stay care<br>Forensic services |
| | 16-bed psychiatric ward within Port Moresby General Hospital, the national teaching and referral hospital | 4 psychiatrists[a]<br>6 psychiatric nurses<br>7 other general clinical health workers | Acute in-patient care<br>Occupational therapy<br>Out-patient clinics |
| | Family Support Centre within Port Moresby General Hospital, the national teaching and referral hospital | Social workers<br>1 psychiatrist[a]<br>Other doctors and nurses<br>Other non-medical agencies | One-stop centre for trauma counselling, child abuse counselling, crisis management, paralegal support and information, overnight emergency accommodation for victims of violence or abuse, liaison with other agencies |
| | Rehabilitation Centre | 1 psychiatrist[a]<br>2 psychiatric nurses<br>1 social worker | Day care<br>Rehabilitation<br>Occupational therapy<br>Family support group |
| Secondary (provincial hospitals) | Psychiatric wards in only two provincial hospitals<br>Most provincial hospitals have only psychiatric clinics | Psychiatric nurses[b] in some hospitals<br>Community health workers<br>Other general health workers<br>Visits once or twice a year by psychiatrists<br>Physicians responsible when psychiatrist is absent | In-patient care where there are units; otherwise, only out-patient clinics<br>Referral to Laloki for admission |
| Primary (district health centres and below) | No psychiatric wards<br>No psychiatric clinics | General nurses<br>Other general health workers | Minimal out-patient care<br>Referral to provincial hospitals |

a. Some psychiatrists work in more than one place: the country has only five practising psychiatrists. b. Psychiatric nurses are often deployed in non-psychiatric sections.

- community-based treatment and rehabilitation shall be established and supported.

# Legislation

Mental health legislation in Papua New Guinea dates back to the Insanity Ordinance of 1912. This was superseded by the Mental Disorders and Treatment Ordinance of 1960. The latter was annulled in 1997 and replaced with a subsidiary chapter (no. 226) of the Public Health Act known as the Public Health (Mental Disorders) Regulation. This is the current mental health legislation in Papua New Guinea, but a review of the legislation is underway to make it more relevant to the mental health needs of 21st-century Papua New Guinea.

# Training

## Undergraduate medical students

There is one medical school in the country, the School of Medicine and Health Sciences of the University of Papua New Guinea, in Port Moresby. The undergraduate curriculum is based on the problem-based learning (PBL) approach and students are exposed to psychiatry from the second year to the final (fifth) year of their MBBS course. During the final year, students undergo a 4-week rotation in psychiatry.

## Postgraduate specialisation

The medical school offers a 4-year degree course (Master of Medicine in Psychiatry, MMed), but psychiatry is a less popular career choice than other disciplines. All the students are required to write a research-based thesis. Students also spend several months of their third year attached to a psychiatric unit in Australia in order to gain exposure to psychiatry in a setting other than Papua New Guinea.

## Psychiatric nurses

In order to specialise in psychiatry, nurses need to undergo a 1-year postgraduate degree course at the medical school.

## Other health workers

Regular mental health workshops are held every 2 years to provide basic mental health training to non-specialists from all over the country to help them manage psychiatric patients. In addition to this, regular VHF radio sessions are broadcast live to all parts of the country, including remote health facilities. The facilitator teaches the topic for that session and health workers participate live and raise questions or seek advice about specific clinical cases. This has been found to be a very convenient and effective way of reaching health workers in remote areas.

# Research

Earlier research in psychiatry, for example by the pioneering psychiatrist Burton-Bradley (1973), identified common forms of mental illness in the country and elicited the public's views about the aetiology of mental illness (often attributed to sorcery). Later research confirmed the occurrence of substance misuse (Johnson, 1991), post-traumatic stress disorder (Johnson, 1989) and so on. However, despite the requirement for all MMed students to carry out research as part of their training, most make no attempt to get their work published after qualifying. As a result, there is still a dearth of research in psychiatry in Papua New Guinea.

# Professional groups

The Papua New Guinea Psychiatric Association comprises all psychiatrists and psychiatric registrars in the country – a total of 11 members.

# Non-governmental organisations

The Mental Health Foundation is a non-governmental organisation that provides support to people who are mentally ill, for example through donations.

The Family Support Group comprises carers of patients with a mental illness who are attending the Rehabilitation Centre. Their functions include education, mutual support, advocacy, fundraising and so on.

# Challenges

The challenges include a shortage of trained staff, frequent shortages of basic psychiatric drugs, the absence of in-patient facilities at the provincial level and an increase in substance misuse, especially cannabis. Cannabis grows readily in the highlands of Papua New Guinea and the number of patients with cannabis-related psychosis has risen greatly over the past 15 years as the cultivation of the plant has increased, both for local consumption and as a cash crop to be smuggled into Australia in exchange for guns, which are then used in tribal fights.

Traditional beliefs about mental illness (e.g. sorcery) also hinder some patients from accessing services or adhering to the treatment prescribed.

An inadequate road network means that patients who need referral to the only psychiatric hospital but who are too disturbed to fly are frequently held not in general hospitals but in local police cells as the only available secure place. They are held until they are stable enough to be transferred by commercial aircraft without posing a risk to others on board.

# References

Burton-Bradley, B. (1973) *Longlong: Transcultural Psychiatry in Papua New Guinea*. Port Moresby: Public Health Department.

Johnson, F. (1989) Post-traumatic stress disorder. *Papua New Guinea Medical Journal*, **32**, 87–88.

Johnson, F. (1991) A comparative study of alcohol-related problems among a group of university students and a group of clerks in the National Capital District, Papua New Guinea. *Medicine and Law*, **10**, 457–467.

Ministry of Health (2000) *Papua New Guinea. National Health Plan 2001–2010: Health Vision 2010. Vol. l: Policy Directions. Vol. ll: Program Policies and Strategies*. Port Moresby: Ministry of Health.

National Statistics Office (2003) *National Census 2000*. Port Moresby: National Statistics Office. Available at http://www.nso.gov.pg/. Last accessed 20 April 2006.

UNICEF (2006) *The State of the World's Children 2006: Excluded and Invisible*. New York: UNICEF. Available at http://www.unicef.org/sowc06/statistics/database.php. Last accessed 20 April 2006.

World Health Organization (2005) *Mental Health Atlas*. Geneva: WHO. Available at http://www.who.int/mental_health/evidence/atlas. Last accessed 20 April 2006.

# Europe

# Albania

Anastas Suli, Ledia Lazëri and Livia Nano

Albania, situated in the western Balkans, has an area of 28 748 km² and a population of 3 069 275 (year 2001), almost one-third of whom are aged 0–14 years. Life expectancy is estimated to be 70.4 years for both sexes (World Health Organization, 2003a). According to the World Health Organization's classification, Albania is a country with low child and low adult mortality rates. The nation's total expenditure on health in 2001 amounted to 3.7% of gross domestic product.

For more than a decade Albania has been undergoing a transitional process of democratisation of its society and decentralisation of its systems, including systems of care in general. However, its relatively recent totalitarian past had created a culture of lack of community initiative, participation and decision-making, and the care system remains prey to financial and regulatory rigidity. The system is still highly centralised and lacks a focus on the social welfare of citizens. Decentralisation and open governance within a framework of comprehensive reform are prerequisites for better services. Furthermore, any intervention to improve the health system will need to take into account the fact that Albania is not a rich country and health is not the top priority when it comes to the allocation of national resources.

## Education in psychiatry

Formal psychiatric education is provided by the only university department of psychiatry in the country; it is part of the Faculty of Medicine of the University of Tirana. Education in psychiatry has had to be transformed in order for it to meet international standards. While psychiatry constitutes 1.4% of the overall training hours in the university curriculum for medical doctors, in 1994 postgraduate psychiatric education was extended from 9 months of internship to 4 years of residency in the university clinic.

Residents annually discuss their training plan with their supervisors. They attend to and follow clinical cases in their charge. The professional qualification for psychiatrists involves several yearly examinations across the entire residency period, and one final examination (oral and written).

While the curriculum offers satisfactory training in biological psychiatry, it is difficult to train young residents properly in the psychosocial aspects of practice, as there are few supervisors with sufficient experience and knowledge in this area. Psychotherapy is taught only theoretically – there is no opportunity for practice and supervision – and psychosocial rehabilitation is missing from formal residency training because the university clinic has no facilities for it.

A curriculum for a residency in child and adolescent psychiatry has recently been approved. This means that the academic year 2004–05 will mark the initiation of a 4-year programme that will cover general paediatrics, neuro-paediatrics, general psychiatry, and child and adolescent psychiatry. It is a step forward in giving to the population better access to more appropriate services.

There are no formal specialisation courses for psychiatric nurses or for clinical social workers, although psychology students in the last year of their undergraduate studies can choose to specialise in clinical psychology or organisational psychology. There is no formal training for occupational therapists.

With an increasing awareness of the need for continuing medical education, including in psychiatry, there are formal negotiations going on between the Ministry of Health and the Ministry of Education in order to establish a responsible body.

# Clinical practice and services

Clinical practice in psychiatry in Albania is exceedingly demanding because so few resources are dedicated to mental illness. For example, within community mental health facilities for children and adults (psychiatric wards in general hospitals, ambulatory clinics, community mental health centres, day centres), there are, nationally, 69 neuropsychiatrists (who have a combined neurology–psychiatry postgraduate qualification, which was abolished in 1974) and psychiatrists (2.2 per 100000 population), of whom 54% are psychiatrists; 130 nurses (4.2 per 100000); 6 psychologists (0.2 per 100000); 12 social workers (0.4 per 100000); and 8 occupational therapists (0.3 per 100000). These figures suggest that psychiatrists (and other professionals) working in ambulatory settings will confront a demand that is impossible to respond to properly in either quantitative or qualitative terms. Except where community mental health centres are already established, the ambulatory clinics are staffed by only one psychiatrist and one nurse, who mostly do diagnostic work and prescribe psychotropic drugs. Psychiatric home care is seldom supported, and visits to a patient's home are made (if at all) only when the patient is not compliant with aspects of psychiatric care.

Albania's in-patient facilities comprise two psychiatric hospitals (Elbasan and Vlora) and two psychiatric wards within general hospitals (Tirana and Shkodra). Except for some administrative/budgetary differences, the approach to service provision is the same for these psychiatric hospitals and wards. The hospitals and wards have a total of 840 beds. This is not a very low figure for the country's population but because half the beds are used for long-stay patients the demand for in-patient services cannot be met.

The two mental hospitals in Elbasan and Vlora have 12 psychiatrists, 93 nurses and 5 occupational therapists. There are no psychologists or social workers at these hospitals.

Psychiatric hospital care involves diagnostic work and free medication – there are few activities available to patients. There is little in the way of rehabilitative work, as it would require a budget and human resources but at present is not a priority.

# Legislation

The Albanian Parliament approved the Mental Health Act in 1996. It provides a framework for compulsory examinations, admissions and treatment, but pays little attention to the establishment of comprehensive, deinstitutionalised services. However, the main problem of the Act is in its implementation. Lack of community services means that institutions continue to be used to segregate people with a mental illness. Efforts are being made to redress the situation, and to build up supportive alternatives, through the drafting of a national mental health policy.

# Developments in mental health

Many actions were taken during the 1990s by international organisations to improve aspects of Albania's psychiatric services, including training and education, day centres and the rehabilitation of institutionalised patients. Unfortunately, these initiatives had little long-term effect. This brought the realisation that it is essential to involve the national authorities in any such work, as this will improve the chances of implementing a break with tradition and estab¬lishing new practices. This would be true anywhere in the world, but is particularly pertinent to the Albanian case, where systems are still managed centrally and so where any important, radical change needs the commitment and influence of central authorities in addition to the initiative and will of local professionals or community groups. Thus, based on the lessons learnt, national professionals have more recently drawn on international expertise in an effort to establish a reform process oriented towards the delivery of comprehensive community mental health services by multidisciplinary teams.

In 1999 the Ministry of Health embraced a proposal by the World Health Organization for a comprehensive reform of the entire psychiatric system. This was made the responsibility of a national organisation when, in 2000, the Minister of Health established the National Steering Committee for

Mental Health. Moreover, the Committee was given the powers necessary to implement the changes required. With technical input from the World Health Organization, the main focus of the Committee has been on elaborating the mental health policy referred to above. This should provide the political framework for change. The Policy for Mental Health Services Development in Albania was approved by the Minister of Health in March 2003. It defines the national goal as the 'establishment and development of a national community mental healthcare system', and describes two main tools to reach the goal: the downsizing of the psychiatric hospitals and the decentralisation of services.

As mandated by the policy document, the National Steering Committee is currently elaborating a strategy for the implementation of the mental health policy, assisted by the World Health Organization.

In addition, pilot projects are now being run to show the feasibility and benefits of community-based mental healthcare.

Considering all the above, there are at present better chances than ever before of achieving comprehensive and accessible mental health services in Albania.

# References

Institute of Statistics (2003) *1993–2001 Statistical Yearbook*. Tirana: INSTAT.

National Steering Committee for Mental Health (2003) *Policy for Mental Health Services Development in Albania*.

World Health Organization (2003*a*) *Atlas: Country Profiles on Mental Health Resources 2001*. Geneva: WHO.

World Health Organization (2003*b*) *The World Health Report 2003*. Geneva: WHO.

World Health Organization Country Office Albania (2003) *Monitoring Mental Health Systems and Services: Case Albania, circulated paper*. Geneva: WHO.

# Austria

W. Wolfgang Fleischhacker and Johannes Wancata

Austria covers an area of some 84000 km$^2$ and has a population of 8.1 million. According to World Bank criteria, Austria is a high-income country. The overall health budget represents 8% of gross domestic product (World Health Organization, 2005). The state of Austria is divided into nine federal provinces, which have significant legislative rights, including in healthcare provision.

Life expectancy at birth is 76.2 years for males and 82.3 years for females (in 2005). The proportion of the population under the age of 15 years is 15% and the proportion above 65 years is 17%. Austria is among the 19 countries worldwide which are projected to have at least 10% of their population aged 80 years or over by the year 2050. Since some mental disorders, such as dementia, increase with age, the number of psychiatric patients will probably rise dramatically.

## Mental health policy and services

The number of psychiatric hospital beds has decreased substantially. In the year 2001 there were 4696 psychiatric beds in total (i.e. 59 per 100000 population), down from nearly 12000 beds in 1974 – a decrease of more than 60%.

The National Hospital Plan includes suggestions for the establishment of psychiatric units in general hospitals. Ten psychiatric units in general hospitals have been established, and several others are planned. Most traditional mental hospitals have been transformed to meet the needs of patients with acut mental illness. In addition, some of them have extended their services to people with physical diseases.

Each of the nine provinces has developed a mental health plan. Although there are regional differences between these, the key points of all plans are: a focus on community psychiatry, the decentralisation of psychiatric services and the social reintegration of persons suffering from mental disorders. The planning and provision of community psychiatric services are the responsibility of the provinces. Although some provinces now have a comprehensive network of community services, others are less advanced. The majority of these services (for vocational rehabilitation, supported housing, counselling, etc.) are provided by private organisations, but are predominantly funded by government agencies. The staff includes a variety of different professions (e.g. psychiatrists, social workers, nurses, psychotherapists, psychologists).

Primary healthcare is usually offered by self-employed general practitioners (GPs), working in solo practices. Most GPs treat patients with psychiatric disorders, but they may decide to refer patients to self-employed psychiatrists or other psychiatric services. Spread between office-based psychiatry, community-based services and psychiatric departments in hospitals, Austria has 11.8 psychiatrists per 100 000 inhabitants. In addition, some GPs have trained in psychosocial medicine/psychotherapy.

In 1991, the Psychotherapy Act established a certified profession of psychotherapists. In Austria, psychotherapy is provided by a variety of different professions. Anyone is allowed to provide it after completing training in psychotherapy and being certified by the Ministry of Health. Nearly all psychiatrists and many psychologists have a certificate in psychotherapy. In the year 2002, overall 5495 persons (i.e. 68 per 100 000 population) were certified psychotherapists.

The healthcare system (including mental healthcare) is predominantly financed via health insurance. This is mandatory for all employed and self-employed persons. There are no specific allocations for mental health within the health budget. The majority of the costs for primary care and secondary care (including psychiatric services) are covered by health insurance. This includes the costs of all psychotropic drugs. Interventions by psychologists as well as by psychotherapists are partly reimbursed. Psychiatric in-patient treatment is fully covered. Disability benefits are available for persons with mental disorders, but local regulations differ.

The fact that psychiatric community services are usually not directly financed by health insurance but via government agencies often complicates overall service provision.

## Mental health legislation

There is no comprehensive mental health act in Austria. Compulsory admissions to psychiatric hospital departments are regulated by the Compulsory Admission Act 1991. According to this law, only persons who pose a threat to their own or other people's health or life because of a mental illness can be admitted compulsorily. Professionals called 'patient advocates' were established by this legislation and they act on behalf of patients in order to protect their rights. The number of compulsorily admitted patients has significantly increased since the new law became effective.

Persons with mental disorders who have committed a crime and are sentenced to jail fall under two main categories: those who are regarded as fit to stand trial; and those who are not. Both groups are detained in special institutions in the prison system, although those who are not regarded as fit to stand trial may also be detained in psychiatric hospitals.

# Research

Psychiatric research is mainly based in universities – three public and one private. The public universities (in Innsbruck, Graz and Vienna) presently receive lump funds from the Austrian government, but there are plans to award at least a proportion of the money based on research output and teaching achievements. All three institutions supplement these funds through third-party funding. The private medical university in Salzburg basically taps into the same funding sources but has no direct support from the Austrian government, although it does receive some from the local government of Salzburg.

The majority of research at these four universities is clinical: Innsbruck focuses strongly on schizophrenia, dementia, neuropsychoimmunology, alcoholism, psycho-oncology and quality of life, whereas Vienna has a strong interest in affective disorders, social psychiatry, genetics and illegal substance misuse. Both centres have neuropsychology/neuroimaging groups. Consultation–liaison psychiatry, forensic psychiatry as well as research in adjustment and somatoform disorders are the stronghold of the Medical University in Graz. Researchers in Salzburg deal mainly with suicidality and bipolar illness. Most academic institutions have close ties to basic science departments with a strong focus on preclinical neurobiology and neuropsychopharmacology.

Some research is also done in non-academic institutions. It includes studies of drug safety and stigma.

# Education and training

Psychiatry is an integral part of the medical curriculum in Austria's universities. Students are first exposed to the field as part of courses on the nervous system in the first year. They also receive some basic training with regard to communication strategies, for which psychiatrists are among the teachers. In the clinical semesters, psychiatry is taught in both theoretical and practical courses, and in the last year students can do a 4-week elective in psychiatry.

Postgraduate training is governed by law in Austria. The Austrian Medical Association (Österreichische Ärztekammer) prepares – after consulting with professional societies such as the ÖGPP – a curriculum, which has to be approved by the Ministry of Health. The latter has passed new regulations, effective as of 27 February 2007. Postgraduate specialist training in psychiatry now comprises 5 years of psychiatry, complemented by a half year each in neurology and internal medicine. Trainees have to take a final examination before being licensed as psychiatrists. The main change to the old curriculum is that the new one includes formalised psychotherapy training as an integral component. This has also led to a change in title from 'Specialist in Psychiatry' to 'Specialist in Psychiatry and Medical Psychotherapy', which is relevant to the question of reimbursement, insofar as specialists who hold a psychotherapy title are also eligible for health insurance coverage for psychotherapeutic services.

Most of the training is provided by hospitals, both academic and non-academic. As most psychiatric departments include both in- and out-patient facilities, trainees are expected to gain experience in different aspects of the field. A training in consultation–liaison psychiatry is also encouraged but, unfortunately, is not available everywhere. In addition, more specialised services, such as alcohol detoxification/rehabilitation, old age psychiatry and the like, are part of the training programme wherever such facilities exist.

Child and adolescent psychiatry has now also been given full specialist status, whereas it used to be a mere add-on specialty to psychiatry, neurology or paediatrics. Training includes 4 years in child and adolescent psychiatry as well as 10 months in paediatrics, 6 in neurology and 8 in adult psychiatry.

## Psychiatric associations

Two major psychiatric associations exist in Austria. The Österreichische Gesellschaft für Psychiatrie und Psychotherapie (ÖGPP, Austrian Association for Psychiatry and Psychotherapy, www.oegpp.at), an association of psychiatrists, has close to 900 members and is the professional forum for most Austrian psychiatrists. It officially represents psychiatry in the Austrian Medical Association and is consulted in most psychiatry-related matters by both government and non-governmental organisations.

Pro Mente Austria (www.promenteaustria.at) is the umbrella organisation of most community psychiatric services in Austria. The focus of Pro Mente Austria is mental health policy, partly in cooperation with ÖGPP. It has many non-psychiatrist members.

Hilfe für Psychisch Erkrankte (HPE, an association for family carers, www.hpe.at) is Austria's largest and best organised transnational advocacy group.

## Sources

Federal Ministry of Health and Women (2001, 2003) *Mental Health in Austria*. Selected Annotated Statistics from the Austrian Mental Health Reports 2001 and 2003.

Österreichisches Bundesinstitut für Gesundheitswesen (1998) *Struktureller Bedarf in der psychiatrischen Versorgung*. (Structural Needs for Organizing Psychiatric Services.)

Österreichisches Bundesinstitut für Gesundheitswesen (2001) *Evaluierung der dezentralen Fachabteilungen für Psychiatrie*. (Evaluation of Psychiatric Units in General Hospitals.)

World Health Organization (2005) *Austria*. In Mental Health Atlas 2005. See http:// globalatlas.who.int/globalatlas/predefinedReports/MentalHealth/Files/AT_Mental_ Health_Profile.pdf

# Republic of Belarus

Natallia Golubeva, Kris Naudts, Ayana Gibbs,
Roman Evsegneev and Siarhei Holubeu

The Republic of Belarus (ROB) covers 207 600 km$^2$ and has a population of about 10 million (Ministry of Statistics and Analysis, 2005). It was a member state of the former Soviet Union until it gained independence in 1991. Belarus is located between Poland, Lithuania and Latvia in the west, Russia in the east, and Ukraine in the south. Seventy-two per cent of the population live in an urban environment and 28% in rural areas. The average life span for men is 63 years and for women 75 years (Ministry of Public Health, 2005).

## Mental health policies and programmes

Historically, psychiatry in the ROB has been strongly influenced by the classical Russian–German school of thought. This implied a biologically oriented approach and an emphasis on hospital in-patient treatment. Over the past 10 years there has been a dramatic shift in ideology, views, priorities, legislation and care models in psychiatry in several former Soviet republics. Many of these countries have welcomed modern Anglo-Saxon approaches to mental health, but have implemented them to varying degrees. In the ROB, ICD–10 (World Health Organization, 1992) was officially introduced in 2002.

Mental healthcare is provided by the Health Service under the auspices of the Ministry of Public Health. The Health Service is funded by the state through general taxation. The country is in the World Bank's lower-middle-income group. The proportion of gross domestic product allocated to the health budget is 5.6%. The per capita total expenditure on health is $464 (all prices here are reported in international dollars, i.e. after adjustment for purchasing power parity), and the per capita government expenditure on health is $402 (World Health Organization, 2005).

There is no private psychiatric system and the state provides psychiatric care free of charge. Psychotropic drugs have increasingly been used since the early 1960s and are the main component of treatment today. In accordance with mental health legislation, people with schizophrenia, epilepsy, bipolar affective disorder and other psychiatric illnesses must receive their medication free of charge. For example, typical antipsychotics and some early atypicals, such as clozapine and sulpiride, are widely and freely available to patients. In recent years, one of the second-generation antipsychotics, risperidone, has also become available.

Mental health policy is set out annually by the Chief Psychiatrist at the Ministry of Public Health. For a few years now, a biopsychosocial model and multidisciplinary teamwork have been advocated, as well as deinstitutionalisation and the development of community-based mental healthcare. However, in practice, the only component that has been realised so far is a substantial reduction in the number of psychiatric beds. The system of psychiatric care none the less remains highly centralised, with often large psychiatric hospitals and almost undeveloped social and community mental health services.

The first port of call for people with mental health problems is the so-called regional dispensary, where predominantly out-patient primary psychiatric care is provided by psychiatrists and psychiatric nurses. Patients receive counselling, are prescribed psychotropic medication or are referred for admission to the hospital. Some dispensaries have a few in-patient beds and some provide ambulatory psychotherapy. In addition, there are also specific dispensaries for children and adolescents, and for people with drug or alcohol addiction.

## In-patient care

There are 14 general psychiatric hospitals, nine psychiatric departments at general medical hospitals, and six in-patient wards in dispensaries. There are 7225 beds available to psychiatric patients, of which 405 are for children. In addition, there are 1285 beds for addiction treatment. Over the past 5 years, the total number of beds has been reduced by about 30% (Ministry of Public Health, 2005). The State Mental Hospital in Minsk (the ROB's capital) is the largest general psychiatric hospital, with almost 2000 beds.

## Day care

An intermediate type of psychiatric care is provided at day hospitals. Usually, this day care takes place on a special ward of a general psychiatric hospital or at a psychiatric dispensary. The patients come in the morning, receive their medications, participate in occupational therapy and return home in the evening.

## Out-patient care

Out-patient psychiatric care is predominantly provided at psychiatric dispensaries by a psychiatrist and a nurse. They are located in cities and towns and cater for a geographically defined catchment area. In addition, some patients who attend the out-patient clinic are occasionally visited at home.

## Long-term care institutions

Institutional care is under the auspices of the Ministry of Social Welfare. People with a chronic mental illness and people with learning disabilities are accommodated in special institutions. The standard of care and comfort is poor.

# Mental health legislation

In 1999 the Mental Healthcare and Civil Rights Guarantee Law, inspired by its Russian equivalent, was adopted. This law stipulates that mental healthcare is guaranteed by the state and based upon the principles of law. It is voluntary and provided free of charge. Diagnoses are made in accordance with ICD–10. Treatment can be started only after written informed consent has been obtained from the patient.

Compulsory admissions of patients with mental disorders who pose a risk to themselves or others are overseen by local courts. These should be dealt with within 3 days of admission, but there is a significant delay in court procedures and patients are often well and fit to be discharged, or competent to consent to treatment, by the time the court attends to their case. Assessments are performed by at least three psychiatrists. Patients have the right to appeal at any time.

In addition, the Ministry of Public Health has made it a requirement that every person diagnosed with a mental disorder is put on a register. Some employers may require a certificate from job applicants to demonstrate that they are not on this register before they consider hiring them. Also, when a person on the register commits an offence a forensic psychiatric assessment is mandatory.

# Workforce and psychiatric associations

In 2004, the incidence of mental disorders was 53 931 and the overall number of people registered at psychiatric services reached 227 300. In the same year, there were 1073 psychiatrists (of whom 328 worked in addiction treatment settings), 162 psychotherapists, 10 clinical psychologists and 7 sexologists (Ministry of Public Health, 2005). There are no statistics concerning the number of psychiatric nurses.

In the State Mental Hospital in Minsk there are about 85 psychiatrists. Typically, two would be responsible for wards containing 50–60 patients. A typical psychiatrist in a dispensary would see more than 5000 patients per year (Ministry of Public Health, 2005).

The Belarusian Psychiatric Association (BPA) was created in 1996; it is a member of the World Psychiatric Association. The BPA initiated the drafting of the Mental Healthcare and Civil Rights Guarantee Law (see above) and implemented it in psychiatric practice. It drives all innovations in education and professional development and clinical practice. The vast majority of psychiatrists hold membership, for a small annual fee.

# Mental health training

## Psychiatrists

It takes 6 years to get a medical degree. There are 12 semesters of 5 months each and 6 weeks of clinical training in the summer. Only the very basics of psychiatry are taught during medical school. This leads to poor psychiatric knowledge among non-psychiatrists, to whom people with mental health problems may present for the first time. To qualify as a psychiatrist takes only 1 year of training in a psychiatric hospital. This 1-year training programme includes a full-time 3-month theoretical course in psychiatry, organised by the Belarusian Medical Academy for Postgraduate Training. At the end of this 1-year programme, trainees have to pass a theory and practical examination before they can start practising independently. Every psychiatrist is required to attend a 2-week refresher course at least once a year.

## Child and adolescent psychiatrists

A division for child and adolescent psychiatry and psychotherapy is being developed at the Belarusian Medical Academy for Postgraduate Training (the project began at the end of 2005). It is envisaged that training will be similar to that for general adult psychiatrists. Previously, people working in this field were general psychiatrists who had gained practical experience in child and adolescent psychiatry or psychotherapy.

## Psychiatric nurses

Any generally trained nurse can work in a psychiatric hospital: there is no specific training for psychiatric nurses, nor are there any particular requirements to work in a mental health setting. However, when they have been working in a psychiatric setting for 3 years, they have to attend a 2-week course in psychiatry.

## Clinical psychologists

Before 1994, psychology training did not involve clinical or psychotherapeutic components. Therefore, most psychologists in clinical posts perform only psycho-diagnostic testing. In 1994, the first faculty of clinical psychology was established, at Hrodno State Medical University. Since 2001, it has produced 30 clinical psychologists per year with advanced knowledge of clinical psychology and psychiatry.

# Research

There has been some participation in a few international projects, such as the Collaborative Study on Alcohol and Injuries by the World Health Organization (2001), but in general research activity has been sparse.

# Human rights

The Mental Healthcare and Civil Rights Guarantee Law states that mental healthcare should be provided by the state on observance of the principles of law, humanity and human rights. It explicitly stipulates that no one can have his or her civil rights restricted solely on the basis of having a mental illness, being on the register or living in a long-term care institution. It also states that methods of treatment should be used only with diagnostic and curative intentions and cannot be applied for punishment.

# Conclusions

Psychiatry in the ROB has undergone major changes in the past decade. Modern mental health legislation has been implemented and deinstitutionalisation has been pursued. However, the latter has not been matched by the implementation of adequate community mental health services. Further development of professional training and research to underpin evidence-based practice are urgently needed.

# References

Ministry of Public Health (2005) *Public Health in the Republic of Belarus: An Official Statistics Collection*. Minsk: Ministry of Public Health.

Ministry of Statistics and Analysis (2005) *Republic of Belarus in Figures: Short Statistical Book*. Minsk: Ministry of Statistics and Analysis.

World Health Organization (1992) *International Classification of Mental and Behavioural Disorders (10th edn) (ICD–10)*. Geneva: WHO.

World Health Organization (2001) *Collaborative Study on Alcohol and Injuries Protocol*. Geneva: WHO.

World Health Organization (2005) *Mental Health Atlas*. Geneva: WHO.

# Belgium

Benjamin J. Baig and Veronique Delvenne

The Kingdom of Belgium is a high-income country in northern Europe with an approximate area of 33 000 km² and a population of 10.5 million. The proportion of the population under the age of 15 years is 17% and the proportion of the population above the age of 60 years is 22%. Life expectancy at birth is 75.2 years for males and 81.5 years for females. As a founding member of what is now the European Union, it hosts the headquarters of the European Commission and the European Parliament, as well as other major organisations, including NATO.

Belgium is divided into the Flemish-speaking region of Flanders, in the north, with 58% of the population, the French-speaking southern region of Wallonia, inhabited by 32%, and the Brussels capital region, officially bilingual, inhabited by 10% of the population. A small German-speaking community exists in eastern Wallonia. Belgium's linguistic diversity is reflected in the organisation of its psychiatric institutions and legislation.

## Mental health policy

In Belgium, as both federal government and communities are in charge of different parts of the mental health service, there is both a national mental health policy, formulated in 1988, and a community mental health policy. A substance misuse policy is present which was initially formulated in 1921 and a national mental health programme was formulated in 1990 and updated in 1999.

Belgium has a suicide prevention policy, implemented by the Mental Health Centre in Brussels. It focuses on the quality of help offered and on the efficacy of the services from the network of providers in mental health and social care. The goals of the policy are: to optimise the care offered to clients at risk of suicidal behaviour; to develop networks to enable follow-up with at-risk patients; to lend support to and to share relevant knowledge with other carers; and to advocate for suicide prevention within local networks.

Belgium has a nationwide data-collection system or epidemiological study on mental health, known as the Minimum Psychiatric Dataset. There are specific programmes for mental health for minorities, refugees, disaster-affected populations, indigenous populations, the elderly and children.

Different organisations subsidised by public authorities exist in Wallonia, Brussels and Flanders. In the not-for-profit sector, organisations include the Wallonia Institute for Mental Health and the Brussels Francophone League for Mental Health. Their objectives are to join the representatives in the field of mental health (via their organisations) with stakeholders, including service users and carers, to regularly evaluate social mental health issues, to encourage critique of mental health practice, to participate in mental health promotion and to work on ethical questions.

There exist 'platforms' of dialogue which group together psychiatric care structures for each region. Their objective is to highlight the study of health service research needs and to open dialogue between the stakeholders in mental health to improve the availability of care.

Belgium has disability benefits for persons with mental disorders. Factors such as degree of autonomy in daily activities, ability to work and degree of handicap are assessed.

## Mental health services

Belgium spends 6% of the total health budget on mental health. There are some 69 psychiatric hospitals in Belgium, with 22.1 psychiatric beds per 10 000 population. There are around 18 psychiatrists per 100 000 population. The primary sources of mental health financing are social insurance, private insurance, out-of-pocket expenditure by the patient or family, and tax-based revenue. The Flemish-speaking and French-speaking communities are in charge of all non-hospital mental healthcare, such as sheltered housing and centres for mental health. The federal government is in charge of hospitals, location of psychiatric care and quality of hospital care. Mental health is a part of the primary healthcare system and so the treatment of severe mental disorders is available at the primary care level. There is regular training in mental health for primary care professionals. Emergency facilities are geographically sectorised across the country, which offers immediate care at low rates, through subsidisation by the local centres.

Patients may also use regional ambulatory centres for a consultation or receive a home visit. Care is offered by a multidisciplinary team able to address the medical, psychiatric, psychological and social aspects of a health problem. The remit of mental healthcare centres is both curative and preventive.

Belgium has a long history of community care. The city of Geel is known for the early adoption of deinstitutionalisation. The earliest Geel infirmary and the model where patients go into town, interact with the community during the day, and return to the hospital at night date from the 13th century. This practice is based on the positive effects that placement in a host family gives. The model continues today, where patients participate in family life and sleep in the family house, but are still considered the responsibility of the hospital; they spend part of the day or all day in hospital doing various activities and can go back to the hospital for observation or in case of crisis. In 2003, there were 770 family accommodation places available in the Flemish region and 192 in the Walloon region.

## Mental health legislation

The royal decision of May 2000 changing the previous one of 1976 fixed a maximum number of beds in psychiatric services. There are specific child and adolescent psychiatric beds in general, paediatric and psychiatric hospitals in Belgium. Since 2002 there have been specific legislative guidelines for child and adolescent psychiatric disorders. The latest legislation was enacted in 2000 and a new piece of legislation regarding the detention of those with a mental disorder was adopted in April 2007. Mental health legislation is uniform across both the Flemish and Wallonia regions.

## Research

Belgium is cited as being in the top ten leading countries for psychiatric research, in terms of both the number of papers and impact. Funding has come primarily from the federal government and European Union framework programmes.

The Department of Psychiatry at Université Libre de Bruxelles, Erasme Hospital, has been involved in initiating and implementing large European consortia (e.g. the GENDEP Consortium) on the genetics of mood disorders and schizophrenia. A European network of clinical and research centres for genetic studies in mood disorders (Biomed I and Biomed II programmes) has been established. The department is now coordinating a European multicentre study on treatment-resistant depression, including prospective work on pharmacogenetics.

Other major research centres include: the Psychoneuroendocrinology Unit, University of Liege, which specialises in affective disorders; the Universitair Centrum Kinder-en Jeugdpsychiatrie, University Hospital, Antwerp, which specialises in child psychiatry; and the University Hospital Brugman, Brussels, which specialises in sleep medicine. The Unit for Suicide Research, University of Gent, studies the epidemiology of suicidal behaviour, the biological and psychological characteristics of suicidal behaviour and prevention strategies.

Pharmaceutical research in Belgium has been led by Janssen and Janssen-Cilag, and resulted in the development of both haloperidol in 1958 and risperidone in 1984.

## Education and training

Belgium has nine medical schools; the oldest, the University of Leuven, dates from the 14th century. Most Belgian undergraduate training takes the form of a 3-year bachelor's degree, encompassing basic sciences, followed by a 4-year masters degree, which includes clinical disciplines. Psychiatry, medical psychology and child and adolescent psychiatry are included during the medical curriculum in the 7 years of study by Belgian medical graduates. They are also trained in aspects of the patient–doctor relationship during small-group sessions.

Postgraduate training and specialisation last 5 years, during which trainees work under the supervision of a 'maître de stage' in adult psychiatry, as well as child and adolescent psychiatry, and they also spend 1 year in neurology, paediatrics or internal medicine.

One year of training can be done in research. At the end of the specialisation, the candidate must publish one paper in an international journal or present at an international conference. Training includes mandatory academic courses and an examination during the third year. Since 2002, specific training in child and adolescent psychiatry has been available. Following specialisation, trainees will have a specific registration number from the Institut National d'Assurance Maladie-Invalidité (National Institute of Illness and Disability Insurance).

## Psychiatric associations

Psychiatric associations in Belgium are divided between adult and child disciplines, and French-speaking and Flemish-speaking organisations. The primary association is the Société Royale de Médecine Mentale de Belgique (Royal Society of Mental Medicine of Belgium), which was founded in 1869. It is responsible for the primary Belgian psychiatric journal, the Acta Psychiatrica Belgica. The Vlaamse Vereniging Voor Psychiatrie (Flemish Association of Psychiatry) represents the Flemish-speaking community of adult psychiatrists. The Société Belge Francophone de Psychiatrie et des Disciplines Associées de l'Enfance et de l'Adolescence (French Belgian Society of Psychiatry and Associated Disciplines of Childhood and Adolescence) represents the French-speaking child and adolescent mental health professionals and the De Vlaamse Vereniging voor Kinder-en Jeugdpsychiatrie is the Flemish equivalent.

These professional societies are responsible for specialist professional standards, education and providing advice on policy. They are responsible for mental health promotion and the organisation of scientific events and congresses each year.

The Belgian College of Neuropsychopharmacology and Biological Psychiatry (BCNBP) was founded in 1974 and represents the scientific body of psychiatrists in Belgium.

## Conclusion

As a high-income European country, Belgium has a modern psychiatric infrastructure comprising policy, legislation, community care, education, training and research. The integration of policy and services may be limited by its linguistic and cultural diversity, and future care programmes and pathways may benefit from a more unified strategy. Community care has historically been seen as a priority and the legislation in 2000 supports this continuing trend.

## Sources

Andriessen, K., Clara, A. & Beuckx, K. (2002) The suicide prevention policy of a mental health centre. *International Journal of Mental Health Promotion*, **4**, 20–23.

Baro F., Prims A. & de Schouwer, P. (1984) Belgium: psychiatric care in a pluralist system. In *Mental Health Care in the European Community* (ed. S. P. Mangen), pp. 42–54. Croom Helm.

Der Minister van Consumentenzaken, Volksgezondheid en Leefmilieu and Aelvoet, M. (2000) *Legislation Concerning Mental Health. Federale databank van de beoefenaars van de gezondheidszorgberoepen.* Public Federal Service of Health, Food Chain Safety and Environment, January, 2004.

Fava, G. A & Ottolini, F. (2004) International trends in psychiatric research. *A citation analysis. Services research and outcomes. Current Opinion in Psychiatry*, **17**, 283–287.

Simoens-Desmet, A. (1998) *Rapport National 1998 du Resume Psychiatrique Minimum.* Ministere des Affaires Sociale, Se la Santè, Publique et de l'Environment.

Van Heeringen, K. (2003) Unit for Suicide Research, University of Gent, Belgium. *British Journal of Psychiatry*, **183**, 260–261.

World Health Organization (2005) Belgium. In *Mental Health Atlas 2005.* See http://www.who.int/globalatlas/default.asp (last accessed August 2008).

# Bosnia and Herzegovina

Osman Sinanovic, Esmina Avdibegovic, Mevludin Hasanovic,
Izet Pajevic, Alija Sutovic, Slobodan Loga and Ismet Ceric

Bosnia and Herzegovina (BH) is located on the western part of the Balkan Peninsula. It has an area of $51210\,km^2$ and a population of 3 972 000. According to the Dayton Agreement of November 1995, which ended the 1992–95 war, BH comprises two 'entities' – the Federation of Bosnia and Herzegovina (FBH) and the Republic of Srpska (RS) – and the District of Brcko. The administrative arrangements for the management and financing of mental health services reflect this. The FBH, with 2 325 018 residents, is a federation of 10 cantons, which have equal rights and responsibilities. The RS has 1 487 785 residents and, in contrast, a centralised administration. Brcko District has just under 80 000 residents.

## Mental health policy and legislation

Healthcare systems in BH are regulated basically by the entities' different laws on healthcare and on health insurance. Each entity and Brcko District is responsible for the financing, management, organisation and provision of healthcare. The health administration is centralised in RS, through the Ministry of Health and Social Welfare, but in FBH is decentralised – each of the 10 cantonal administrations has responsibility for healthcare through its own ministries. The central Ministry of Health of the FBH, located in Sarajevo, coordinates cantonal health administrations at a federal level. The District of Brcko provides primary and secondary care to its citizens. The mental health policies and national programmes for mental health were created in 1999 and adopted in 2005. A law on the protection of persons with mental disorders was adopted in 2001 and 2002 in FBH (*Official Gazette of BH*, Nos 37/01 and 40/02), and in 2004 in RS (*Official Gazette of RS*, No. 46/04). These laws define the rights of people and regulates the procedure for voluntary or involuntary admission to a psychiatric hospital.

## Mental health service delivery

There are no private mental health institutions. Psychiatric services are available for all citizens, paid from a special national fund for healthcare, financed by mandatory health insurance. The reform of mental health services began in 1995. The focus has been on care in the community, limiting the use of psychiatric hospital beds, establishing a network of community mental health centres (CMHCs), and developing other services in the community, a multidisciplinary approach and teamwork, as well as cooperation between sectors. Each CMHC is responsible for general mental health in a catchment area of 50 000–80 000 inhabitants; each has 10 psychiatric beds, intended for the acute admission of patients (these beds are in fact on neuropsychiatric wards of regional general hospitals). The CMHCs have many different functions, including the promotion of mental health, early detection of mental disorders, and the provision of multidisciplinary care (Ceric *et al*, 2001).

Psychiatric services are provided throughout BH through the network of 55 CMHCs and family medicine services at primary care level. Secondary and tertiary mental health services are provided in three psychiatric clinics, one department of a university clinical centre, two general psychiatry hospitals, two institutions for the treatment, rehabilitation and social care of patients who are chronically mentally ill, and neuropsychiatric wards in general hospitals in major cities. In the reform of the mental health services, mentioned above, new out-patient services were established, the existing primary care services were adapted to mental healthcare and, in addition to the CMHCs, sheltered housing services for patients with a chronic mental illness were established.

The reform of mental health services had a direct impact on the development of users' initiatives in BH: there are now several user associations, which are provided with professional support and education from CMHCs and psychiatry clinics.

There are only two wards and two specialists for child and adolescent psychiatry within the psychiatry clinics. There are four institutions for the care of adults and children with special needs and chronic mental disorders, mainly financed from social welfare. Persons with drug addiction are treated in a specialist institute and two other centres for addiction; methadone is the predominant form of treatment.

There are no specific programmes for the mental healthcare of minorities and the elderly in BH. There are programmes for refugees and war victims of torture, through a network of non-governmental organisations developed during the war.

The provision of forensic psychiatry services is insufficient. Individuals with mental health problems who commit criminal acts are treated in one forensic ward of a general psychiatry department of a prison psychiatry hospital.

According to the Regional Office of the Mental Health Project for South Eastern Europe (2004), in 2002 in FBH there were 159 neuropsychiatrists, in RS 67 and in Brcko District 6. The number of psychiatric beds in FBH was 632, in RS 640 and in Brcko District 30. These data differ from those in Table 1, from the World Health Organization (2005) and based on data collected from 2001 to 2004.

# Treatment of traumatised persons

At the beginning of the war (1992) knowledge about the psychological consequences of war and therapeutic approaches to post-traumatic stress disorder (PTSD) in BH was rather poor. The therapeutic approach was based on the experience of psychiatrists and their receptiveness to the ideas suggested by the foreign literature and the many foreign workers (Jensen & Ceric, 1994; Hasanovic *et al*, 2006). At the end of the war, various psychosocial programmes were organised by the government and international non-governmental organisations (de Jong & Stickers, 2003; Nelson, 2003). The psychosocial approach to trauma aimed to reduce not only the risk of serious mental disorders but also stigma, through mass education about the psychological consequences of trauma. Working with traumatised people during the war, we perceived that religious people coped more successfully with difficulties than those who were not religious. In selected cases, spirituality and religion are therefore used in the process of healing, and so they found their place in educational programmes and psychotherapeutic treatment. In hospitals, adequate rooms for the spiritual and religious needs of patients were allocated (Pajevic *et al*, 2005).

# Psychiatric training

There are five medical faculties, two in RS and three in FBH, with different education programmes, all lasting 6 years. At four medical faculties, the undergraduate courses include only two semesters of psychiatry, while at one medical faculty the undergraduate course has only a neuropsychiatry element. Medical schools are associated with psychiatric clinics. After

**Table 1** Numbers of psychiatric beds and staff

|  | Federation of Bosnia and Herzegovina | Republic of Srpska | Brcko District |
|---|---|---|---|
| Total number of psychiatric beds per 10 000 residents | 3.6 | 3.93 | 3.5 |
| in psychiatry hospitals | 2.4 | 0.91 |  |
| in general hospitals | 1 | 0.68 | 3.5 |
| in other institutions | 0.2 | 2.33 |  |
| Numbers of professionals per 100 000 residents |  |  |  |
| psychiatrists[a] | – | 2.3 | – |
| neuropsychiatrists[a] | 1.8 | 1.2 | 7.0 |
| nurses in psychiatry | 10 | 19.4 | 21.8 |
| psychologists | 0.5 | 0.86 | 1.8 |
| social workers | 0.03 | 0.66 | 1.8 |

a. In Bosnia and Herzegovina until 1992 there was education in 'neuropsychiatry' only; during the war (1992–95), medical doctors from the Republic of Srpska were trained in Belgrade (Serbia), where they could gain a qualification in 'psychiatry'.

Source: World Health Organization (2005).

graduation from the medical faculty and a 1-year internship, specialisation in neuropsychiatry/psychiatry is available, authorised by the entity's Ministry of Health.

Specialist training is different in the two entities. In FBH there is specialisation in neuropsychiatry, which takes 4 years, with 20 months of psychiatry, while in RS there is a programme of education in psychiatry only, which also lasts 4 years. There is no unified national programme of psychiatric education for residents.

## Psychiatric subspecialties and allied professions

The educational programme for the specialisation in neuropsychiatry/psychiatry does not include psychotherapy. Residents from neuropsychiatry/psychiatry are familiar with the theoretical basis of psychotherapy mainly from their undergraduate education. There are no institutions for education in psychotherapy in BH, and there is no regulation of psychotherapy licences. Education in psychotherapy is organised from psychiatry clinics and by psychologists' associations, in cooperation with psychotherapist educators from other European countries.

The only recognised sub-specialisations are in social psychiatry and alcoholism and drug addiction, each taking 1 year. There is undergraduate education in psychology, but no specialisation in clinical psychology. Furthermore, there is no specialist training for psychiatric nurses. Additional psychiatric education for nurses is provided through special education programmes organised at the psychiatric hospitals.

# Main areas of research

Psychiatric research in BH is insufficiently developed. There is no professional psychiatry journal, nor a particular institute for research in psychiatry. Existing research projects are undertaken at the psychiatric hospitals and medical faculties. The main areas of research are currently related to the psychosocial consequences of war trauma. Lack of a uniform database and insufficient development of entity and cantonal public health services represents big problem for research, particularly epidemiological studies.

# References

Ceric, I., Loga, S., Sinanovic, O., *et al* (2001) Reconstruction of mental health services in Bosnia and Herzegovina. *Medicinski Arhive*, **55 (suppl. 1)**, 5–23.

de Jong, K. & Stickers, R. (2003) Early psychosocial interventions for war-affected populations. In *Early Interventions in Emergencies* (eds R. Orner & U. Schnyder), pp. 184–192. Oxford University Press.

Hasanovic, M., Sinanovic, O., Pajevic, I., *et al* (2006) Post-war mental health promotion in Bosnia and Herezgovina. *Psychiatria Danubina*, **8**, 74–78.

Jensen, B. S. & Ceric, I. (1994) *Community-Oriented Mental Health Care in Bosnia and Herzegovina: Strategy and Model Project*. WHO Office for Bosnia and Herzegovina.

Nelson, B. S. (2003) Post-war trauma and reconciliation in Bosnia and Herzegovina: observations, experiences, and implications for marriage and family therapy. *American Journal of Family Therapy*, **31**, 305–316.

Pajevic, I., Sinanovic, O. & Hasanovic, M. (2005) Religiosity and mental health. *Psychiatria Danubina*, **17**, 84–89.

Regional Office of the Mental Health Project for South-Eastern Europe (2004) *Mental Health Policies and Legislation in South-Eastern Europe*. Available at http://www.euro.who.int/document/E88509.pdf (last accessed November 2008).

World Health Organization (2005) *Mental Health Atlas, Bosnia and Herzegovina*. Available at http://www.who.int/globalatlas/predefinedReports/MentalHealth/Files/BA_Mental_Health_Profile.pdf (last accessed November 2008).

# Croatia

## Sladjana Strkalj Ivezic, Martina Rojnic Kuzman and Maja Silobrcic Radic

The Republic of Croatia is in central Europe, on the Mediterranean. A large majority of its 4 440 000 inhabitants are Croats (89.6%). The main religion is Roman Catholicism (88%). Sixteen per cent of the population is aged over 65 years. Croatia was a part of Yugoslavia after the Second World War until 1991, when Croatia declared independence. Following the declaration, Croatia was attacked by the Yugoslav army and by Serbia and suffered a devastating war (1991–95). The transition had consequences for mental health, for example a dramatic rise in the prevalence of post-traumatic stress disorder, especially among soldiers. The majority of soldiers received appropriate psychiatric treatment; there has, however, been an increase in claims motivated by secondary gain, as a result of government policy.

Croatia is a member of the United Nations, the Council of Europe and the North Atlantic Treaty Organization (NATO), and has applied to join the European Union (EU). The EU application is expected to help Croatia shift the focus of its mental health system to community psychiatry.

## Mental health policy and legislation

Mental health policy is a construct of the overall health policy, under legislation from the Croatian Ministry of Health and Welfare (CMHW). Currently, two initiatives to define mental health policy are being developed by the CMHW and the Croatian National Institute of Public Health (CNIPH): the Croatian Alcohol Action Plan (2006) and the National Mental Health Strategy (2009).

The legislation stipulates that mental healthcare is to be provided at primary, secondary and tertiary levels. The primary level comprises general practitioners (GPs), school medicine specialists and mental health professionals in mental health centres and in public health institutes. The secondary level comprises mental health professionals, mainly psychiatrists. The tertiary level – the prevention of mental illness, the promotion of mental health, epidemiology and mental health statistics – is the reponsibility of mental health professionals, the Croatian Institute for Mental Health and the CNIPH, and incorporates the Croatian Psychosis Registry, the Croatian Suicide Registry, and the Croatian National Registry of Treated Psychoactive Drug Addicts.

Other potential creators of the mental health policy, such as mental health professionals and mental service users' organisations, are only marginally involved.

The health budget is covered by social insurance and is tax based. There is no separate budget allocation for mental health, except for drug addictions. Basic healthcare is obligatory for all and is provided by the Croatian Health Insurance Institute. This covers the treatment of all mental illnesses and the cost of antipsychotic drugs. Supplementary and private insurance are possible but uncommon.

## Mental health service delivery

Although GPs are highly accessible, psychiatric diagnoses comprised only 4.8% of all GP diagnoses in 2007 (CNIPH, 2008) and most service provision for serious mental illness is restricted to psychiatrists (Gater *et al*, 2005; Rojnic Kuzman *et al*, 2009*a*). For years, mental disorders have accounted for 6–7% of the overall hospital morbidity rate in Croatia. Most of these hospital admissions are for people aged 20–59 years, which makes mental illness one of the leading causes of hospital morbidity in the occupationally active age group and therefore one of the top health priorities (Fig. 1) (CNIPH, 2008).

Patients with a mental illness are largely cared for within hospital; 1 in 4–5 days of treatment provided in hospitals is for mental disorders (CNIPH, 2008). The therapeutic community movement has promoted the organisation of in-patient programmes and day hospitals. Today, the majority of psychiatric wards and hospitals also offer day programmes for patients with various diagnoses. Unfortunately, this has not facilitated the

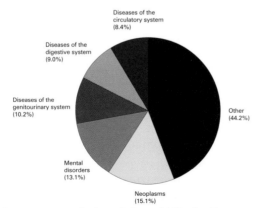

**Fig. 1** Leading disease groups in hospital morbidity for the age group 20–59 years, Croatia, 2007.

deinstitutionalisation of patients as it did in the USA and Europe. After hospital discharge, the majority of patients are treated as out-patients; they generally visit a psychiatrist once a month, or more frequently in psychotherapy sessions. Group psychodynamic psychotherapy, for patients with various diagnoses, including psychosis, is practised in the majority of psychiatric institutions.

There are a total of 3421 psychiatric beds in psychiatric hospitals, plus 426 in psychiatric wards in general hospitals and 428 in university psychiatric departments. The average duration of hospital treatment is 48.8, 12.1 and 17.0 days in these institutions, respectively (CNIPH, 2008).

There are very few rehabilitation and employment programmes for those with severe mental illness. The exceptions include initiatives at the Mental Health Centre and the Community Rehabilitation Centre in Zagreb, some hospitals with programmes for patients in a first episode of psychosis, self-help groups for patients and interventions for the involvement of patients' families in therapy and case management programmes (Gruber *et al*, 2006; Ivezic *et al*, 2009). There are several active user groups for persons who are severely mentally ill and people with addiction problems, which may be able to offer more comprehensive programmes on housing and employment in the near future.

Child and adolescent psychiatry (CAP) services lack both infrastructure (adequate centres and hospitals) and specialists. Preventive work in the field of mental health and mental health promotion was delegated to the National Programme for the Prevention and Treatment of Drug Addiction and the Croatian National Programme Against Stigma (CNIPH, 2008; Ivezic, 2002), but the latter was never applied (Ivezic, 2002).

Overall, there is poor collaboration between care providers at the three levels of healthcare. Unfortunately, one of the most comprehensive mental health programmes, which was supported by the majority of mental health policy makers, was never implemented (Croatian Psychiatric Association *et al*, 2001).

# Workforce issues

In Croatia, there are currently 389 psychiatrists, 47 neuropsychiatrists and 105 psychiatric trainees. Psychiatrists work mainly in hospital in-patient and out-patient services. The few private psychiatrists in Croatia do not work additionally in the public health sector. Other mental health professionals include 1669 nurses, 130 psychologists, and 26 social workers and occupational therapists, working mainly in hospitals.

# Education

The undergraduate medical programme is offered at four state medical schools; it lasts 6 years. After medical school and a 1-year internship, doctors obtain their licence by passing the state examination. Residency training usually follows. While waiting for a place on a residency programme, doctors usually work as GPs in specialised institutions or on scientific projects as research assistants. Postgraduate studies last 3 years.

Residency training in psychiatry follows the national programme developed by the Ministry of Health and Welfare. It lasts 4 years and comprises several parts: introduction (6 months), clinical psychiatry (18 months), alcoholism and addictions (3 months), psychological medicine (9 months), community psychiatry (5 months), forensic psychiatry (2 months), CAP (3 months) and neurology (3 months).

In two studies (Strkalj Ivezic *et al*, 2003; Rojnic Kuzman *et al*, 2009*b*), this programme was rated as generally unsatisfactory by the majority of residents. This is due to the lack of correlation between the training provided and the official programme outline, the inefficiency of the mentoring system, the lack of practical psychotherapy and funding issues. Together with training recommendations from the Union Européenne des Médecins Spécialistes (UEMS, European Union of Medical Specialists), these issues were addressed in the new residency training programme developed by an independent commission formed from representatives of the UEMS, academic staff and the Croatian Medical Chamber. This new programme was due to start in 2009.

To become a subspecialist, a psychiatrist enrols in subspecialty training, according to a programme designed by the CMHW. There are five subspecialties in Croatia: biological psychiatry; child and adolescent psychiatry; forensic psychiatry; psychotherapy; and social psychiatry. In addition, national psychiatric associations continually organise education for the subspecialties.

The ability of nurses to specialise in psychiatry during their undergraduate study represents an advancement of the education system for mental health professionals.

# Research and publications

Croatian residents show an interest in science – about a third of them attend postdoctoral studies and publish scientific papers during their residency training (Fig. 2) (Rojnic Kuzman *et al*, 2009*b*). However, research activities are somewhat discouraged among residents; for example, the majority of residents rarely go abroad for scientific education. Also, the cost of doctoral studies is high compared with salaries (Rojnic Kuzman *et al*, 2009*b*).

Research projects in the field of mental health are mostly funded by the Ministry of Science, Education and Sport and recently by international funding sources. As judged by the type of ongoing scientific projects and published scientific papers, the main areas of psychiatric research in Croatia include addiction, war-related anxiety disorders and post-traumatic stress

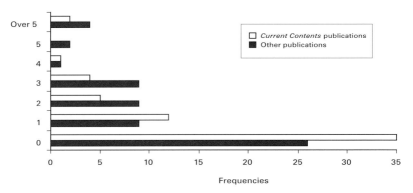

**Fig. 2** Number of publications by Croatian residents, 2006 ($n = 66$, 89% of all psychiatric trainees in Croatia).

disorder, pharmacogenetics and genomics, suicidality, pharmacotherapy, neuroscience, education and social psychiatry.

There are two professional scientific journals in the field of mental health: *Social Psychiatry* and *Psychiatria Danubina*.

## International collaboration

Croatia is an associate member of the UEMS Board and Section of Psychiatry. The Croatian Psychiatric Association is a regular member of the World Psychiatric Association (WPA). In addition, Croatian residents and young psychiatrists are actively involved in the work of the European Federation of Psychiatric Trainees and thus the UEMS, and in the existing networks of young psychiatrists within the WPA and the European Psychiatric Association.

The World Health Organization (WHO) has an office in Zagreb. Croatia has a mental health representative in the WHO and collaborates with the WHO on many joint programmes, such the Stability Pact Initiative for the Development of Community Mental Health Centres, which resulted in the opening of the aforementioned Mental Health Centre and the Community Rehabilitation Centre in Zagreb.

On the other hand, few non-governmental organisations working in the field of mental health have participated in international programmes on stigma and human rights.

## Conclusion

Despite the initiatives for the improvement of overall mental healthcare in Croatia in the past two decades, there is a need for organised mental health services in the community.

# Sources

*Naroden Novine* (*People's Newspaper*) is the official gazette of the Republic of Croatia. The following are available in Croatian:

Zakon o zdravstvenoj zaštiti [Health care law]. *Narodne Novine* (2008), **150**.

Plan i program mjera zdravstvene zaštite [Healthcare measure plan and programme]. *Narodne Novine* (2006), **126**.

Zakon o obveznom zdravstvenom osiguranju [Obligatory health insurance law]. *Narodne Novine* (2008), **150**.

Croatian National Institute of Public Health (2008) *Croatian Health Service Yearbook 2007*. CNIPH.

Croatian Psychiatric Association, Croatian Medical Association, Croatian Society for Clinical Psychiatry, Psychiatric Department, University of Illinois, USA (2001) *Plan reorganizacije službe za mentalno zdravlje u RH*. [The re-organization plan for the mental health services based on the model of community pychiatry.]

Gater, R., Jordanova, V., Maric, N., *et al* (2005) Pathways to psychiatric care in eastern Europe. *British Journal of Psychiatry*, **186**, 529–535.

Gruber, E. N., Kajevic, M., Agius, M., *et al* (2006) Group psychotherapy for parents of patients with schizophrenia. *International Journal of Social Psychiatry*, **52**, 487–500.

Ivezic, S. (2002) *Nacionalni Program borbe protiv Stigme Psihicke Bolesti*. 42. [National programme against the stigma associated with mental illnesses.] Medunarodni neuropsihijatrijski simpozij.

Ivezic, S., Muzinic, L. & Vidulin, I. (2009) Program koordiniranog lijecenja (case managment) u rehabilitaciji osoba s psihoticnim poremecajem. [The program of coordinated treatment (case management) in the rehabiliation of people with psychotic disorders.] *Socijalna psihijatrija* (in press).

Rojnic Kuzman, M., Bolanca, M. & Rojnic Palavra, I. (2009a) General practice meeting the needs for psychiatric care in Croatia. *Psychiatria Danubina* (in press).

Rojnic Kuzman, M., Jovanovic, N., Vidovic, D., *et al* (2009b) Problems in the current psychiatry residency training program in Croatia: residents' perspective. *Collegium Antropologicum*, **33**, 217–223.

Strkalj Ivezic, S., Folnegovic Smalc, V. & Bajs Bjegovic, M. (2003) Procjena programa specijalizacije iz psihijatrije [The evaluation of the psychiatry residency programme]. *Lijec Vjesn*, **125**, 36–40.

# Czech Republic

Jirí Raboch

The profound political, social and economic changes that occurred after the end of communist rule in Central Europe in 1989 had a profound influence on Czech psychiatry. In the socialist Czechoslovakia the healthcare system was fully owned, financed and organised by the state, in so-called regional institutes of healthcare. These had obligatory catchment areas of about 100 000 inhabitants and comprised in-patient as well as out-patient care facilities, including psychiatry. The main trends after 1989 were decentralisation of the healthcare system, rapid privatisation, especially of out-patient services, and financing through the newly established health insurance corporations.

## Medical education

In the Czech Republic the system of education is similar to systems in other European states: there are 9 years of primary and 3 years of secondary education; doctors do 6 years of study in medical school. Psychiatry is usually taught during the 4th, 5th or 6th year, mainly in a 3- to 4-week course, totalling about 60–100 hours. Classes typically have about 10 students. There are also obligatory courses in medical psychology and ethics and electives in psychotherapy and in communication skills.

Postgraduate training of physicians was until recently centralised and organised by the Institute of Postgraduate Studies of Physicians, an organ of the Ministry of Health. A law regulating the postgraduate training of healthcare workers, passed by the Czech Parliament at the beginning of 2004, has substantially changed these procedures. Medical schools as well as other accredited institutions are allowed to participate in postgraduate training. Training in psychotherapy became a common part of physicians' education.

Specialisation in general adult psychiatry includes 5.5 years of practising psychiatry at accredited departments, with rotation in various types of ward and out-patient facilities. Internships in internal medicine and neurology lasting 3 months each are obligatory. There are also special separate courses and specialisations in child psychiatry, old age psychiatry, drug addiction and sexology.

## Service provision

We estimate that less than 3.9% of the healthcare budget has been allocated to mental healthcare, which is one of the lowest rates in the European Economic Area (Commission of the European Communities, 2005). In recent years the number of physicians working in psychiatry (Health Statistics, 2004) has been increasing and in the year 2002 there were 1210 (11.8/10000 population), most (49.8%) working in out-patient clinics. Since 1995 about 80% of psychiatric ambulatory clinics have been in private hands. There is free access to these specialists, who have no catchment areas.

There was no period of rapid deinstitutionalisation in the Czech Republic but the number of psychiatric beds was substantially reduced in the 1990s (from 14/100000 in 1990 to 11.1/100000 in 2002). However, in recent years this trend has stopped. In the year 2002 there were 21 psychiatric hospitals with a total of 10045 beds (four of those hospitals specialise in child psychiatry and have a total of 368 beds) and 33 psychiatric units in general hospitals, with 1546 beds (Health Statistics, 2004).

Every psychiatric hospital has a catchment area of about 1 million inhabitants. The distance from a patient's home is sometimes up to 200 km. Officially, only chronic patients should be hospitalised in these facilities. However, owing to the lack of acute beds in general hospitals about a third of their capacity is occupied by acute admissions. The average length of hospital stay, despite its decline in the last decade, remains high, at 80 days in psychiatric hospitals and 22.5 days in general hospitals. Almost all psychiatric beds (99%) are state owned.

The relatively high number of beds in the Czech Republic can be explained both by the tradition of in-patient care in central Europe and by the fact that psychiatry is substituting for a lack of social care and community services. It is estimated that up to about one-third of the patients are hospitalised for social reasons; these include patients with a learning disability, some with chronic schizophrenia, as well as elderly patients who have no accommodation, relatives or other social support (Raboch, 2003).

There are no official statistics regarding community psychiatry but from the European research project EDEN (European Day Hospital Evaluation) we know more about the functioning of day care centres in the Czech Republic (Kallert et al, 2002). There are 35 members of the association of day care and crisis intervention centres. They are located mainly in larger cities; for example, the capital, Prague, has eight. They concentrate on psychotherapy for patients with various types of neurotic disorder and on the rehabilitation of patients with chronic psychiatric illnesses, such as schizophrenia or alcohol and drug dependencies. Programmes for older adults with dementias are still lacking. In the treatment of acute psychiatric disorders, day care centres are not very frequently employed as an alternative to hospitalisation.

## Legislation and patients' rights

Under Czech law there is neither a specific act on mental health nor a comprehensive act regulating involuntary admission, involuntary treatment or use of coercive measures concerning persons with a mental illness. As a principle, diagnostic and therapeutic measures may be carried out only with the consent of the person concerned or if the consent can be anticipated. According to the Healthcare Act, diagnostic and urgent measures without the patient's consent may be carried out or a patient may be admitted to a medical establishment if, besides other conditions, a person with signs of a mental disorder or intoxication threatens him- or herself or others.

The Czech Republic has recently been criticised by various European bodies and authorities (e.g. the Committee for the Prevention of Torture and Inhuman or Degrading Treatment or Punishment of the Council of Europe) for using cage and net beds. Cage beds are not used any more in Czech healthcare facilities. Net beds, of which there are about 100–200 in the whole country, are still used (and not only in psychiatric facilities), especially in the treatment of emergency states in patients with a learning disability or psychosis and as a safety measure for patients with dementia with night-time confusion. In recent years their number has decreased rapidly.

Every psychiatric institution has transparent and strict rules on how to use restrictive measures, in what situations they should be used, how to document their use and how to supervise these. However, the number of auxiliary nurses and other healthcare personnel is very low in Czech psychiatric facilities (on average 0.36 per bed) and frequently no other technical support, such as modern seclusion rooms, is available (Commission for the Realisation of Reform of Psychiatric Care, 2004).

In order to stress the international and European involvement of Czech psychiatry in this very sensitive part of mental healthcare, we should mention that two Prague psychiatric facilities are participating in the EUNOMIA project (European Evaluation of Coercion in Psychiatry and Harmonisation of Best Clinical Practise) (Kallert *et al*, 2005). This was set up under the 5th Framework Programme of the European Commission. In the 3-year study period the use of coercive treatment measures in psychiatry in 11 member states of the European Union and in Israel will be mapped on the basis of data collected on two groups of psychiatric patients: those involuntarily admitted and those voluntarily admitted but who feel coerced.

## Professional associations and collaboration

The Czech Psychiatric Association is one of the oldest Czech medical societies. It was founded in 1919, after the formation of the independent

Czechoslovakia (Czech Medical Society, 2000). More than 1000 of the 1200 physicians working in psychiatry are members. It has 16 sections, the most active of which are biological psychiatry, psychopharmacology, forensic psychiatry, child and adolescent psychiatry, social psychiatry, psychosomatics, eating disorders and hospital psychiatry. The Association has monthly meetings and regular working days at the Psychiatric Department of Charles University in Prague.

A taskforce of the Association has prepared a report on the reform of psychiatric care, which has been approved by the Ministry of Health. This pointed to the need to strengthen the continuity of care for patients with severe mental disorders, to widen the system of community care and acute hospital care, and to find adequate and functional boundaries between chronic psychiatric and social care (Commission for the Realisation of Reform of Psychiatric Care, 2004). A special advisory commission to the Minister of Health was recently established for the realisation of the reform and will push for the advice of the January 2005 meeting of European Ministers for Mental Health in Helsinki to be put into practice.

Czech psychiatrists are also very active internationally, especially in hosting various major international congresses. Prague hosted the regional meeting of the World Psychiatric Association (WPA) in 1993, the conference of the Association of European Psychiatrists (AEP) in 2000, the European Congress on Cognitive Behavioural Therapy in 2003, and a meeting of the European College of Neuropsychopharmacology in 2003. A regional meeting of the Collegium Internationale Neuropsychopharmacologicum (CINP) in 2004 was held in Brno. The World Conference for Social Psychiatry in 2007 and World Congress of Psychiatry in 2008 will take place in Prague.

## Conclusion

After 1989, psychiatric care provided in the Czech Republic started to change. New social phenomena appeared that required action (more stressful life, an increasing number of people seeking psychiatric care, drug issues, homelessness, unemployment, etc.) but positive modern trends also emerged, as well as new ways of problem-solving and new programmes. The prevailing institutional psychiatric care is already being complemented by community services and by user and family member programmes. At present, we are looking for political and financial support to be able to realise our very concrete plans.

## References

Commission of the European Communities (2005) *Improving the Mental Health of the Population (green paper)*. COM 484 final. Brussels: CEC.

Commission for the Realisation of Reform of Psychiatric Care (2004) *Reform of Mental Healthcare*. Praha: Ministry of Health. [In Czech]

Czech Medical Society (2000) *History of Czech Medical Society*. J. E. Purkyne. Praha: CLS JEP. [In Czech]

Kallert, T., Priebe, S., Kiejna, A., *et al* (2002) The European Day Hospital Evaluation (EDEN) study: an example of EC-funded mental health services research. In *Psychiatry in Medicine and Medicine in Psychiatry* (eds J. Raboch, P. Doubek & I. Zrzavecká), pp. 103–108. Praha: Galen.

Kallert, T. W., Glöckner, M., Onchev, G., *et al* (2005) The EUNOMIA project on coercion in psychiatry: study design and preliminary data. *World Psychiatry*, **4**, 168–172.

Health Statistics (2004) *Psychiatric Care 2002*. Praha: ÚZIS CR, Ministry of Health. [In Czech]

Raboch, J. (2003) The position of psychiatry among other medical disciplines. In *Transformation of Psychiatry. Praha: Academia Medica Pragensis*. [In Czech]

# Estonia

## Anne Kleinberg

Estonia is a small country (45000 km$^2$) with a population of 1.3 million people. It has undergone rapid change since it gained independence from the Soviet Union in 1991. It has achieved some economic success, although there is a suggestion that this has been at the expense of the mental health and general emotional well-being of the people. In the Estonian Health Interview Survey, depressive symptoms were observed in 11.1% of respondents and their presence was strongly correlated with socio-economic status (Aluoja et al, 2004).

## Health system

The Estonian health system is funded via a national social insurance scheme. The Health Insurance Fund is provided from taxes on incomes of the working population, but it also covers those who have no income from employment. It is a universal scheme, under which medical institutions are reimbursed for treatments provided to all patients.

The first point of contact for the patient is the family doctor. Where necessary, the family doctor can refer the patient to a specialist for consultation or can transfer the patient to hospital. Emergency medical cover is provided to all persons staying in the territory of the Republic of Estonia, regardless of nationality, citizenship or possession of a health insurance card. Psychiatry belongs to the sphere of specialist medical care.

## Mental health policy

There is no mental health policy in Estonia, although attempts have been made to draft one. The first of these was made as early as 2001, when the Ministry of Social Affairs ordered the compilation of a source document of mental health policy from the Praxis foundation. The project was ended in December 2002. The intention had been to gather together all the important organisations and different interest groups in the mental health area, and to draft a well-balanced mental health policy centred on the client's perspective.

The policy document was to have included a hierarchical listing of the most important mental health problems in Estonia, together with their possible solutions. Options for the development of mental health services for Estonia were described, alongside the existing plans for their development. This document was never adopted. There is, though, a Mental Health Act that regulates the provision of mental health services, and this is described below.

While no substantive national progress has been made in the area of mental health policy, the Estonian government, under the supervision of Commission of the European Communities, made a valuable contribution to the European Green Paper (2005) entitled Improving the Mental Health of the Population. Towards a Strategy on Mental Health for the European Union. Furthermore, Estonia has signed the Helsinki Declaration of the World Health Organization.

# Mental health services

Estonia's mental health services have improved considerably over the past 10–15 years. The old system had been modelled on Soviet psychiatry; services are now more centred on the patient and are essentially targeted at improving clients' quality of life.

The Mental Health Act regulates the organisation of psychiatric care and defines the financial obligations of the state and local government in that respect. Under the Act, only those healthcare institutions, physicians and other specialists with appropriate licences may provide psychiatric care. Local governments must guarantee access to social services for people with mental disorders. The law also provides that in order to get psychiatric care the patient may turn directly to a specialist for out-patient consultation, that is, without referral from a family doctor.

Mental illness prevention is the responsibility of the Ministry of Social Affairs. Other legislation relevant to mental health includes the Social Welfare Act.

Psychiatric care is mainly provided on an out-patient basis in Estonia. In-patient psychiatric care is mainly used to help patients through a short-term crisis or for solving complex differential diagnostic and treatment problems. Hospital admission is resorted to only where a period of continuous monitoring is necessary for diagnosis, medical treatment or rehabilitation, or when patients are deemed to be a danger to themselves or others, or are unable to cope without assistance outside hospital. People can be admitted to the psychiatric department of a hospital for emergency psychiatric care or otherwise treated without their consent (or that of their legal representative) only if all of the following circumstances exist:

- they have a severe mental disorder which restricts their ability to understand or control their behaviour
- without in-patient treatment, they endanger the life, health or safety of themselves or others as a result of the mental disorder
- other psychiatric care is not sufficient.

Persons in involuntary treatment may not be subject to clinical trials, or the testing of new medicinal products or treatment methods. The Healthcare Board supervises involuntary treatment.

Biological treatment methods predominate in comparison with psychotherapy. Indeed, the availability of psychotherapy and counselling or emergency help services – for example emergency counselling for family crisis or school violence – is limited. Emergency help on the basis of in-patient hospitalisation is guaranteed. There was little in the way of community-based services during the Soviet period, but these have been expanded year on year. As this process is ongoing, it is difficult to give actual figures.

The provision of rehabilitation services is ensured by the Social Insurance Board.

## Training and numbers of specialists

Psychiatric training is available to graduates of Tartu University's Faculty of Medicine who have spent 1 year in training as a general doctor and who have passed an examination to become a specialist trainee. Training starts at Tartu University Psychiatric Clinic. After 4 years of 'common trunk' training and a final examination in psychiatry, doctors will have the specialty of psychiatry accredited to them by the Healthcare Board. A psychiatrist can apply for the subspecialty status of child and adolescent psychiatrist or psychotherapist from the Estonian Psychiatric Association.

As of 1 January 2002, the structure and quality of the healthcare professions have been governed by specialty and professional associations, such as the Estonian Nurses' Union. For example, these bodies carry out periodic assessment of the competency of their members, although these assessments are voluntary for the professionals. The certification system of the Estonian Psychiatric Association was established in 2004.

Based on workload standards and training requirements, the Ministry of Social Affairs has suggested that the optimal number of psychiatrists in 2015 will be 260. The model takes into account working hours, training sessions, vacations, the numbers of patients and the numbers of episodes of illness, as well as the age and potential migration of doctors currently working in the system. Based on this estimate, the Ministry has submitted a government order for employment contracts for at least eight additional psychiatry residents (including one resident in children's psychiatry) each year. The Estonian Psychiatric Association broadly concurs with these Ministry estimates, on the basis of the numbers shown in Table 1.

## Professional association

The Estonian Psychiatric Association was established in 1989. It has three specialist sections – child and adolescent psychiatry, biological psychiatry and eating disorders – and a section for young psychiatrists and trainees.

**Table 1** Estonia's national requirements for psychiatrists

| Area of work | Basis for estimate | Numbers required |
|---|---|---|
| Out-patient psychiatrists | 1 psychiatrist per 10 000 inhabitants | 130 |
| Child psychiatrists | 1 child psychiatrist per 40 000 inhabitants | 30+ |
| In-patient psychiatrists | Dependent on the number of beds and shifts | 90–100 |
| Other fields – education and research, forensic psychiatry, prison psychiatry | | 5–10 total |

In recent years the members of the Association have been increasingly active. Some important campaigns have related to:

- price rises in connection with mental health services
- the need for a mental health policy
- the need to re-establish child and adolescent psychiatry as a specialty, and in particular the need for more child and adolescent psychiatry centres.

# Research

The main areas of research in Estonian psychiatry are the epidemiology of depression and biological markers of anxiety disorders. In recent years there has been increasing interest in research on the part of psychiatric trainees and young doctors. One obstacle is a national lack of research supervisors, but consequently there has been a trend to work with foreign colleagues.

# Stigma and human rights

A pre-conference meeting on mental health at the World Health Organization's European Ministerial Conference took place in Estonia in October 2004. The matters raised included mental health issues in the workplace, especially stigma and the need of those with a mental disability to find appropriate employment. Stigma was also discussed in the document on mental health policy (see above).

Institutions which mainly deal with human rights in relation to mental health include the Estonian Chamber of Disabled People, the Estonian Mentally Disabled People Support Organisation, the Estonian Patients' Advocacy Association, the Estonian Psychosocial Rehabilitation Association and the Estonian Psychiatric Association.

# References and sources

Aluoja, A., Leinsalu, M., Shlik, J., *et al* (2004) Symptoms of depression in the Estonian population: prevalence, sociodemographic correlates and social adjustment. *Journal of Affective Disorders*, **78**, 27–35.

Habicht, T. & Thetloff, M. (2003) *Financing of Mental Health Services in Estonia. Praxis Working Paper No. 3/2003*. Praxis. Available at http://www.praxis.ee/data/WP_03_20030.pdf (last accessed March 2008).

Healthcare Association (2005) *An Overview of the System of Mental Health Services in Estonia*. Healthcare Association in collaboration with Ministry of Social Affairs in Estonia and World Health Organization.

Statistics Estonia (2006) *Annual Report*. Available at http://www.stat.ee (last accessed March 2008).

# Finland

## Eero Lahtinen

The prevalence of mental illnesses in Finland generally reflects global trends, with a clear increase in the occurrence of depression and anxiety. At any time, between 4% and 9% of the population of 5.2 million suffer from major depressive disorders. Some 10–20% of the population experience depression during their lifetime. Bipolar depressive disorders affect 1–2% and schizophrenia 0.5–1.5% of the population. The prevalence of alcoholism is 4–8%.

The incidence of depression has increased over the past 15 years, in part reflecting better diagnostic practices and more widespread antidepressant treatment but also the altered living and psychosocial environment. Depression has been a growing cause of sickness absenteeism and work disability pensions – although the overall level of work disability has dropped.

Stress and burnout are common among employees, and are experienced in some form by over 50% of the workforce. The recession of the 1990s, the subsequent changes in the labour market, job insecurity and persistent long-term unemployment are all part of the national context for increasing mental ill health, although mental health trends parallel those of other countries. There is also concern about the growing extent of psychosocial problems among children and young people.

## Policy, programmes and preventive work

Finland deployed the first comprehensive national suicide prevention programme between 1986 and 1996. There have since been several other national programmes to develop preventive and early intervention measures in mental health. They include the National Depression Programme, Mental Health in Primary Services, and the Meaningful Life, Early Interaction and the Effective Family programmes.

A mental health policy was initially formulated in 1993. It focused on advocacy, promotion, prevention, treatment and rehabilitation. Part of the mental health policy has been the de-institutionalisation of psychiatric care. A substance misuse policy was initially formulated in 1997.

The Ministry of Social Affairs and Health produced quality guidelines for mental health services in 2001 and is working on quality guidelines for supportive housing for people with mental health problems. The government has also adopted a Drug Policy Action Programme for 2004–07. The national Alcohol Programme was launched in 2004. Comprehensive quality guidelines for health promotion at the local level are in preparation, linked with the updating of the Primary Healthcare Act.

National strategies such as the Health 2015 public health programme and the government's Goal and Action Plan for Social Welfare and Healthcare 2004–07 stress mental health and mental health promotion. Both policy strategies also highlight the need to improve mental health among young people and children.

Ongoing programmes (e.g. in occupational health) to encourage people to extend their working lives emphasise better intervention to safeguard mental health.

Two interlinked national projects, the National Healthcare Project and the National Development Project for Social Services, make mental health and the improvement of mental health services integral to the development of the health and welfare systems.

Prevention to forestall mental ill health is crucial to programmes to develop child welfare. Efforts are under way to boost cooperation between schools, day care centres and healthcare services for the prevention of mental health problems among children and young people, and for identifying problems and providing help at an early stage.

## Mental health services

The healthcare system in Finland is decentralised. It is organised at local level within the country's 432 municipalities spread over five provinces. Some municipalities contain very small and scattered populations. The country has 21 hospital districts and specialised healthcare is provided at this level.

Municipalities are responsible for organising out-patient mental healthcare and rehabilitation through the primary healthcare system provided at health centres and through social services. Specialised mental healthcare comprises in-patient services arranged through hospital districts, as well as out-patient services provided by hospital districts and health centres.

As municipalities have taken a greater share of the responsibility for arranging health services, the role of primary healthcare in organising mental health services has increased.

Since the early 1990s there has been a major shift away from institutional in-patient care for psychiatric patients towards out-patient community care. In 1980, there were 4.2 beds for psychiatric patients per 1000 inhabitants. By 1994, the ratio was 1.3 per 1000 inhabitants. Correspondingly, out-patient visits rose from 520000 in 1980 to 1290000 in 1997.

A challenge for mental healthcare is to reduce regional disparities in quality and availability of services and ensure comprehensive mental health planning at local level. Programmes seek to develop supportive out-patient services for long-term patients, with more supported housing, day centres, support staff and guided leisure activities, and improved support for carers.

## Rehabilitation

Occupational healthcare focuses on vocational rehabilitation in addition to preventive work. The Social Insurance Institution and labour authorities have responsibility for organising vocational rehabilitation. The Ministry of Social Affairs and Health has focused on the need for increased support for rehabilitation services. An active approach to rehabilitation in general, and that relating to mental health problems in particular, is a characteristic of Finnish health policy.

The report of an expert group appointed by the Ministry of Social Affairs and Health (Lehto *et al*, 2005) highlighted various needs in the area of rehabilitation that are being addressed in current work. They include:

- the crucial role of psychotherapy and the need to link it to other activities promoting functional capacity and social interaction
- an emphasis on rehabilitation services, and especially vocational rehabilitation, for example by increasing the training and skills of rehabilitation professionals
- cooperation between occupational health services, workplaces and rehabilitation providers.

## Organisations

In addition to local authorities, numerous non-governmental organisations play a central role in providing mental health services and rehabilitation. The largest include:

- the Finnish Association for Mental Health
- the Finnish Central Association for Mental Health
- the VATES Foundation (which promotes the employment of people with disabilities)
- the Rehabilitation Foundation.

The main state authorities and related agencies dealing with mental health are:

- the Ministry of Social Affairs and Health
- the National Research and Development Centre for Welfare and Health (STAKES)
- the Finnish Institute for Occupational Health
- the Ministry of Labour.

Mental health also features in the activities of other branches of government, including the Ministry of Education, Ministry of Defence and the development programmes of the Ministry for Foreign Affairs.

# Changing profile

Psychiatric care in Finland has been transformed over the last quarter of a century, from a system focused on in-patient institutional care and treatment, when Finland had one of the highest ratios of hospital beds to population in Europe, to one essentially based on community services. Finland's deep economic recession in the 1990s (the most dramatic ever seen in an industrialised country) disrupted the smooth transition to community-based care. Resources were cut and the tight financial situation of the municipalities meant that greater priority was given to somatic, general health services.

Now, additional allocations to mental health services have been granted by the government to support the development of the sector, for example in the context of the National Healthcare Project and the National Development Project for Social Services.

Despite the autonomy of municipalities in arranging services, a large number of municipalities have adopted central government recommendations on mental health and interventions promoting mental health for children. Efforts are under way to tackle regional disparities in service availability.

At the same time, population ageing and the need to encourage a longer working life have raised the profile of good mental health as integral to people's capacity to lead active and rewarding lives.

# Reference

Lehto, M., Lindström, K., Lönnqvist, J., *et al* (2005) *Mielenterveyden häiriöt työkyvyttömyyseläkkeen syynä – ajatuksia ehkäisystä, hoidosta ja kuntoutuksesta.* [Mental disorders as a cause of disability pensions – ideas about prevention, treatment and rehabilitation.] Helsinki: Ministry of Health.

# France

Michel Botbol

French psychiatry is currently facing a period of profound change, as many of what were considered its most specific characteristics and traditions have been called into question. It is therefore difficult to draw a profile of French psychiatry, because it has to take into account a radical splitting between, on the one hand, what is still the common profile of most French psychiatrists and, on the other, the new model imposed by stakeholders and policy makers who want French psychiatry to take on a more Anglo-Saxon profile, with evidence-based practice coming to the fore, for instance.

## Staffing

In this context workforce issues are becoming a major concern for French psychiatrists. Until very recently France was ranked second in the world in terms of the per capita provision of psychiatrists (nearly four times higher than that in the UK, for example), with, at its peak, about 13 500 psychiatrists for a general population of some 60 million. Nevertheless, around 20% of public hospital positions remain vacant, which reflects a growing preference for private practice. There is also a marked geographical disparity: the population density of psychiatrists is 10 times higher in Paris than in the north-east of the country.

Most stakeholders wish to correct the French figure for psychiatrist density. There is a trend to reduce the number of all types of doctor to the European average, but psychiatry is particularly affected in this regard, and since 1990 the number of psychiatry students has dropped by 37%. Accordingly, the number of psychiatrists will be 40% lower in 2020. If there is no significant increase in the number of psychiatric students, or if psychiatrists' freedom to choose their type of practice is maintained, the present disparity in the provision of psychiatric resources will be exacerbated, and a large part of the French population will have very limited access to psychiatric services.

The same disparity also exists for allied professions: France has 58 000 nurses working in psychiatry. Their number is set to decrease with the recent termination of a specific psychiatric nursing diploma. There are also

35 000 psychologists and psychoanalysts, but for historical reasons they are still not officially considered health professionals (the idea was opposed by both medical and psychological organisations for ideological or economic reasons). The psychologist's role in both the public health sector and private practice is limited, because it is not recognised by the national social security system.

## Education

In France, psychiatric specialisation follows a 4-year national diploma programme, which is open to students who have passed the 6-year general medicine programme. Access to medical schools is very tightly regulated. These training programmes are offered by at least one public university in each of the country's 12 regions. At the end of the programme for general medicine the number of positions available for each specialty is decided nationally; for psychiatry (including child and adolescent psychiatry) this number has been recently increased slightly, to 200. Medical students choose their specialisation in accordance with their rank in a national competitive examination at the end of the programme for general medicine.

The specialisation programme includes 4 years of residency training in psychiatric wards with at least 1 year in child psychiatry for future general psychiatrists and 1 year of general psychiatry for future child psychiatrists. Each student has to take a number of 'education units'; most are optional and particular to each university, but some are compulsory, including diagnosis and treatment using different techniques and theories. At most universities this allows prominence to be given to psychotherapeutic techniques and theory, especially psychodynamics and psychoanalysis. However, there is no specific training in any of the psychotherapeutic techniques, the specifics of training being left to each student to choose, through non-governmental scientific associations. Most of the psychiatric wards receiving residents give them supervision for their psychiatric practice rather than specific training in a particular psychotherapeutic technique. There is currently a debate concerning which psychotherapeutic techniques should be included within undergraduate training, and which of the scientific associations should be involved in it. The strength and diversity of French psychoanalytic movements (Freudian and Lacanian) add to the complexity of the problem.

## Mental health policy and programmes

French psychiatry is also facing a crisis over the organisation of its public mental health services. This organisation is still very much based on le secteur, the division of the country in géo-démographique zones of 60 000–80 000 inhabitants for general psychiatry, and of 150 000–200 000 inhabitants for child and adolescent psychiatry. Within each sector a multi-disciplinary team is in charge of all the mental health needs of the population, from prevention through to rehabilitation and different treatment modalities (from ambulatory consultation to in-patient units or day care), under the direction of a psychiatrist. Private hospitals in psychiatry are not very numerous compared with other developed countries. They are generally used for less severe or less acute disorders and for patients of higher socio-economic status, even if in most cases they do not cost patients more because the national social security system reimburses much of the expense.

This sectoral model is valued by most public psychiatrists, who see it as well adapted to the treatment of patients with a psychosis, especially in reducing the burden of chronic psychosis. It has allowed the modernisation of hospital treatment, which was once limited to old asylums.

The problem is that the public service is required to take charge of an ever-growing range of problems, many of them worsened by the disengagement of social agencies with the end of the welfare state model. As a consequence, most of the *secteurs* are no longer able to give adequate attention to many psychiatric patients, either because of waiting lists for ambulatory early treatments or because of a drastic shortage of psychiatric beds (a reduction of 41% between 1987 and 1997, with the mean length of hospital stay dropping from 86 days in 1989 to 52 days in 1997). There has been a corresponding decrease in the medical supervision of psychiatric in-patient units and an increasing use of compulsory and urgent hospital admissions because they are becoming the only way to obtain a bed in overbooked public hospitals.

The future of the sectoral system is therefore being debated and new trends are emerging to try to improve its functioning:

- complementarities between the sectors need to be recognised to take into account the specific psychiatric needs of, for example, the homeless, elderly, emergencies, adolescents and young adults, and infants
- network strategies are needed for specific pathologies (sexual delinquency, schizophrenia, bipolarity, eating disorders, suicidality, etc.)
- rehabilitation programmes are required for the patient with chronic impairment in collaboration with specific social non-psychiatric public or private agencies
- better links with users and their associations are needed.

## Legal issues

The French Mental Health Act gives priority to medical considerations and a limited role for judicial power in respect of compulsory hospitalisation. When things are working properly, priority is given to the psychiatric aspect of the hospitalisation needs of the patient. With the reduction in hospital resources and the growing need to protect users from medical abuse, this model has to be revised, at least in some respects. The Health Democracy

Law passed in 2002 increased the power of users and of users' associations, and has given them the right to be informed and to have free access to their medical files.

Nevertheless, since 1992, under a new law governing compulsory hospitalisation (the French Mental Health Act of 1990, which replaced La Loi de 1838, written under the influence of Esquirol) involuntary hospitalisations have nearly doubled (even if these still represent no more than 13% of hospitalisations in psychiatry). At the same time, the number of mentally ill prisoners has never been so high, partly because of a growing tendency to limit the use of sentence reductions for psychiatric reasons.

To deal with both these problems and increasing public concern, special units for dangerous patients were recently developed, changing the type of relationship between psychiatric wards and penal institutions for these patients.

## Scientific issues

Most French research and publications in psychiatry are based on clinical studies. Standardised research studies based on evidence-based methods are still relatively rare. For this reason French psychiatric literature has a low international impact factor. Linguistic considerations may account for some of this under-representation but most of it arises for both theoretical and material reasons.

The French psychiatric tradition values a global, humanistic approach rather than a symptom-focused one. It rejects theoretical reductionism and, as a consequence, is hesitant to adopt the methodological reductionism required by standardised evidence-based approaches. Many French psychiatrists consider that this type of approach is an artefact and does not account for psychiatric subjective reality. The same sort of ambivalence appears when one looks at nosographic issues: most French psychiatrists consider DSM–IV to be a purely research classification that is inadequate for clinical work, and which therefore serves to increase the split between research and clinical reality.

French psychiatry is relatively under-resourced in terms of research. There is no specific research institute in psychiatry comparable to the Institute of Psychiatry in London. There are twice as many researchers at the Institute of Psychiatry as there are in all of France, despite the density of psychiatrists being, nationally, four times higher.

Epidemiological and outcome studies as well as aetiological research are thus relatively rare in all psychiatric fields. However, things are changing, with young psychiatrists placing a growing value on publication in international journals with a high impact factor (i.e. in English-language journals) for academic advancement. Genetic and cognitive work on schizophrenia, autism, eating disorders, bipolar disorders and borderline personality disorders is currently emerging but has yet to be published.

The abundant French-language literature contains valuable theoretical and clinical work on infant and adolescent mental health, bridges with social sciences, attachment and separation theory, developmental approaches in work with children and adolescents, the therapeutic alliance and community treatments. Much of this work adopts a psychodynamic perspective and refers to psychoanalytic or phenomenological psychopathology. Current leading topics are psychodynamic and cognitive approaches to schizophrenia and borderline personality disorders, and psychodynamic and systemic approaches to addiction, eating disorders and infant–mother interactions.

## Professional organisations

Another specific feature of French psychiatry is that there is a division between psychiatric scientific organisations and the professional 'syndicate' bodies. Another uncommon feature is the number of these organisations. French psychiatry has nearly 40 active scientific associations and six specific syndicates. Syndicates are related to different types of practice, whereas the scientific associations were established on the basis of theoretical differences or are closely linked with one of the syndicates. The associations are of unequal importance: some have fewer than 100 members, whereas the larger ones have nearer 2000; some are of historical or symbolic value, but others are directly dependent on a syndicate; some issue a journal whereas others do not; some have only an annual scientific meeting, whereas others have monthly business or scientific meetings. None the less, all of them are federated on an equal basis in the French Federation of Psychiatry (FFP), which was created 10 years ago to try to overcome the weakness of such divided psychiatric scientific representation. International representation is still quite scattered, however. Six of the French scientific associations are members of the World Psychiatric Association (WPA) – the French Association of Psychiatry, the Psychiatric Evolution Society, the Medico-Psychological Society, the French Association of Psychiatrists of Private Practice, the Psychiatric Information Society (public sector psychiatrists) and the French Society of Expression Psychopathology – but it has been impossible to unify this representation under the FFP banner, and French psychiatrists are still rather under-represented in the WPA, as they are in most international and even European psychiatric societies.

# Germany

Wolfgang Gaebel, Jürgen Zielasek and Ulrich Müller

Germany has an approximate area of 357 000 km$^2$. Its population is 82 526 million. The life expectancy at birth is 75.6 years for men and 81.6 years for women (World Health Organization, 2005). The proportion of gross domestic product allocated to the health budget is 10.8%. The per capita total expenditure on health is $2820 (international dollars here and below) and the per capita government expenditure on health is $2113 (World Health Organization, 2005). A major factor in recent German history was reunification, which had a pronounced effect on the German healthcare system.

## History

The term 'psychiatry' was coined by Johann Christian Reil in 1808. In the 19th century, German psychiatry began to develop into a scientific discipline under the influence of Wilhelm Griesinger (1817–68), who focused on a holistic but differentiated approach, covering biological and psychological methods. At the beginning of the 20th century, psychiatrists like Emil Kraepelin, Alois Alzheimer, Kurt Schneider and Carl Wernicke founded the basis of current psychiatric classification systems.

In the period of the National Socialists (1933–45), German psychiatry was partially instrumentalised for political purposes, especially for the programme of 'euthanasia'. This terrible period has been intensively analysed. The review by Seeman (2005) is a useful English introduction to this topic.

In the late 18th and early 19th century, large psychiatric institutions were founded, mainly outside the metropolitan areas. In the last part of the 20th century, the advent of psychopharmacotherapy and social psychiatry changed the picture of German psychiatry. Following the *Psychiatrie Enquête* report of 1975 (see under 'Mental health policy', below), many smaller psychiatric departments were set up in community hospitals but the total number of psychiatric hospital beds declined.

# Epidemiology

The lifetime prevalence for any psychiatric disorder in Germany is 42% and the 12-month prevalence rate is 31% for the adult population, not much different from the prevalence rate in the European Union (EU) as a whole, of 27% (Wittchen & Jacobi, 2005). In Germany, only about 25% of the population with a mental illness are in contact with mental health services, compared with 26% in the EU. Mental disorders are responsible for about 40% of all sick leave from work and 28% of all early retirements (Roth-Sackenheim, 2005). Mental disorders comprise the only growing group of disorders among all cases and days of sick leave in Germany, with an increase of approximately 70% from 1994 to 2004 (DAK Gesundheitsreport, 2006).

There are about 55 000 general practitioners in Germany. Given the 12-month prevalence rate of mental disorders in Germany of 31%, there should be, annually, some 24 million people presenting with mental disorders, but general practitioners treat only about 10 million patients with mental disorders per year.

# Mental health policy

In 1975 a Federal Commission of the Bundestag submitted a report (Psychiatrie Enquête) about the situation of psychiatry in Germany. The Commission defined the targets of a reform of psychiatry. The number of psychiatric hospital beds was reduced from 118 000 in 1970 to 56 392 in 1998. The number of psychiatric hospitals decreased from 216 in 1994 to 195 in 1998 (Fritze *et al*, 2005). There was a considerable increase in the provision of community-based care as part of the psychiatric reforms. The involvement of family members and former patients gained more importance.

Several laws and regulations govern psychiatric medicine in Germany, with the most important being the state laws concerning forensic psychiatry and the federal ordinance determining the staffing of psychiatric hospitals. Furthermore, there is federal support for the prevention of addiction, and the German Health Ministry has issued an agenda regarding addiction research and management, with an emphasis on prevention.

In 1996, the World Psychiatric Association (WPA) started the Global Programme against Stigma and Discrimination because of Schizophrenia – 'Open the Doors' (Sartorius & Schulze, 2005). In 1999, this public education programme was established in Germany and is now being implemented successfully in six project centres nationally. The National Programme to Reduce Stigma of Mental Disorders (chaired by Professor W. Gaebel) is an initiative of the German Society for Psychiatry, Psychotherapy and Nervous Diseases (DGPPN) and a non-governmental organisation, 'Open the Doors' (Baumann & Gaebel, 2006).

There is no federal mental health act.

# Organisation of mental health services

Mental health services in Germany are mainly community based. In-patient services are provided by university hospitals, state or local hospitals. Out-patient psychiatric services are mainly provided by private practitioners and hospital out-patient departments. In addition, specialised psychiatric out-patient services are arranged by local welfare organisations.

# Medical education

Undergraduate medical education in Germany includes a 4-month course in psychiatry and psychotherapy. Although it is a separate medical specialty in Germany, child and adolescent psychiatry is often taught within the general psychiatry course. For historical reasons, psychosomatic medicine is a separate clinical specialty. However, the topics which are found under the heading 'psychosomatic medicine' in Anglo-American countries are found within the general psychiatry curriculum in Germany. Medical students in their final (sixth) year of undergraduate medical school may choose a 4-month elective in psychiatry as one of three clinical specialties in which they receive specialist training.

Postgraduate medical education, to become a board-certified psychiatrist, comprises 5 years of full-time employment in a psychiatric hospital, including 1 year in neurology.

Clinical psychiatrists need to participate in continuing medical education (CME) to achieve a minimum of 250 CME credit points within each 5-year term.

Forensic medicine has been established since 2004 as the only psychiatric clinical subspecialty in Germany.

Psychotherapy is part of the compulsory clinical training in the specialty fields of 'psychiatry and psychotherapy', 'psychosomatic medicine and psychotherapy' and 'child and adolescent psychiatry'. Board certification requires knowledge in psychotherapy in all these specialties. Medical doctors who have obtained one of these specialty certifications may addition-ally acquire a further specialisation in psychoanalysis. Additional board certifications may be obtained by any medical doctor in Germany in the field of addiction disorders, and by any already specialised medical doctor (in any field) or psychologist in the field of psychotherapy.

# Psychiatric workforce

Care for psychiatric patients in Germany is mainly centred on in- and out-patient settings in hospitals and private practices. In addition, rehabilitation programmes, sheltered workplaces and day-care facilities play a large role. Psychosocial counselling is also provided by the states, municipalities, churches and private facilities.

There are about 13 800 specialists in the fields of 'psychiatry and psychotherapy', including the former specialisation in *nervenheilkunde* (nervous disorders). About 4500 psychiatrists in private practice are treating approximately 2.5 million patients per year. Thus, a large proportion of Germans may not have the necessary contact with the mental health system. The results of some surveys indicate that many patients with psychiatric diagnoses are not treated by psychiatrists, but by general practitioners or psychologists.

There are 7.5 psychiatric beds per 10 000 population (4.5 in mental hospitals and 3.0 in general hospitals). The number of psychiatrists per 100 000 population is 2.9 (World Health Organization, 2005).

# Research

In Germany, each of the 36 university hospitals of psychiatry supports research activities. Additionally, the Max Planck Society has a research institute for psychiatry in Munich.

The Ministry of Education and Research established a number of 'networks of competence in medicine' in 1999, among which were research networks for schizophrenia, depression and suicide, and dementia. In addition, the German Research Council and the Federal Ministry of Research and Education fund mental health research. In the major current research funding lines of the German Research Council, few psychiatric topics are included. A complete list would be beyond the scope of this report.

The Ministry of Education and Research supports three psychiatric Networks of Excellence and Brain-Net (total funding approximately c66 million for a 5-year period; Brain-Net is a collection of clinical data and brain autopsy tissues). It also supports addiction research (c33 million over 1991–2004; the current emphasis is on the transfer of research results into clinical practice with an additional funding of c9 million for 2004–07). Smaller-scale research funding is currently being initiated in special research programmes for cognitive science and clinical research.

The German Health Ministry has identified both major depression and nicotine addiction as targets for health intervention, besides type 2 diabetes and breast cancer, among others (Weber, 2006).

# Professional organisations

The DGPPN is the scientific organisation of psychiatrists in Germany (www.dgppn.de). Its objectives are to provide CME, to support legislation, administration concerning all aspects of mental disorders, and the development of international relations. Currently, it has more than 3500 members. The DGPPN has developed treatment guidelines for clinical practice. For example, the guidelines for schizophrenia were developed as evidence-based consensus guidelines (S3 level) (Gaebel & Falkai, 2006).

There are also professional societies for psychiatrists in private practice (Bundesverband Deutscher Nervenärzte, Bundesverband Deutscher Psychiater), senior psychiatrists in hospitals (Bundesdirektorenkonferenz), for practitioners of psychosomatic medicine (Deutsche Gesellschaft für Psychosomatische Medizin und Ärztliche Psychotherapie), and for child and adolescent psychiatry, psychosomatics and psychotherapy (Deutsche Gesellschaft für Kinder- und Jugendpsychiatrie, Psychosomatik und Psychotherapie). In addition, there are many regional and local associations of psychiatrists, plus approximately 30 societies governing special aspects of psychiatry or psychotherapy.

## Outlook

A more extensive report on the current state and trend of mental healthcare in Germany was recently published by Salize *et al* (2007). Some topics have an international background; these include the development of ICD–11 and DSM–V. Furthermore, the new insights from genetic and neurobiological studies will increasingly be transferred to clinical practice. The integration of neurobiology, social sciences and psychology with psychopathology will clearly become a major issue.

German clinical psychiatry is facing tremendous challenges because of the demographic changes resulting in an increased proportion of older patients and an increasing demand from patients from immigrant families. Clinically, topics like somatic comorbidity (among others, the metabolic syndrome in patients treated with atypical antipsychotics), evidence-based assessment of psychotherapeutic practices (including novel approaches to relate clinical effects of psychotherapy to functional magnetic resonance imaging) and the development of evidence-based therapy guidelines are gaining importance, to name just a few.

## References

Baumann, A. & Gaebel, W. (2006) Entstigmatisierung seelischer Erkrankungen. Ein nationales Programm. [Destigmatisation of mental disorders. A national programme.] *Nervenheilkunde*, **25**, 69–72.

DAK *Gesundheitsreport* (2006) See http://www.dak.de/content/filesopen/ Gesundheitsreport_2006.pdf (last accessed 17 April 2007).

Fritze, J., Saß, H. & Schmauß, M. (2005) Befragung der Fachgesellschaften durch den Sachverständigenrat. Stellungnahme der Deutschen Gesellschaft für Psychiatrie, Psychotherapie und Nervenheilkunde (DGPPN) aus dem Jahre 2001. [Questioning of the societies of medical specialties by the board of experts. Statement from the German Society for Psychiatry, Psychotherapy and Nervous Disorders (DGPPN).] In *Die Versorgung psychischer Erkrankungen in Deutschland. Aktuelle Stellungnahmen der DGPPN 2003–2004* (eds M. Berger, J. Fritze, C. Roth-Sackenheim, *et al*), pp. 83–176. Springer Verlag.

Gaebel, W. & Falkai, P. (2006) *S3 Praxisleitlinien in Psychiatrie und Psychotherapie. Band 1: Behandlungsleitlinie Schizophrenie*. [Practice Guidelines in Psychiatry and Psychotherapy. Volume 1: Treatment Guideline for Schizophrenia.] Deutsche Gesellschaft für Psychiatrie, Psychotherapie und Nervenheilkunde. Steinkopff Verlag.

Roth-Sackenheim, C. (2005) Qualifizierte ambulante Versorgung psychisch Erkrankter durch fehlgeleitetete Ressourcenverteilung nur noch Utopie. [Qualified out-patient care of patients with mental disorders only a utopia due to misguided allocation of resources.] In *Die Versorgung psychischer Erkrankungen in Deutschland. Aktuelle Stellungnahmen der DGPPN 2003–2004* (eds M. Berger, J. Fritze, C. Roth-Sackenheim, *et al*), pp. 29–38. Springer Verlag.

Salize, H. J., Rössler, W. & Becker, T. (2007) Mental healthcare in Germany. *Current state and trends. European Archives of Psychiatry and Clinical Neuroscience*, **257**, 92–103.

Sartorius, N. & Schulze, H. (2005) *Reducing the Stigma of Mental Illness. A Report from a Global Programme of the World Psychiatric Association*. Cambridge University Press.

Seeman, M. V. (2005) Psychiatry in the Nazi era. *Canadian Journal of Psychiatry*, **50**, 218–225.

Weber, I. (2006) Nationale Gesundheitsziele zu Depressionen. [National health goals for depression.] *Deutsches Ärzteblatt*, **103**, B1408.

Wittchen, H. U. & Jacobi, F. (2005) Size and burden of mental disorders in Europe – a critical review and appraisal of 27 studies. *European Neuropharmacology*, **15**, 357–376.

World Health Organization (2005) *Mental Health Atlas. Country Profile Germany*. WHO. See http://globalatlas.who.int/globalatlas/predefinedReports/MentalHealth/Files/DE_Mental_Health_Profile.pdf (last accessed 17 April 2007).

# Greece

George Christodoulou, Dimitris Ploumpidis,
Nikos Christodoulou and Dimitris Anagnostopoulos

Since the mid-1980s, a profound reform in the organisation of mental health provision has been taking place in Greece (Madianos & Christodoulou, 2007; Christodoulou, 2009). The aim has been to modernise the outdated system of care (Christodoulou, 1970), which was based on in-patient asylum-like treatment, the beginning of which can be roughly dated to the second half of the 19th century (Christodoulou *et al*, 2010).

Two major programmes of financial and technical assistance from the European Union, Regulation 815/1984 (1984–94) and Psychargos I and II (1999–2007), greatly contributed to the implementation of the reform. Their main targets were the following:

1   the provision of community psychiatric services in sectors ('sectorisation')
2   a progressive reduction in the number of traditional hospitals, in parallel with the creation of a network of housing units
3   the creation of psychiatric units in general hospitals
4   the creation of mobile units in rural areas and the islands
5   the establishment of a network of units for psychosocial rehabilitation
6   the establishment of pilot units for psychogeriatric patients and people with autism.

## Mental health policy and legislation

Law 1397 of 1983 on the National Health System provided the legal framework for the psychiatric reform.

Law 2071 of 1992 aimed to modernise the conditions of care in Greece, especially regarding involuntary hospitalisation, and introduced the principle of 'sectorisation' (the establishment of sectors of 250 000–280 000 inhabitants) in the provision of services.

Law 2444 of 1996, especially articles 1666–88, offers broad legal guarantees to persons under court protection orders.

Law 2716 of 1999 defined the principles of mental health practice in Greece (article 1) and identified the 'units of mental health' (articles 4–12).

Sectorisation was again a key principle. This law also introduced the concept of 'social cooperative units' (Κοι.Σ.Π.Ε.), which give people with mental health problems and other disabilities the opportunity to engage in work.

# Mental health service delivery

Mental health services are provided by the public sector, by non-profit units and by the private sector.

Sectorisation has yet not been systematically organised. There are also deficiencies in primary care and in follow-up, creating increased demand for beds (because the filters that would prevent admission to hospital do not work well).

The dysfunctional aspects of the system are manifest in:

1    the high rates of involuntary hospital admissions (over 50% of admissions in public psychiatric hospitals and 35–40% of those to psychiatric units in general hospitals in Athens, although in other cities the rates are lower – Tables 1 and 2)

2    the frequent use of 'auxiliary beds' in public units, especially in the psychiatric units of general hospitals in the Athens area.

## *Sectorisation – networking of psychiatric services*

There are 13 sectors for the Athens area and three for the area of Thessaloniki. Each sector has in principle the responsibility for out-patient and in-patient care within the sector, but few of them are sufficiently developed to satisfy this requirement. Each sector is regulated by a sectoral committee of mental health (Τ.Ε.Ψ.Υ.), a body whose responsibility it is to

**Table 1** Public psychiatric hospitals in Greece

| | Number of beds for acute patients[a] | Number of admissions per year[b] | Proportion of admissions that are involuntary |
|---|---|---|---|
| Psychiatric Hospital of Athens | 250 | 2800 | 52–55% |
| Dromokaition Psychiatric Hospital (Athens) | 180 | 1560 | 50–52% |
| Psychiatric Hospital of Thessaloniki | 120 | 3300 | 26–29% |
| Psychiatric Hospital of Tripolis | 100 | 1015 | 59–63% |
| Psychiatric Hospital of Leros | 20–22 | 190 | 31–32% |

a. There are additional beds occupied by chronic patients and also in housing units outside the hospitals.

b. The Psychiatry Department of Athens University (Eginition hospital) additionally admits approximately 500 voluntary patients per year.

**Table 2** Psychiatric units in general hospitals[a]

| | Number of units | Total number of beds | Number of admissions per year (approximate) | Proportion of admissions that are involuntary |
|---|---|---|---|---|
| Athens | 8 | 150–160 | 2700 | 35–40% |
| Other cities | 12 | 200 | 5200 | 22–23%[b] |

[a]They generally have 20 beds, but some of these are not always in use, mainly due to insufficient nursing staff.

[b]This figure is approximate and we have not included six units that do not admit involuntary patients.

coordinate the out-patient and in-patient units, which usually belong to a variety of mental health facilities run by various organisations. It is felt that in order to fulfil their mission, the sectors must be adequately funded and be entrusted with sufficient authority for decision making.

## Hospital admissions

Data from 2006 and 2007, collected by a committee established by the Hellenic Psychiatric Association (Ploumpidis *et al*, 2008), indicate the following:

### Public psychiatric hospitals

Admissions to the nine public psychiatric hospitals have steadily diminished since the late 1970s (Madianos & Christodoulou, 2007). Four of them (the psychiatric hospitals of Petra-Olympus, Corfu, Crete and the child psychiatric hospital of Attiki) have practically closed down, although they still provide administrative services to the hostels, out-patient units and psychosocial rehabilitation centres in their areas.

The five fully functioning public psychiatric hospitals maintain many hostels, rehabilitation units and out-patient units. There is a high rate of involuntary admission to them.

### Psychiatric units in general hospitals

Fifty-four hospitals have out-patient facilities and liaison psychiatry, but only 20 of them also have in-patient units. Six more units in general hospitals will start admitting patients as soon as they resolve their staff shortages (mainly nursing).

The majority of these units have been created in the last 25 years. Their contribution to the implementation of psychiatric reform has been substantial. Many of them house university departments of psychiatry.

In the Athens area, many of these psychiatric units are overcrowded and 'auxiliary beds' are used to accommodate the patients. In the rest of the country, conditions are better.

**321**

## Out-patient care

The largest social security organisation (I.K.A.) offers primary care through its out-patient services. Practically all in-patient psychiatric facilities also offer out-patient services.

There are nine mental health centres in Athens, three in the Thessaloniki area and 22 in the rest of the country (a total of 34). These facilities offer the possibility of combining primary mental healthcare, psychotherapy and day hospital services.

Primary psychiatric care is carried out by general practitioners, healthcare centres and psychiatrists and physicians in private practice, especially in rural areas.

Sectorisation is certainly a prerequisite for the meaningful organisation of services, but in spite of efforts this has not been achieved to the desired extent.

## Housing units

The programme of deinstitutionalisation has been based on the creation of a network of housing units. In 2005 there were 377 housing units, 269 state-owned and 108 run by non-governmental organisations (NGOs). These units served 2695 users and employed 3061 professional staff. Recent budgetary problems have affected the operation of these units, especially those run by NGOs.

## Rehabilitation units

In the 1990s, psychosocial rehabilitation developed remarkably in Greece. Social and pre-vocational rehabilitation programmes are still active but vocational rehabilitation has regressed, following increasing difficulties in the labour market. The social cooperative units mentioned above have yet to be fully developed.

## Private facilities

In the Athens area there are 12 private psychiatric hospitals, with a total of approximately 1700 beds. They have a high proportion of chronic patients and bed occupancy approaching 100%. In Macedonia (northern Greece) there are nine units with a total of 1430 beds and in Thessaly (central Greece) there are nine units with a total of 1175 beds.

# Psychiatric training

Undergraduate psychiatric training is carried out in the six medical schools of the country.

There are several available postgraduate degree programmes related to mental health. Postgraduate training is carried out in university and state hospital settings. Specialty training in psychiatry lasts for 5 years and consists of 6 months of training in general medicine, 12 months in neurology and 42 months in psychiatry. There are more than 2000 psychiatrists in Greece.

Child psychiatry was established as a specialty in 1980. Training lasts 4 years 6 months (18 months in adult psychiatry, 6 months in neurology and 30 months in child psychiatry). More than 300 child psychiatrists practise in Greece.

For both specialties, the certificate of specialist training is provided after an oral (and sometimes a written) examination by a committee of psychiatrists appointed by the Ministry of Health. The Hellenic Psychiatric Association has requested greater involvement of the Association in training and examinations as well as harmonisation with the recommendations of the European Board of Psychiatry of the Union Européenne des médecins spécialistes (EUEMS; European Union of Medical Specialists).

# Psychiatric subspecialties and allied professions

Psychiatrists regularly collaborate with other mental health professionals (especially psychologists, psychiatric nurses and social workers).

## Child and adolescent psychiatry

Law 2716 of 1999 introduced sectorisation of child and adolescent psychiatric services, which was implemented only in the Athens and Thessaloniki areas.

One of the main targets of psychiatric reform in child psychiatry was the closure of the Child Psychiatric Hospital of Attiki, which had operated since 1960, mainly with children with severe intellectual difficulties. Reform was achieved with the creation of modern community services.

There are nine child and adolescent mental health centres – eight in the Athens area and one in the Thessaloniki area. Also, three units (of 10 beds each) are hosted in paediatric hospitals (one in Athens and two in the Thessaloniki area). There has been an adolescent psychiatry unit in Athens since 1985 and one in Thessaloniki since 2009.

Six psychiatric hospitals and 20 paediatric hospitals run child guidance clinics. In addition, eight child guidance clinics are run by the Hellenic Centre for Mental Health and Research and two are run by other non-profit organisations.

## Psychiatric nursing and psychotherapy

There are too few nursing staff in the public sector, mainly due to budgetary restrictions. There is a postgraduate, 1-year national training programme for psychiatric nursing, which leads to the Certificate of Psychiatric Nursing.

Training mainly in psychoanalytic, behavioural and cognitive psychotherapies is available at private and university units, affiliated to international organisations.

Budgetary deficits are evident in relation to psychiatric nursing and psychotherapy.

# Research

Research is carried out mainly in clinical psychiatry, biological psychiatry, social psychiatry, community-based psychiatry, psychosocial rehabilitation and psychotherapies. Research is also carried out by non-medical professionals, mainly psychologists.

# Human rights

There has been progress with respect to the human rights of service users. Ethics committees in research programmes are obligatory. Law 2716 of 1999 introduced the Special Committee for the Control and Protection of the Rights of Persons with Psychological Disorders. Its annual reports of 2007, 2008 and 2009 pointed out omissions in several units.

A wide-ranging anti-stigma programme has been implemented since 2000 (Economou *et al*, 2005; Ploumpidis *et al*, 2009) and mental health promotion programmes are being implemented by a number of agencies, notably the Hellenic Psychiatric Association and the Psychiatry Department of Athens University.

# International initiatives

The Hellenic Psychiatric Association has representation on many international organisations (e.g. the WPA, EPA, ICPM, PAEEB, WFMH, RCPsych) and is active in initiatives that aim to increase scientific collaboration with psychiatric societies in Eastern Europe, the Balkans (see /www.paeeb.com) and the Middle East. The Association has mediated locally in Israel, Lebanon and Palestine for the production of anti-war statements, in collaboration with the relevant task forces of the World Psychiatric Association, and has undertaken mental health promotion initiatives in Serbia, Albania, Iraq and Cyprus. Recently it has begun collaborating with the World Health Organization on an 'advanced psychiatry' course in Palestine.

# Conclusion

The Greek mental healthcare system is now largely based on prevention, community care and limited in-hospital care (Thornicroft *et al*, 2008). However, there are serious problems, stemming mainly from funding difficulties and the resulting staff shortages.

# References

Christodoulou, G. N. (1970) Psychiatry in Greece. *International Journal of Social Psychiatry*, **16**, 314–316.

Christodoulou, G. N. (2009) Psychiatric reform revisited. *World Psychiatry*, **8**, 121–122.

Christodoulou, G. N., Ploumpidis, D. N. & Karavatos, A. (eds) (2010) *Anthology of Greek Psychiatric Texts*. Beta.

Economou, M., Gramandani, C., Richardson, C., *et al* (2005) Public attitudes towards people with schizophrenia in Greece. *World Psychiatry*, **4 (suppl. 1)**, 40–44.

Madianos, M. G. & Christodoulou, G. N. (2007) Reform of the mental healthcare system in Greece. *International Psychiatry*, **4**, 6–19.

Ploumpidis, D., Garani-Papadatou, T. & Economou, M. (2008) Deinstitutionalisation in Greece: ethical problems. *Psychiatriki*, **19**, 320–329.

Ploumpidis, N. D. (coordinator), Karavatos, A., Ploumpidis, N. D., *et al* (2009) *Report of the Committee of Psychiatric Reform, Years 2006–2008*. Hellenic Psychiatric Association. Available at http://www.psych.gr (in Greek).

Thornicroft, G., Tansella, M. & Law, A. (2008) Steps, challenges and mistakes to avoid in the implementation of community mental health care. *World Psychiatry*, **2**, 87–92.

# Hungary

Tamás Kurimay

The Republic of Hungary is a landlocked country of 93 000 km² in central Europe; it is bordered by Austria, Slovakia, Ukraine, Romania, Serbia, Croatia and Slovenia. Its official language is Hungarian. Hungary joined the European Union (EU) in 2004. About 90% of the population of c. 10 million is ethnically Hungarian, with Roma comprising the largest minority population (6–8%). Currently classified as a middle-income country with a gross domestic product (GDP) of $191.7 billion (2007 figure), Hungary's total health spending accounted for 7.4% of GDP in 2007, less than the average of 8.9% among member states of the Organisation for Economic Co-operation and Development (OECD, 2009). The proportion of the total health budget for mental health is 5.1%, which is low when compared with, for instance, the UK (England and Wales 13.8%, Scotland 9.5%) (World Health Organization, 2008, p. 118, Fig. 8.1).

Hungary has long been a major contributor to the development of psychiatry, psychology and psychotherapy, through the works of Sándor Ferenczi, Géza Róheim, Melanie Klein, Michael Bálint, Lipót Szondi, Ferenc Mérei, Iván Böszörményi-Nagy, Kálmán Pándy, László von Meduna, Pál Juhász, Mihály Arató and the recently deceased István Degrell (Bánki, 1991; Rihmer & Füredi, 1993).

## Status of general and mental health in Hungary

The average life expectancy for a Hungarian citizen at birth is only 73.3 years, more than 5 years below the OECD average of 79 years. The mortality rate presently exceeds the birth rate, which means the population is declining. More than half the mortality is due to cardiovascular disease (coronary heart disease is the leading cause of death). As elsewhere, drinking, smoking, obesity, unhealthy eating habits and lack of physical activity undermine the health of the population (Skrabski et al, 2005; Tringer, 2005).

The prevalence of both mental disorders and substance use disorders is on the rise. About 300 000–400 000 people (around 4% of the population) experience depression, but only 40 000 of them have a medical diagnosis

(European Commission, 2008). A study applying DSM–IV criteria found the current rate for depression to be 18.5% among people attending primary care, while the rate for major depressive episode was 7.3% (Torzsa *et al*, 2008).

The suicide rate in Hungary remains the highest (after Lithuania) in the EU despite the fact that between 2000 and 2005 the decrease in Hungary's suicide rate was the second largest after Denmark's, not only in Europe but in the world (Rihmer & Akiskal, 2006).

Hungary has among the highest rates in the world of alcohol-related mortality and morbidity (chronic liver disease, cirrhosis and alcoholism). After Moldavia, Hungary has the second highest mortality rate of liver disease and cirrhosis. This rose from 5.0 per 100000 in 1950 to a peak of 83.9 in 1994, although it has fallen since, to 54.8 per 100000.

Between 2003 and 2008, the numbers of patients entering treatment for addiction varied from 13500 to 15500, with between 4000 and 6300 new patients per year. The most common illicit drug was cannabis, followed by opiates, amphetamines and fewer cases of cocaine usage (OSAP, 2008).

# Healthcare system and mental health resources

Hungary's healthcare system is primarily financed through the Health Insurance Fund. The current system of insurance-based funding has contributed to the ongoing funding problems of most mental health programmes and has impaired the ability of psychiatry departments and universities across Hungary to function.

There is no specific law regulating mental health services in Hungary but, on the whole, legislation regarding mental health issues, including protection of the human rights of mental patients, conforms to EU requirements (Tringer, 2005).

In terms of government policy, whereas both the National Programme for the Prevention and Treatment of Cardiovascular System Diseases and the National Cancer Programme have been recently revised, the National Programme for Mental Health was accepted in 2009 but has yet to be financed. In addition, with the Hospital Law of 2006, the government further reduced the number of psychiatry beds (from the previous 4.8 to 3.1 active/acute psychiatry beds per 10000 population) and the same law also closed the National Psychiatry and Neurology Institute, which was the country's largest in-patient mental hospital, as well as an essential research, information-gathering and training centre.

Attempts to strengthen the mental health of children and adolescents have been made, under the National Infant and Children Health Programme (2007–2013). In addition, a Substance Misuse Policy was formulated in 2000 that ran until the end of 2009. The National Psychiatry Centre was established in 2009 to collect accurate, scientific data about the mental health of the population. Since 2008 the Ministry of Health has made greater efforts to participate in EU partnership programmes, including the European Pact of Mental Health (2008); it also hosted the EU Prevention of Depression and Suicide Thematic Conference in December 2009. The Hungarian College of Psychiatry and the Hungarian Psychiatric Association have been working in collaboration with the EU Directoriate General for 'Health and Consumers' and the WHO Europe Regional Office to get through the National Programme of Mental Health (NPMH).

## Activities in priority areas

Two successful current programmes should be noted: the Suicide Prevention Programme in Regions with a Very High Suicide Rate, which aims to determine the effectiveness of an educational programme on the management of depression for general practitioners (Szántó *et al*, 2007); and a programme in Szolnok, which is part of the European Alliance Against Depression collaborative project (Hegerl *et al*, 2008).

Civil organisations have begun to play a more significant role in both health services and social care. The Hungarian Alzheimer Society, representing the interests of relatives of persons with Alzheimer's disease and other forms of dementia, is an example of an effective organisation supporting mental health in Hungary.

## Research

Hungary has no central body coordinating mental health research. Major research centres include: Semmelweis University Budapest's Psychiatric and Psychotherapeutic Clinic (Simon *et al*, 2009); the Mental Hygienic Department, Institute of Behavioral Medicine; the Institute of Psychology of the Hungarian Academy of Science; Eötvös Lóránt University; Budapest University of Technology and Economics Research Centre for Cognitive Science; the University of Szeged; the Albert Szent-Györgyi Medical and Pharmaceutical Centre's Department of Psychiatry; the University of Pécs; the University of Debrecen; the University of Gáspár Károli; and Péter Pázmány Catholic University.

One of the major national sources of finance for scientific research is the National Scientific Research Fund (OTKA). In 2004, Hungary was second in terms of indexed impact factor for scientific publications on neuropsychiatry and psychology (Scheffler & Potucek, 2008, p. 236).

The Hungarian Psychiatric Association organises a congress every year, and over 2000 professionals from the mental health field participate. Its member societies (e.g. the Psychoanalytical Society, the Psychopharmacological Society and the Hungarian Family Therapy Association) also have annual meetings.

# Training

## Medical undergraduate training

There are four medical universities in Hungary, located in Budapest, Debrecen, Szeged and Pécs. Although undergraduate training in psychiatry is based on a national curriculum, the medical universities develop their own programmes. The 6-year medical training includes medical psychology, behavioural medicine and elective courses in psychotherapy.

## Postgraduate training in psychiatry

Hungary is an active member of the European Union of Medical Specialists.

Postgraduate training in psychiatry is a 5-year programme with obligatory theoretical courses. Because of new EU regulations, child and adolescent psychiatry training has been a basic 5-year course in Hungary since 2005.

A secondary specialisation in psychotherapy is available only for medical doctors and psychologists. Psychotherapeutic training is efficiently organised in Hungary, and since 1990 a non-governmental organisation, the Hungarian Psychotherapeutic Council, has been coordinating the standards of training and practice. The Council is an accredited member of the European Association of Psychotherapy.

## Allied professions

Basic training for nurses (BSc) consists of 4600 hours in 3 years and for masters training in a specialty (MSc) another 3 years of training. Postgraduate psychology training for clinical psychology requires 4 years of training and clinical practice. There are accredited postgraduate courses for psychiatric social work.

# Human rights issues

In terms of patient rights, Hungary follows international norms and the EU directives. There are few violations and those that do arise are, in general, a consequence of inadequate infrastructure, or more especially the low numbers of nurses and therapists.

Issues surrounding the treatment of high-risk and violent patients, their legal regulation and forensic management remain unresolved. Hungary has no high-security wards or units, nor does it have a forensic psychiatry institute. The profession has prepared concrete plans for the introduction of both, but these have yet to be officially endorsed.

Current obstacles, future challenges

Key areas for mental health policy and services are:

- integration with primary care
- the skills mix of the workforce

- the implementation of community services
- the collection of adequate information.

Although the National Programme for Mental Health addresses all of these challenges, there are still systemic problems to solve. For instance, community mental health services (community psychiatry, mobile teams, in-home treatment) – an essential part of the Programme, with an emphasis on civil and user-led services – have been introduced in only a few areas.

The overall number of mental health professionals is low and they are unevenly distributed across the country. Many psychiatrists and psychiatric nurses are leaving for jobs in the UK, Sweden and Denmark. As a consequence, there are places in Hungary where basic mental health services are in jeopardy.

# Conclusions

Mental health must overcome party politics and become a government priority in Hungary. This is crucial in light of Hungary's comparatively poor mental health indexes. The programmes need adequate funding for training and research, otherwise the mental well-being of the population will deteriorate further. In addition, there needs to be a willingness to find new and creative ways to strengthen prevention and make treatment more effective.

# References

Bánki, M. C. (1991) Hungary: new horizons in psychiatry? *Lancet*, **338**, 176.

European Commission (2008) *Mental Health Briefing Sheets. Facts and Activities in Member States. Hungary*. Available at http://ec.europa.eu/health/ph_determinants/life_style/mental/docs/Hungary.pdf (last accessed February 2010).

Hegerl, U., Wittmann, M., Arensman, E., *et al* (2008) The 'European Alliance Against Depression (EAAD)': a multifaceted, community-based action programme against depression and suicidality. *World Journal of Biological Psychiatry*, **9**, 51–58.

OECD (2009) *OECD Health Data, 2009*. OECD. For briefing note on Hungary see http://www.oecd.org/dataoecd/43/20/40904982.pdf (last accessed February 2010).

OSAP (Országos Statisztikai Adatgyüjtési Program; National Statistical Data-Gathering Programme) (2008) *Adatok a magyarországi kábítószer helyzetrol (OSAP 1627)*. [Data on the drug situation in Hungary.] Available at http://www.szmm.gov.hu (last accessed February 2010).

Rihmer, Z. & Akiskal, H. (2006) Do antidepressants threaten depressives? Toward a clinically judicious formulation of the antidepressant–suicidality FDA advisory in light of declining national suicide statistics from many countries. *Journal of Affective Disorder*, **94**, 3–13.

Rihmer, Z. & Furedi, J. (1993) Psychiatry in Hungary: past, present and future. *Psychiatric Bulletin*, **17**, 667–669.

Scheffler, R. M. & Potucek, M. (2008) *Mental Health Care Reform in the Czech and Slovak Republics, 1989 to the Present*. Karolinum Press.

Simon, V., Czobor, P., Balint, S., *et al* (2009) Prevalence and correlates of adult attention-deficit hyperactivity disorder (ADHD): meta-analysis. *British Journal of Psychiatry*, **194**, 204–211.

Skrabski, Á., Kopp, M., Rózsa, S., *et al* (2005) Life meaning: an important correlate of health in the Hungarian population. *International Journal of Behavioral Medicine*, **12**, 78–85.

Szántó, K., Kalmár, S., Hendin, H., *et al* (2007) A suicide prevention program in a region with a very high suicide rate. *Archives of General Psychiatry*, **64**, 914–920.

Torzsa, P., Rihmer, Z., Gonda, X., *et al* (2008) A depresszió pervalenciája az alapellátásban Magyarországon. [Prevalence of major depression in primary care practices in Hungary.] *Neuropsychopharmacologia Hungarica*, **10**, 265–270.

Tringer, L. (2005) Hungary. In *Mental Health Atlas 2005*. Department of Mental Health and Substance Abuse, World Health Organization.

World Health Organization (2008) *Policies and Practice for Mental Health in Europe*. WHO.

# Ireland

Zahid Latif

Ireland is the third largest island in Europe and the twentieth largest island in the world, with an area of 86 576 km$^2$; it has a total population of slightly under 6 million. It lies to the north-west of continental Europe and to the west of Great Britain. The Republic of Ireland covers five-sixths of the island; Northern Ireland, which is part of the United Kingdom, is in the north-east. Twenty-six of the 32 counties are in the Republic of Ireland, which has a population of 4.2 million, and its capital is Dublin. The other six counties are in Northern Ireland, which has a population of 1.75 million, and its capital is Belfast. In 1973 both parts of Ireland joined the European Economic Community. This article looks at psychiatry in the Republic of Ireland.

## Health spending and organisation

The Health Service Executive (HSE) is responsible for managing and delivering health and personal social services in the Republic of Ireland. It is the largest employer in the state. The €12.4 billion budget in 2006 was the largest of any public sector organisation (Health Service Executive, 2008). In Ireland, nearly 80% of health spending is funded by government revenues, above the average of 73% among member states of the Organisation for Economic Cooperation and Development (OECD). In 2001, public spending accounted for roughly 78% of all money spent on healthcare. Spending has been increasing in recent years on a per capita basis but is lower as a percentage of gross domestic product (GDP) (7.1%) or gross national product (GNP) (8.5%) than the OECD average (8.9%) (Health Research Board, 2008). The 2004 Health Strategy estimated that Ireland's health spending per capita in 2004 was US$2596 and thus slightly above the average in the rest of the European Union (EU) (US$2550) (Health Research Board, 2008).

In Ireland, as in the UK, general practitioners (GPs) act as gatekeepers of the psychiatric services and specialists can generally be approached only through GPs. As of 1 January 2003, there were 276 permanent consultant psychiatrist posts (171 general adult, 49 child psychiatry, 21 old age psychiatry, 30 learning disability and 5 forensic psychiatry) and 439 non-consultant hospital doctors (NCHDs) (40 senior registrars, 164 registrars and 235 senior house officers) in the public sector and it was proposed that a national target of 421 consultant psychiatrists by the year 2009 and 596 by the year 2013 should be achieved to implement the European Working Time Directive (Department of Health and Children, 2003). This target has not yet been reached.

Irish psychiatry is organised around sectors or catchment areas, based on zones of 25 000–30 000 inhabitants for general psychiatry. Within each sector a multidisciplinary team is in charge of all the mental health needs of the population, from prevention through to rehabilitation, under the direction of a consultant psychiatrist.

## Government policies and planning

In the modern era there have been only two national planning documents for mental health, one a report of a commission of inquiry into mental illness (1966) and another entitled Planning for the Future (1984). Both promoted a move to community care. Planning for the Future, in particular, was a prescriptive document, describing in detail the mechanisms for phasing out traditional mental hospitals and placing considerable emphasis on the relocation of acute units in general hospitals. That, though, is a quarter of century old and can no longer respond to new developments in psychiatry such as advanced community models of care.

A *Vision for Change* is a strategy document which sets out the direction for mental health services in Ireland (Department of Health and Children, 2009). It describes a framework for building and fostering positive mental health across the entire community and for providing accessible, community-based, specialist services for people with mental illness.

## Mental health legislation

Mental health legislation in Ireland has not been given priority. A replacement for the 1945 Mental Treatment Act has only recently been implemented: the Mental Health Act 2001, signed into law in July 2001, was implemented on 1 November 2006. The purpose of this Act is to provide a modern framework within which people who are mentally disordered and who need treatment or protection, either in their own interest or in the interest of others, can be cared for and treated (Mental Health Commission, 2008). The Act brings Irish legislation in relation to the detention of patients with a mental disorder into conformity with the European Convention on the Protection of Human Rights and Fundamental Freedoms (Mental Health Commission, 2008).

The Act also has a second purpose, which is to put in place mechanisms by which the standards of care and treatment in mental health services can be monitored, inspected and regulated. The main vehicle for change will be the Mental Health Commission, which was established on 5 April 2002 under the terms of this Act. Mental health tribunals, operating under the aegis of the Mental Health Commission, will conduct a review of each decision by a consultant psychiatrist to detain a patient on an involuntary basis or to extend the duration of such detention. The Inspector of Mental Health Services, as provided by the Act, will be putting in place a system of annual inspections and reports (Mental Health Commission, 2008).

## Mental health service delivery

We have seen major changes in the delivery of mental health services in Ireland in recent years. Enormous strides have been made and continue to be made in developing a service that is comprehensive, community based and integrated with other health services. This shift in the delivery of services from predominantly hospital-based care has been extremely successful. Under the National Development Plan, approximately €190 million in capital funding has been made available for the provision of acute psychiatric units attached to general hospitals, additional day care, mental health centres and community residences throughout the country.

The development of psychiatric services in Ireland has mirrored the developments taking place internationally. There has been a move from institutional to community care and a marked decline in hospitalised morbidity. This decline has resulted primarily from a reduction in the number of long-stay patients. At the same time, however, admissions to mental hospitals have risen substantially, placing considerable pressure on acute psychiatric beds. A phenomenon has developed of rapid turnover, with a cycle of readmission, short length of stay and often premature discharge, leading to further readmissions (Health Research Board, 2007).

In Ireland, the rate of private health insurance has increased steadily over time, from around 22% in 1979 to around 50% currently (Health Research Board, 2008). Private hospitals in psychiatry are not very numerous in Ireland compared with other high-income countries: there are in fact only two, St Patrick's Hospital and St John of God Hospital, both in Dublin. Very few psychiatric patients with severe and long-term illness have private insurance.

Central Mental Hospital is probably the oldest forensic secure hospital in Europe, having opened in 1850. The hospital admits approximately 150 patients per year, from the criminal justice system and also from the psychiatric services under the provisions of the Mental Health Act. It also provides a consultative assessment service for the prison service and for hospitals throughout the country. As the prison population has expanded in recent years, the services of the Central Mental Hospital have come under increasing pressure, resulting in delays in the transfer of prisoners with a mental illness to the hospital (National Forensic Mental Health Services, 2008).

The voluntary sector plays an integral role in the provision of health and personal social services in Ireland. The Commission on Health Funding in 1989 highlighted the immensely important role of voluntary organisations in Ireland. A recently published Amnesty International report acknowledged the funding which is being made available by the Department of Health and Children to support groups and organisations such as Schizophrenia Ireland, Mental Health Ireland, GROW and AWARE to heighten awareness and develop support services for mental health service users and carers (Department of Health and Children, 2008).

## Training and education

The academic departments of psychiatry in all medical schools have undergraduate training programmes, which feature 6 weeks of clinical attachments as well as classroom teaching of psychiatry.

In Ireland, psychiatric specialisation follows the Royal College of Psychiatrists' guidelines in terms of training and assessment. There is no specialisation examination in Ireland at present, except the Diploma in Clinical Psychiatry (DCP), which is designed for GPs. There is the possibility of an MD, which is usually research based, and which most psychiatrists do after they have passed the membership examination. After an overhaul of training, assessment and accreditation in the UK, Ireland has to develop its own system of psychiatric specialisation before 2011, but work is very slow, probably owing to lack of financial resources for educational research.

The All Ireland Institute of Psychiatry arranges two scientific meetings every year.

Since 1 January 2009, the College of Psychiatry of Ireland has been fully operational as the sole body responsible for continuing professional development (CPD), postgraduate training, mental health policy and external relations.

## Research and publications

Lack of indigenous research has been a major hindrance to the rational planning and allocation of resources; however, over the past few years a number of research papers have been published.

*Reach Out – A National Strategy for Action on Suicide Prevention*, a 10-year strategy, was launched on September 2005, which was developed by the HSE and National Suicide Review Group (Department of Health and Children, 2008). The National Office for Suicide Prevention is committed to supporting research in the areas of suicide research/prevention and mental health promotion (National Office for Suicide Prevention, 2009).

The Health Promotion Research Centre is located at the National University of Ireland, Galway. The Centre was established in 1990 to conduct research on health promotion in an Irish context. It is the only designated research centre in Ireland dedicated to health promotion. The Centre collaborates with regional, national and international agencies on the development and evaluation of health promotion strategies and has published widely in the field of mental health promotion (National University of Ireland, Galway, 2009)

The quarterly *Irish Journal of Psychological Medicine*, Ireland's only peer-reviewed psychiatric journal, has been supporting and encouraging original Irish psychiatric and psychological research. Irish psychiatric literature has a low international impact factor and Irish psychiatry is relatively underresourced in terms of research.

# References

Department of Health and Children (2003) *Report of National Task Force on Medical Staffing (Hanly report)*. Available at http://www.dohc.ie/publications/pdf/hanly.pdf (last accessed 12 January 2009).

Department of Health and Children (2008) *Latest Publications: Press Releases*. Available at http://www.dohc.ie (last accessed 20 December 2008).

Department of Health and Children (2009) *'A Vision for Change'*. Report of the Expert Group on Mental Health Policy. Available at http://www.dohc.ie/publications/vision_for_change.html (last accessed 11 January 2009).

Health Research Board (2007) *NPIRS – National Psychiatric Inpatient Reporting System*. Available at http://www.hrb.ie/health-information-in-house-research/mental-health/information-systems/npirs-national-psychiatric-in-patient-reporting-system (last accessed 29 October 2007).

Health Research Board (2008) *Health Information and In-house Research*. Available at http://www.hrb.ie (last accessed 2 December 2008).

Health Service Executive (2008) *Annual Report 2006*. Available at http://www.hse.ie (last accessed 29 October 2008).

Mental Health Commission (2008) *Information: Publications*. Available at http://www.mhcirl.ie (last accessed 28 December 2008).

National Forensic Mental Health Services (2008) *Introduction: Background*. Available at http://www.centralmentalhospital.ie/en/AboutUs/Intro-Backround (last accessed 20 December 2008).

National Office for Suicide Prevention (2009) *Research*. Available at http://www.nosp.ie/html/research.html (last accessed 13 January 2009).

National University of Ireland, Galway (2009) *Health Promotion*. Available at http://www.nuigalway.ie/health_promotion/research/index.htm (last accessed 13 January 2009).

# Italy

Angelo Fioritti, Mariano Bassi and Giovanni de Girolamo

Italian psychiatry is probably more debated than known in the international arena. Law 180 of 1978, which introduced a radical community psychiatry system, has drawn worldwide attention and debate, with comments ranging from the enthusiastic to the frankly disparaging (Mosher, 1982; Jones et al, 1991). More recently, this interest was marked by a well-attended symposium 'Lessons Learned from Italian Reforms in Psychiatry' held at the 2003 annual meeting of the Royal College of Psychiatrists in Edinburgh.

Historical analyses of how the reform movement took momentum, produced a law and how it was enacted can be found elsewhere (Perris & Kemali, 1985; Saraceno & Tognoni, 1989; Mangen, 1989; Fioritti et al, 1997). In this article we try to outline the general social context in Italy, its health and psychiatric services, their organisation, functioning and culture.

## Italian communities at a glance

Italy is a country of 56995744 inhabitants (census of 21 October 2001) and its economy is the world's seventh largest in terms of gross domestic product (GDP) (World Bank, 2003). It has the world's fifth highest life expectancy at birth (76.9 years for men and 83.3 years for women) (World Health Organization, 2003).

Administratively, the country is divided into 20 regions and 109 provinces. Because of its historical fragmentation until reunification in 1870, striking social and economic differences persist across the nation. Per capita income, economic activities, distribution of wealth, rates of unemployment and the development of welfare services are still very different in northern-central compared with southern regions. In acknowledgement of this, a policy of devolution is now transferring most administrative powers to regional councils; notably, this includes all functions related to planning and management of health services. This explains the remarkable differences in models and implementation of psychiatric services, whose landscape has been described as 'patchy and confused' (Freeman et al, 1985).

Although rapid demographic changes are occurring (in particular, massive immigration is compensating for a decrease in the native population, which presently has a low birth rate), Italian society is still based on strong family links and demographic stability. Recent comparative studies (Warner *et al*, 1998; Fioritti *et al*, 2002) have shown that over 70% of patients with psychosis live with their family, in accommodation they own and in which they have typically lived for about 20 years. Patients are usually well protected from certain psychosocial stresses (e.g. housing and financial problems) but quite dependent on significant others, whose involvement in the care process is almost always required. Families are fundamental stakeholders in health administration and their associations have become very influential on national and regional mental health policies (e.g. becoming providers of mental health services or supporting bills to reform current legislation).

## Healthcare and psychiatric services

Italy has had a National Health Service (NHS) since 1978, when a comprehensive public health policy was adopted. The NHS absorbs about 6% of the nation's GDP, while an additional 2–3% of it is spent on private health services. About 5% of NHS resources are allocated to child and adult psychiatry, excluding services for drug misuse and learning disabilities. It is generally held that the implementation of the NHS has achieved good results in the northern regions but failed most of its promises in the south, mostly because of pre-existing social and economic factors (Putnam, 1993).

The NHS is organised through 401 local health trusts (aziende unità sanitarie locali – AUSL), each caring for a geographically defined population of 200000–500000 inhabitants. They have full economic accountability and reasonable autonomy in planning, managing and evaluating services. Each AUSL has one mental health department (dipartimento di salute mentale – DSM), which provides comprehensive psychiatric care for the local population and manages on a unitary basis the full set of necessary services (as stipulated within national policy documents):

- community mental health centres (CMHCs)
- day-hospital/day-care rehabilitation centres
- psychiatric wards within a general hospital (servizio psichiatrico di diagnosi e cura – SPDC)
- non-hospital residential medium- and long-term facilities (NHRF).

Regional and local differences can be found as to standards (i.e. number of beds, allocation of resources to each unit within the department), integration of private services within the DSM and integration with child psychiatry, drug misuse and learning disabilities services.

This system is the end-point of a process started by Law 180 of 1978, which had five key effects:

1 all mental hospitals were gradually phased out, with a halt to all new admissions
2 general hospital psychiatric wards (SPDCs) were established, each with a maximum of 15 beds

3    severe limitations were set on procedures for compulsory admissions and on their length (maximum 7 days, renewable weekly)

4    the CMHCs were established to provide psychiatric care to geographically defined areas

5    all new and old public psychiatric services were integrated within the NHS.

The 1980s saw the establishment of the CMHCs, the deinstitutionalisation of patients from the mental hospitals, who were usually moved into small NHRFs, and the establishment of the network of SPDCs by the general hospitals. The 1990s saw the establishment of the coordination of all these facilities under the DSM and the adaption of existing services to the new chronic population that was emerging. Only in 1999 were the last mental hospitals closed, thereby bringing a 21-year process to an end. A critical issue of the 1990s was also the integration of economic and quality assurance elements within the management of clinical teams, as required by policies and laws affecting all health services. Throughout that decade, the actual number of professionals employed by the NHS in psychiatry decreased by about 10% (from 34 000 in 1992 to 30 711 in 2002) and so did the number of psychiatrists (from 6276 in 1992 to 5561 in 2002).

Italian psychiatry today represents a multifaceted and complex system (Table 1). CMHCs are well established all over the nation; their multi-professional teams ensure general psychiatric evaluation and care, and often good assertive outreach. These services are grounded in an interesting mix of phenomenology, psychodynamics, and clinical and social psychiatry. The actual number of hospital beds and facilities is among the lowest in Europe.

**Table 1** The composition of Italian mental health services

|  | Number | Rates per 100 000 population |
| --- | --- | --- |
| Community mental health centres | 707 | 1.24 |
| Psychiatric wards in the general hospital |  |  |
| Number | 321 | 0.56 |
| Beds | 3997 | 7.01 |
| Private clinics |  |  |
| Number | 56 | 0.09 |
| Beds | 3950 | 6.92 |
| Non-hospital residential facilities |  |  |
| Number | 1370 | 2.40 |
| Beds | 17 138 | 30.06 |
| Day centres | 921 | 1.61 |

Data from Ministero della Salute (2001) and, for the non-hospital residential facilities, de Girolamo *et al* (2002) (these facilities comprise supported housing with four or more beds with any degree of staff supervision, therapeutic communities and facilities set up as alternative to mental hospitals).

One recent comparison of the psychiatric laws of all European Union countries acknowledged that the Italian law and system pose the lowest level of formal coercion over the patient (Fioritti, 2002). In seven regions, additional hospital beds are acquired from private clinics under 'allowance schemes', but the total number of beds in hospitals remains low. The area of medium- to long-term NHRFs saw a large expansion during the 1990s and now accounts for more beds than the hospital sector (de Girolamo *et al*, 2002).

Challenges currently on the agenda include: collaboration with primary care; the integration with drug misuse services; and the integration (or reform) of the forensic psychiatry sector, which is still a separate system, run by the Ministry of Justice, with very few points of contact with the NHS (Fioritti & Melega, 2000).

## Education and training

Psychiatry is part of the compulsory undergraduate training of every medical student on a degree course in medicine and surgery at any Italian university. It is usually organised as formal teaching (i.e. lectures and seminars), and it is then followed by an oral examination.

Psychiatry is now taught in its own right at postgraduate level as well, having been separated from neurology in the mid-1970s, but still in the 1980s the psychological sciences had little place in medical curricula. At the beginning of the 1990s Italy had to conform to European educational standards and universities adapted very rapidly to these requirements. To become a psychiatrist, the student (who has already registered with the Medical Council before applying to the Psychiatry Residency School) must attend courses for four academic years and must discuss his/her own dissertation at the end of training. Today, residents are fully integrated within the teams of teaching psychiatric clinics or of public health services. They attend theoretical lessons and receive a broad range of practical experiences in general hospital and community psychiatry, consultation–liaison, psychotherapy, rehabilitation and research.

Other mental health professionals do not receive specific training before employment and their education is based on practical experience and educational programmes set up by their employers. In 2000 a formal system of continuing medical education based on credits was set up and has served to greatly improve local educational programmes at both public and private psychiatric institutions.

## Research

Research in mental health has achieved mixed results. Italian psychiatry ranks ninth internationally in terms of the number of papers published and eleventh in terms of their impact (Fava & Montanari, 1998); these contributions largely come from a few distinguished centres (Verona for social psychiatry and epidemiology, Pisa, Milan and Cagliari for biological psychiatry, Bologna for psychotherapy) (Fava & Tansella, 2002). This is not an adequate representation of the intensive national and international scientific life of Italian universities, scientific societies and DSMs. Some research projects whose formal bibliometric impact is low have none the less yielded very significant results and shown that good organisation and commitment can produce good research within very limited budgets (e.g. the 'Progres Project'; de Girolamo *et al*, 2002). Finally, Italian research teams are currently involved in all major collaborative studies financed by the European Union in psychiatry (e.g. EUNOMIA and EQOLISE).

## Professional bodies

The Italian Psychiatric Association (Società Italiana di Psichiatria – SIP) has about 6000 members and has 25 thematic sections. It is very active and supports several educational and research programmes.

Important acknowledgements to Italian psychiatry have come from appointments to international bodies of highly representative psychiatrists: Dr Benedetto Saraceno is currently Director of Mental Health and Substance Dependence at the World Health Organization in Geneva; and Professor Mario Maj is President of the European Association of Psychiatrists.

## Conclusions

As early as 1950, Italian psychiatry was mentioned in international scientific papers for its obsolete and repressive institutions (Lemkau & de Sanctis, 1950). This went on until the reform law of 1978. Deinstitutionalisation has probably met in Italy its more radical form and produced a complex and multifaceted system of community psychiatry which is now actively looking for international comparison.

## References

de Girolamo, G., Picardi, A., Micciolo, R., *et al* (2002) Residential care in Italy: national survey of non-hospital facilities. *British Journal of Psychiatry*, **181**, 220–225.

Fava, G. A. & Montanari, A. (1998) National trends in behavioural sciences. *Psychotherapy and Psychosomatics*, **67**, 281–301.

Fava, G. A. & Tansella, M. (2002) Gli autori ed i lavori italiani più citati nelle riviste internazionali di Psichiatria e Psicologia. *Epidemiologia e Psichiatria Sociale*, **11**, 298–302.

Fioritti, A. (2002) *Leggi e Salute Mentale: Panorama europeo delle legislazioni di interesse psichiatrico*. Torino: Centro Scientifico Editore.

Fioritti, A. & Melega, V. (2000) Psichiatria forense in Italia, una storia ancora da scrivere. [Italian forensic psychiatry: a story to be written.] *Epidemiologia e Psichiatria Sociale*, **9**, 219–226.

Fioritti, A., Lo Russo, L. & Melega, V. (1997) Reform said or done? The case of Emilia-Romagna within the Italian psychiatric context. *American Journal of Psychiatry*, **154**, 94–98.

Fioritti, A., Burns, T., Rubatta, P., *et al* (2002) Impact of the community on intensive community care: A comparative study of patient characteristics and inpatient service use in Bologna and London. *International Journal of Mental Health*, **31**, 66–77.

Freeman, H. L., Fryers, T. & Henderson, J. H. (1985) *Mental Health Services in Europe*. Ten Years On. Geneva: WHO.

Jones, K., Wilkinson, G. & Craig, T. K. (1991) The 1978 Italian mental health law – a personal evaluation: a review. *British Journal of Psychiatry*, **159**, 556–561.

Lemkau, P. V. & de Sanctis, C. (1950) A survey of Italian psychiatry. *American Journal of Psychiatry*, **107**, 401–408.

Mangen, S. (1989) The Italian psychiatric experience. *International Journal of Social Psychiatry*, **35**, 3–6.

Ministero della Salute (2001) *Assistenza Psichiatrica in Italia*. Rome: Ministero della Salute.

Mosher, L. R. (1982) Italy's revolutionary mental health law: an assessment. *American Journal of Psychiatry*, **139**, 199–203.

Perris, C. & Kemali, D. (1985) Focus on the Italian psychiatric reform: an introduction. *Acta Psychiatrica Scandinavica Supplementum*, **316**, 9–14.

Putnam, R. D. (1993) *Making Democracy Work: Civic Traditions in Modern Italy*. Princeton, NJ: Princeton University Press.

Saraceno, B. & Tognoni, G. (1989) Methodological lessons from the Italian psychiatric experience. *International Journal of Social Psychiatry*, **35**, 98–109.

Warner, R., de Girolamo, G., Belelli, G., *et al* (1998) The quality of life of people with schizophrenia in Boulder, Colorado, and Bologna, Italy. *Schizophrenia Bulletin*, **24**, 559–568.

World Bank (2003) Data from the website www.worldbank.org.

World Health Organization (2003) Data from the website www.who.int.

# Lithuania

Dainius Puras

Lithuania is a country with an approximate area of 65 000 km². Its population is 3.422 million, and the gender ratio (expressed as men per 100 women) is 87. The proportion of the population under the age of 15 years is 18%, and the proportion above the age of 60 years is 20%. The literacy rate is 99.6% for both men and women. The country is in the higher middle-income group (by World Bank 2004 criteria).

The health budget represents 6% of the country's gross domestic product. The per capita total expenditure on health is $478 (international $) and the per capita government expenditure on health is $337. Life expectancy at birth is 66.2 years for males and 77.6 years for females. Healthy life expectancy at birth is 59 years for males and 68 years for females (World Health Organization, 2005).

## Cultural context

Lithuania has undergone a marked transition in its economic, social and cultural life. After economic decline in the 1990s, the economy started to grow significantly after 2000. Similar trends can be observed in the dynamics of public health indicators: they reached their worst in 1994; after that a gradual improvement in the indicators of mortality and general morbidity was observed. However, high levels of social pathology remain (including violence, suicides, alcohol misuse and other self-destructive behaviours); this is combined with a stigmatising approach by the general population towards people with a mental disturbance and other vulnerable groups. Lithuania is among the countries with the highest rates of suicide in Europe, and indeed the world (42–44 per 100 000 per year during the last 10 years), with middle-aged rural males the group at highest risk (among whom the rates of suicide exceed 100 per 100 000). According to a World Health Organization (2002) report, youth homicide rates in Lithuania (5.4 cases per 100 000 of the population aged 10–29 years) and other Baltic countries are several times higher than those in 'old' member states of the European Union (EU) and Central European countries, but none the less are three times lower than those in Russia. Recently the problem of bullying in schools has been recognised as a serious issue (it appears that more than half of all schoolchildren in Lithuania are involved in bullying).

## Psychiatric services

Analysis of existing data about financial and human resources invested in the mental healthcare system has raised questions for policy makers about the effectiveness of the traditional investments. Lithuania, like other countries of Eastern Europe, does not have a problem with a lack of psychiatrists and psychiatric services. The largest proportion of physical and human capital is concentrated in psychiatric institutions, with large numbers of beds, psychiatrists and increasing funding for reimbursement for the new generation of psychotropic medications. However, the other components of care are lacking, such as community-based housing, psychosocial and vocational rehabilitation, psychotherapy, community-based child mental health services, and supportive services for families at risk. The political will is needed to develop these as priorities and as alternatives to the powerful system of residential institutions and psychiatric hospitals.

In 1997 a new network of municipal out-patient psychiatric services (municipal mental health centres) was launched; the total number of such centres throughout the country was 64 in 2004. It was a very important first step in the development of community-based services and mental health promotion. However, the composition of staff in the centres is too 'medicalised': the 617 staff members in 2002, for example, comprised 32% psychiatrists, 33% nursing staff, 22% social workers and 13% psychologists. The annual general cost of reimbursement of psychotropic medications prescribed by psychiatrists attached to these municipal mental health centres is two times higher than the sum of the running costs of all the mental health centres (including salaries for mental health teams and other staff).

The number of beds in psychiatric hospitals has steadily decreased, from 5380 in 1991 to 2996 in 2003. However, this has been achieved to a certain extent through the transfer of patients with a chronic mental illness from psychiatric hospitals (which are under the Ministry of Health and funded from obligatory health insurance funds) to psychiatric long-stay care institutions (which fall under the system of social welfare). In these centralised large residential institutions (of which there are over 20 throughout the country) the number of clients is more than 6000. The new network of municipal mental health centres (mentioned above) is not currently able to start the process of deinstitutionalisation, and there are waiting lists for placement in residential institutions, in the absence of alternative community-based services.

Another gap which was identified during an analysis of resources and processes is a lack of sustainable and effective activities in the field of mental health promotion and the prevention of mental disorders. There are many new initiatives by municipal authorities and non-governmental organisations (NGOs) in the field of mental health promotion and prevention; however, these lack a tradition of measuring their effectiveness and sustainability of funding. Also, general practitioners (GPs) are not involved in mental health issues, partly because it was planned that the municipal mental health centres would take care of all people who are in need of out-patient mental healthcare. Now it is becoming obvious that GPs need to be involved as gatekeepers in primary mental healthcare, as the municipal mental health centres are receiving too many referrals of common cases.

These findings may be useful for the development of modern mental health policies in the countries of Eastern and Central Europe, which were deprived for decades of the possibility of introducing evidence-based mental health policies and services.

During an analysis of the performance of the national mental healthcare system, it became clear that existing policies and programmes do not include economic or social outcomes, which should be monitored as criteria by which to measure the effectiveness of resources and processes (services). However, there are some indicator targets which the Lithuanian Health Programme and the State Programme on Prevention of Mental Disorders have been planning to reach, for example to reduce the suicide rate to 25 per 100 000 and to reduce morbidity from alcoholic psychosis to 10 per 100 000 by 2005. It is obvious now that these goals have not been reached; neither has a primary goal of the State Programme on Prevention of Mental Disorders: 'to create an effective community-level network of social psychiatric structures by including NGOs in service provision'.

## Psychiatric training and education

The system of training in psychiatry and other mental health and allied professions is undergoing changes towards harmonisation with EU standards. After 6 years of undergraduate medical education and 1 year of general internship, graduates of medical schools (there are medical faculties at Vilnius University and at Kaunas Medical University) may choose 4 years' residency in two psychiatric specialties – general psychiatry and child and adolescent psychiatry. Courses of continuing medical education are also available in these medical schools. Training courses in psychotherapy are available for both medical doctors and psychologists. Social work is developing as a new specialty.

## Research

Research in the field of psychiatry and mental health is not very well developed, mainly because of a lack of research capacity and the absence of research institutions in these fields. It is difficult to compete for national and international research funds against fields like cardiology, oncology, rheumatology and other traditional priorities in health research, which have separate state-funded research institutes from Soviet times. Most of the research in the field of psychiatry and mental health is carried out at Vilnius University and Kaunas Medical University, by PhD doctoral fellows and teaching faculty. Recently PhD theses have been defended on subjects such as eating disorders, autistic spectrum disorders, depression and suicide. In 2004 the first epidemiological study in Lithuania in the field of mental health was completed – the prevalence of child mental health problems was evaluated by a joint research team at Vilnius University with the use of validated instruments. The first attempts at the evidence-based assessment of mental health systems have been provided by the research team in Vilnius University. The problems of research capacity in the field of mental health and unsustained funding remain unsolved.

# The future

Completion of a 'country profile' (Puras *et al*, 2004) was a very important exercise in the country, which is looking forward to developing and implementing an evidence-based mental health policy and improving both the performance of the mental health system and indicators of population mental health. The country profile revealed a phenomenon common to most Eastern European countries, whereby statistical accounts keep the tradition of presenting processes as outcomes, while the modern assessment of outcomes of services, programmes and policies is lacking. This tradition of monitoring the amount of processes as if they were outcomes creates a vicious circle in which a system of services that do not meet the modern requirements of a public mental health approach and the needs of patients becomes a serious obstacle to the formulation, development and implementation of new mental health policies.

Analysis of the findings from the country profile identified the gaps in the existing mental healthcare system and raised the question of the need for a national evidence-based mental health policy. After a World Health Organization ministerial conference on mental health, the Lithuanian Minister of Health appointed the Committee for Mental Health, which has prepared a draft of a new mental health policy. This draft new mental health policy is currently being debated.

In conclusion, there is an obvious need to establish a modern culture of evaluation, independent assessment and research within the mental health sector in the countries of Central and Eastern Europe (Jenkins *et al*, 2001). These countries fall into two groups economically, with some (e.g. the Baltic states) seeing an improving economy but others experiencing greater economic difficulties. It is the case, however, that both groups have problems in the field of mental health. In this context there is a need for responsible, transparent and evidence-based decisions over the allocation of resources. An improvement is required in the governance of the systems in order to make mental health systems accountable and effective and to enable them to meet the needs of patients. Lithuania could be a good candidate as a demonstration country, with its improving economy and quality of life, in the development of modern mental health services as an alternative to the traditional system of centralised psychiatric institutions.

# References

Jenkins, R., Tomov, T., Puras, D., *et al* (2001) Mental health reform in Eastern Europe. *Eurohealth*, **7**, 15–21.

Puras, D., Germnanavicius, A., Povilaitis, R., *et al* (2004) Lithuania mental health country profile. *International Review of Psychiatry*, **16**, 117–125.

World Health Organization (2002) *Violence and Health*. Geneva: WHO.

World Health Organization (2005) *Mental Health Atlas 2005*. Geneva: WHO.

# Malta

Susanna Galea and John Mifsud

The Maltese Islands are located in the Mediterranean Sea and have a total area of 316 km$^2$. They consist of three inhabited islands – Malta (the largest of the group), Gozo and Comino – and two uninhabited islands – Filfla and Cominotto. Malta is a democratic republic. Since its independence in 1964, Malta has played a more significant part in international relations. It became a member of the Commonwealth, the United Nations, the World Health Organization and several other organisations. In May 2004, Malta also became a member of the European Union.

The organisation and delivery of mental health services, and access to them, are influenced by Malta's sociocultural specifics. Most (98%) of the Maltese population is Catholic and the Church plays an influential role in Maltese society. It contributes to the Maltese perception of mental illness and its aetiology and consequences, as well as to the nature of presentation and the utilisation of services. It also affects the community support network and rehabilitation. The geographical proximity of the populace and the predominance of the extended family also play a significant role in the perception, nature and progression of mental illness.

## Population

The population of the Maltese Islands in 2002 was recorded at 394 000. Since 1974, the population has grown linearly and in 2001 the natural population growth was estimated at 2.5 per 1000 population (World Health Organization, 2003). The total number of births in 2002 was 3805, giving a crude birth rate of 9.7 per 1000 population. In the same year, the total number of deaths was 3031, giving a crude death rate of 7.7 per 1000 population. The main causes of death among the Maltese population are non-communicable diseases, mainly circulatory disease and cancers. The life expectancy at birth in 2002 was 75.8 years for males and 80.5 years for females (National Statistics Office, 2003; Ministry of Health, 2004a).

# The organisation of healthcare

The Maltese government provides a free national health service, for which the Minister of Health has overall responsibility. Residents receive comprehensive care, funded from general taxation (Ministry of Health, 2004b). The proportion of Malta's gross domestic product allocated to the health budget is 6.3%. Residents are not obliged to have health insurance in order to be entitled to health services, and those determined by means-testing to have a 'low income' and those suffering from chronic conditions (e.g. schizophrenia) are entitled to free drug treatment. Means-tested social assistance benefits are offered to some of those who have a mental health disorder, including those with severe learning disabilities, schizophrenia, certain neurological conditions (e.g. epilepsy) and substance misuse (World Health Organization, 2002).

Private health services run alongside the national health service. Private general practitioners as well as specialist practitioners offer community health services. There are three private hospitals on Malta.

# Mental health resources

The provision of mental healthcare falls under the same organisational system as general health. Of the overall healthcare budget, 9% is allocated to mental health (World Health Organization, 2002). Most of the services are offered as part of the national health service, although private services also offer community specialist care. Two non-governmental organisations, the Friends of Attard Hospital Society and the Richmond Foundation, run alongside the public and private provision.

The Ministry of Health gives its mission statement as follows: 'to promote and provide for the healthcare needs of the Maltese people and to deliver appropriate services' (Ministry of Health, 2004c). The mental health policy aims to promote a healthy environment within Maltese society, and to empower individuals to cope better with mental health issues. The policy's objectives are to deliver a wide range of services, and to facilitate advocacy, promotion, prevention, treatment and rehabilitation (World Health Organization, 2002).

The public mental health service falls under eight consultant-led firms. In-patient facilities are offered at two sites: St Luke's Hospital, which has a short-stay psychiatric unit (with 11 beds); and Mount Carmel Hospital, which has beds for acute, rehabilitation and long-stay patients, as well as beds specifically for older people, children and adolescents and people with learning disabilities, and a forensic ward. Mount Carmel Hospital provides for 520 beds in total, accounting for 143.3 beds per 100 000 population (World Health Organization, 2003). When compared with other European countries, Malta has one of the highest numbers of psychiatric beds per 1000 population (World Health Organization, 2003). However, when considering the provision for acute admissions, each consultant firm is entitled to only four beds (two for men and two for women), which makes acute in-patient care difficult to access.

Mount Carmel Hospital also offers para-clinical services, electroconvulsive therapy and a consultation–liaison service to other government hospitals. Community care facilities are offered at other sites and include:

- psychiatric out-patient facilities at St Luke's Hospital and Gozo Psychiatric Hospital, as well as within community-based health centres
- a child guidance clinic
- a clinical psychology service
- electroconvulsive therapy at the St Luke's site
- occupational therapy day services.

Other community care facilities include day centres, sheltered homes, long-stay hostels, respite centres and independent living, offered by both the governmental and non-governmental organisations, including the church. Community care, principally in the form of out-patient follow-up, is also offered by the private sector, by a psychiatrist or a general physician. Mount Carmel Hospital coordinates the overall mental health provision. Non-governmental organisations' main roles are advocacy, promotion and rehabilitation for individuals with mental illness and their families.

The eight consultant-led firms operate within all the mental health facilities; some teams offer some specialist care, depending upon the relevant consultant's training and special interests. For example, the team led by the consultant author offers specialist provision for eating disorders and sexual disorders, as well as general psychiatric provision. Fifty psychiatric nurses, eight generic occupational therapists, six generic social workers and four psychologists work alongside the eight consultants, with the aim of implementing a multidisciplinary approach. In-patient and community care facilities also aim to function through holistic approaches, according to individual needs, which may involve engaging the whole family in treatment. However, partly because of the limited human resources, in-patient care still operates in a largely custodial manner. Similarly, a multi-disciplinary approach within community care facilities is limited, with provision mainly consisting of follow-up by a physician.

Provision for substance misuse falls under the Ministry of Family and Social Solidarity. Most of the substance misuse services are provided by a government-funded autonomous agency, the National Agency against Drug and Alcohol Abuse (Sedqa). The objective of the Agency is:

> '[to] plan and recommend developments and updates of the National Policy in the field of drug and alcohol abuse and to provide services in health promotion, prevention, treatment and rehabilitation to persons with drug and/or alcohol problems and to their families so as to help them live a stable life and to integrate better [into] society' (Sedqa, 1994).

The services principally employ a multidisciplinary approach, and provide a range of treatment modalities, including out-patient and in-patient detoxification, community-based one-to-one as well as group psychosocial interventions, family therapy facilities and longer-term residential rehabilitation facilities. Other community-based provision includes prevention programmes and a parental skills programme (Bell, 1997; Bugeja, 2000). Acute provision for substance misuse, however, falls under the Department of Psychiatry within the main psychiatric hospital. A non-governmental organisation, Caritas, works alongside the National Agency; its main roles are prevention and community-based rehabilitation. The Department of Psychiatry also provides for psychiatric care within the criminal justice system.

## Training

Basic undergraduate training in the field of psychiatry forms part of the MD curriculum. This is in the form of formal lectures as well as clinical placement within the various mental health facilities (University of Malta, 2003). Opportunities for postgraduate training in psychiatry include clinical placements at the levels of house officer (four posts) and senior house officer (seven posts), under the supervision of the consultant psychiatrists. Formal training in psychiatry leading on to full qualification as a psychiatrist is not provided in Malta and hence doctors must acquire formal training abroad.

The National Agency against Drug and Alcohol Abuse provides basic training in substance misuse for those involved in service provision. It also offers a 'Voluntary Action Training Programme' for leading figures in the community, to facilitate a preventive approach with youths (Bugeja, 2000).

Membership of the Association of Maltese Specialists in Psychiatry provides the specialist registration of psychiatrists. Following recent developments, all psychiatrists will have recognition and registration of their specialty only if they are approved by the Association. There is no specialist registration for the other disciplines.

## Research activities

Mental health research activities are conducted by each consultant on some practical aspect of psychiatric care. The aim of such research is the improvement of psychiatric care and its delivery. Research projects are usually conducted over a 12-month period and are funded in part by the Merit Award Scheme. Other research activities are conducted by undergraduate and postgraduate students at the University of Malta.

## Conclusion

Mental health services in Malta are tailored to the sociocultural needs of the population. Provision of care tends to be personalised and holistic, with specialist care being an integral part of general psychiatric care. The national health service and services provided by both non-governmental organisations and the private sector function together, which allows individuals to choose their preferred option of care, and it is easy to switch between each mode of provision. The number of beds available for acute admissions is insufficient for the population, despite the relatively high number of psychiatric beds per 100 000 population. This is likely to be a consequence of the custodial care approach employed and of ineffective community care. Although services have actively been trying to move away from institutionalisation to a more community-based setting, the limited number of fully qualified mental health professionals makes this move difficult. Investment in and upgrading of training and research among all disciplines would provide the basis for a more modern, community-based, multi-disciplinary approach to the delivery of mental healthcare.

# References

Bell, A. (ed.) *(1997) Sedqa Annual Report*. Malta: Union Print Company.

Bugeja, S. (2000) A profile of Sedqa – the National Agency Against Drug and Alcohol Abuse, Malta. *Substance Misuse Bulletin*, **13**, 6.

Ministry of Health (2004a) *The Health of the Maltese Nation*. Available at www.gov.mt. Last accessed 27 April 2004.

Ministry of Health (2004b) *The Health Care System in Malta*. Available at www.gov.mt. Last accessed 27 April 2004.

Ministry of Health (2004c) *The Ministry*. Available at www.gov.mt. Last accessed 27 April 2004.

National Statistics Office (2003) *Demographic Review 2002*. Valletta: National Statistics Office.

Sedqa (1994) *Sedqa Mission Statement*. Available at www.sedqa.org.mt. Last accessed 27 April 2004.

University of Malta (2003) *Psychiatry Lecture Programme, MD Course Vth Year*. Faculty of Medicine and Surgery. Available at http://home.um.edu.mt/med-surg/courses/vthyear/psychiatry1.html. Last accessed 27 April 2004.

World Health Organization (2002) *Atlas: Country Profiles on Mental Health Resources. Project Atlas: Country Profile: Malta*. Geneva: WHO.

World Health Organization (2003) *Atlas of Health in Europe*. Geneva: WHO.

# The Netherlands

R. J. A. ten Doesschate and P. P. G. Hodiamont

The Netherlands borders the North Sea and is located between Belgium and Germany. Its total area is about 41 500 km², nearly 34 000 km² of which is land area. The country consists mostly of coastal lowland and land reclaimed from the sea (polders). An extensive system of dykes and dams protects nearly one-half of the total area from being flooded.

The Netherlands is one of the most densely populated countries in the world, at around 480 persons per km² of land area (total population of 16 299 000 as of 1 January 2005). About 20% of the population have a foreign background. Of the total number of jobs available, about one-sixth are in trade, one-sixth in industry, one-eighth in business and one-eighth in health and social care. Agriculture and fisheries account for only 1.5% of the workforce, so it is fair to call The Netherlands an advanced post-industrial society (Metz & Poorter, 1998).

According to the Healthcare Budgetary Framework (Ministry of Health, Welfare and Sport), the cost of healthcare was c45 billion in 2004, representing 9.2% of gross domestic product (GDP). Healthcare expenditure as a percentage of GDP in The Netherlands is on a level with the middle group of European countries.

The annual prevalence rate of mental conditions (excluding alcohol and substance misuse) in the Dutch population is 16%. Over 40% of the Dutch population have at one time had a mental condition (including alcohol and substance misuse). In the period 2000–4 one in every three Dutch adults with a mental condition sought help.

## Mental health policy

Mental healthcare is part of the portfolio of the Minister of Health. Since the late 1990s, government policy has been based on principles such as continuity of care. Collaboration between clinical and ambulatory care resulted in the establishment of integrated institutes for mental healthcare.

Mental healthcare is mainly financed through the Exceptional Health Expenses Act (Algemene Wet Bijzondere Ziektekosten, AWBZ), but this mechanism is due to change over the next few years. A substantial part of mental healthcare will be transferred to the health insurance system and be financed in a manner similar to physical healthcare. Payments will be based on 'diagnosis treatment combinations' (diagnose behandel combinaties, DBCs). Only hospitalisation exceeding 12 months will be paid through the Exceptional Health Expenses Act.

Government policy on mental healthcare is also changing. Mental healthcare is now integrated into general healthcare. The introduction of evidence-based programmes and guidelines will improve the diagnosis and treatment of psychiatric disorders, both in primary care and in specialist care; a system of 'stepped care' will also be introduced. Competition between care providers will be promoted and new mental healthcare organisations are being persuaded to enter the (mental) health market. The purpose of this competition is to keep costs down and to improve the quality of care.

## Mental health service delivery

Mental healthcare is delivered by some 40 integrated institutions (hospital, day hospital, out-patient and community care) for children, adults and elderly people, of which ten are for children and adolescents, nine for people with addictions and seven for forensic psychiatric care. The total number of beds is 29 000. Mental healthcare uses 8% of the total healthcare budget of c45 billion and employs about 40 000 people.

## Psychiatric training

Undergraduate medical training takes 6 years and ends with the final licensing examination, after which the student obtains the formal qualification to practise medicine. Nearly all graduates continue their studies with specialty training. Dutch specialist training is elaborately regulated and closely monitored; there is no final examination. Regulations for specialist training specify the requirements for the specialists in charge of the training, the teaching institutions and the duration, content and conditions of training.

Candidates for training in psychiatry apply for a place on an acknowledged specialist training programme. If accepted by the trainer, they are required to notify the Committee for the Registration of Medical Specialists (MSRC) and to submit a training schedule for approval. This schedule must accord with the regulations for psychiatry. The trainee works as a resident under the supervision of a specialist trainer within the framework of specific teaching rules. Residents are evaluated annually and feedback is sent to the MSRC. In case of concerns about the resident's progress, the MSRC is empowered to prolong, or even terminate, the training. Once the resident has completed training, the MSRC may, on receipt of the trainer's final statement, enter them as a psychiatrist on the Dutch register of specialists. The resident must provide the MSRC with detailed information on the training, in the form of a logbook. As one of the requirements for registration, doctors must publish a paper in a peer-reviewed journal or present a lecture at a peer-reviewed scientific meeting. In 2006, 664 (266 male, 398 female) doctors were trained to become psychiatrists. The 2616 (1649 male, 967 female) registered psychiatrists constitute around 15% of the total number of medical specialists in The Netherlands (17030).

Training for psychiatrists in The Netherlands complies with most requirements of the Board of Psychiatry of the Union Européenne des Médecins Spécialistes (UEMS; see www.uemspsychiatry.org/board/reports/Chapter6-11.10.03.pdf). The only departure from this guidance provided by the UEMS is in the duration of training, which in The Netherlands is 4.5 years instead of the recommended 5.

Training in community psychiatry and psychotherapy is an integral part of the programme. Also, 50 sessions of psychotherapy undergone by the trainee (i.e. as a client) is a mandatory part of training.

Most training in psychiatry is carried out in the integrated mental health institutes (27 of these offer training), but it is also done in seven of the university clinics and in one psychiatric department at a general hospital.

Assessment visits to every training scheme are mandatory at least every 5 years. The assessment team includes a trainee who speaks independently to the trainees on that scheme.

There are no formal subspecialties in psychiatry in The Netherlands, although there is a register of child and adolescent psychiatrists.

## Re-registration

Every medical specialist has to be re-registered every 5 years. To meet the revalidation criteria, psychiatrists are required to work at least 16 hours a week in psychiatry for 5 years and to accumulate 40 hours of continuing medical education (CME) a year. In addition, psychiatrists should take part every 5 years in the assessment visit scheme of the Dutch Psychiatric Association (Nederlandse Vereniging voor Psychiatrie, NVvP).

## Allied professions

All healthcare professionals providing direct patient care must, by law, be registered under the Individual Healthcare Professions Act – that is, on the wet Beroepen Individuele Gezondheidszorg (BIG) register. The legislation covers both general medical doctors and specialists.

An estimated 16000 nurses work in mental healthcare, 30% of whom are graduates and 2% of whom have achieved a professional qualification at a masters or specialist level. About 5500 generalist psychologists and an estimated 1100 specialist psychologists (clinical psychologists, klinisch psycholoog) work in mental healthcare. As in psychiatry, psychotherapy is an integral part of the professional training of specialist psychologists.

Furthermore, there are about 1400 psychotherapists and an estimated 600 medical doctors working in mental healthcare.

## Main areas of research

Research in psychiatry in The Netherlands is concentrated around the seven university clinics, although the efforts of the integrated mental health institutes are growing. An important impetus to mental health research in general has been given by the ZonMw (the national health council appointed by the Ministry of Health; www.zonmw.nl/programmas/geestkracht) and The Netherlands Organisation for Scientific Research (NOW) to promote quality and innovation in the field of health research and care. An ambitious long-term programme, with a budget of c24 billion, under the name 'Geestkracht' (Mental Power), has three specific objectives:

- to promote application-oriented research, knowledge transfer and implementation
- to facilitate PhD research and to promote the availability and uptake of adequate educational opportunities for mental health researchers
- to strengthen research and knowledge infrastructure through cooperation between different scientific institutes and institutions providing healthcare.

GROUP (www.groupproject.nl) is a national consortium of 39 university and non-university institutes that concentrates its research on psychotic disorders. 'Generation R and Trails' and NESDA (Netherlands Study on Depression and Anxiety, www.nesda.nl) are both engaged in research concerning children and young adults, and anxiety and depression respectively.

## Human rights issues

Although there are no exact data available, the general view is that seclusion rooms are used more frequently in The Netherlands than in neighbouring countries. One of the reasons for this is that treatment against the patient's will is restricted by law. Only when there is acute danger to the patient or others is carefully monitored forced medication allowed. Fortunately, the growing feeling of discomfort among professionals, psychiatrists and nurses is slowly contributing to the re-evaluation of the use of seclusion rooms. Furthermore, there are initiatives to change mental health legislation in The Netherlands which would lead to (involuntary) treatment being sometimes used as an alternative to seclusion and restraint.

## Challenges

Further implementation of multidisciplinary guidelines is one of the challenges for the healthcare professions. Psychiatrists, supported by their scientific association, will play an important part in this implementation process.

Although prevention is not neglected at the moment, primary and secondary prevention, in cooperation with public healthcare, should receive more emphasis in the near future.

As mentioned above, a reduction in the use of restraint, supported by scientific research, will be one of the major challenges for psychiatrists in the coming decade.

It is not unlikely that psychiatric patients with chronic illness will fall victim to greater competition in the healthcare market. It is reasonable to expect that the attention of the insurance companies, healthcare organisations and professionals will be focused on the less complicated cases (typically patients with Axis I disorders). The challenge for psychiatrists and other professions will be to ensure that patients with chronic illness receive adequate (community) mental healthcare in the future.

# Reference

Metz, J.& Poorter, J. (1998) The Netherlands. In *Medicine and Medical Education in Europe* (ed. G. Eysenbach). Thieme.

# Norway

Jan Olav Johannessen, Bjarte Stubhaug and Jan Skandsen

Few countries (if any) have experienced the abundance of material welfare Norway has had for the last decades. The report of the Organisation for Economic Co-operation and Development (OECD) for 2004 places Norway on the very top of the list of 'best countries to live in'. One might therefore expect that mental disorders would not thrive in Norway, but this is not so.

Norway is a constitutional monarchy: its parliament decides new laws; a government with a parliamentary basis executes political decisions; and the judicial system interprets and enforces the laws.

The total population is about 4.5 million, approximately 1 million of whom are under 18 years of age. The population is concentrated around the major cities in the southern part of the country, Oslo, Bergen and Stavanger; large areas of the country feature only small towns and villages and a scattered population. This creates challenges for the provision of an equal health service to all the country's inhabitants.

The predominant political ideology throughout the last 50 years has been based on social democratic ideas of equality in health and social services and education. Therefore most health services are in the public sector, in which hospital treatments are free and most out-patient services are financed by public means. Patients pay a small amount, not exceeding 150 euros per year. Over the last decade, the number of private services have increased, some of which are purchased by the public healthcare system. In the mental health services, this has given rise to private services for people with less severe disorders, who would otherwise fall outside the priorities of the public system.

## History of mental healthcare

Norway passed a Law of the Treatment and Care of the Insane in 1848. It declared that the responsibility for the care of the insane was the government's. A Control Commission was established to inspect the asylums and the private residencies that lodged people with a mental illness, and it looked after patients' legal rights. The law stated that isolation and restraint should be kept to a minimum.

This law underwent only minor amendment until it was replaced by the 1961 Law on Mental Healthcare. The major change was that the new law introduced the possibility of admission for observation when there was doubt about the mental state of the patient, that is, whether the patient suffered from a psychosis. This observation period could last up to 3 weeks. In 2001 this law was revised and the maximum observation period reduced to 10 days. The revised law allows more use of compulsory treatment for out-patients.

The mental asylums established from 1865 to 1920 have gradually been replaced by smaller hospitals and psychiatric wards in general hospitals. Over the last 10–20 years, however, decentralisation and deinstitutionalisation have taken place, with a dramatic decline in the number of hospital beds and far greater provision of out-patient services. There is presently an intense discussion – political, professional, in the media and in the public – of whether this has proceeded too quickly. The critics say more time is needed to establish new services and establish professional competence locally, and that the psychiatric patients most in need of welfare and treatment are paying the price of an ideologically driven process of decentralisation. The supporters advocate the local design and implementation of mental health services, with patients living in their homes or in small community health centres. There is agreement, however, that there are too few professionals, principally psychiatrists and clinical psychologists, to assure the professional quality of the many local services. This is indeed a great challenge for the structure of services.

## Today's mental health system: economy and personnel

There is broad political agreement in Norway that the mental health services need to be improved, both quantitatively and qualitatively, especially the services for those under 18 years of age. In 1997 the Norwegian parliament approved a plan for better, and more decentralised, mental health services, the so-called Escalation Plan for Mental Health (EPMH). In 1996 the total expenditure on mental health services was about 1.16 billion euros. Over the period 1999–2008 this annual figure is due to increase by some 0.7 billion euros, and an additional investment of around 1 billion euros will be made.

### Services for children and adolescents

It has been estimated that 5% of the population under 18 years, or a total of 54 000 young people, require treatment in specialised child and adolescent services, almost entirely on an out-patient basis. In 2003 this number was 33 000. Some 3000 people work in the services for children and adolescents;

as of 2003, there were 340 in-patient beds, but expansion to 500 by 2008 is planned. There are 154 doctors working in the out-patient units, 120 of whom are child psychiatrists. There are 450 psychologists working in these out-patient units. Consultations per 'professional year' (i.e. how many consultations each doctor or psychologist has annually) total about 380. This level of 'productivity' is a very much debated subject, as some politicians find this number far too low, given that the norm established by some health trusts is 450.

## Adult services

There are about 1050 psychiatrists and 500 residents working with adults; 1525 clinical psychologists work within adult psychiatry. Hospital beds total 5600; the norms set out by the EPMH are 9 hospital beds per 10000 inhabitants and 6 beds per 10000 in local district psychiatric centres (an equivalent to community-based mental health centres). The average length of stay is about 42 days (averaged over acute wards as well as long-stay departments).

For out-patient units the norm is one professional health worker per 1500 inhabitants aged over 18 years, and the suggested norm for productivity is 500 consultations per professional year.

# Training

The training period for a resident to become a specialist in psychiatry is 5 years (with an extra half year's training for child and adolescent psychiatry). There are clinical programmes of training in specified fields and areas (acute, long-term, out-patient etc.), and educational (theoretical) programmes covering therapy, service models and the client–therapist relationship, leadership and judicial matters. One year of residency might be in another relevant medical specialty (e.g. in child psychiatry or in research). Psychotherapy education, practice and supervision are for a minimum of 3 years: 2 years with psychodynamically based therapies, and one year with cognitive or group analytic treatment (a minimum of 110 hours). Most psychiatrists go on to further training in cognitive or psychodynamic psychotherapy; group analysis has declined in popularity and training in classical psychoanalysis is undertaken only by the dedicated few. In child and adolescent psychiatry, everybody has 40 hours of psychodynamic therapy and some have a 2-year programme in psychotherapy training. There are also training programmes within psychopharmacology, family therapies and community-based treatment of psychosis.

Fifty per cent of residents start training directly after internship, and 50% after 4–10 years of clinical work, mainly in general practice. There is no examination before approval as a psychiatrist, but the clinical training and the clinical supervisors evaluate personal suitability. Training for child and adolescent psychiatry involves 6 months of paediatric practice.

# Main areas of research

The universities and colleges, together with the Department of Health and Social Affairs, support a vast range of research activities. There are major programmes on early intervention in first-episode psychosis and extensive programmes of psychotherapy research, including studies of its effects, patient compliance and combined treatments. A national network is examining the efficacy of group analysis for personality disorders. Epidemiological research is undertaken at both regional and community level. Other important fields of interest are genetics, brain imaging, dementia, neuropsychiatry and neurophysiology, psychophysiology, psycho-pharmacology, sleep disorders, trauma and forensics. In child and adolescent psychiatry the major areas of research are autism, epidemiology, transcultural psychiatry, eating disorders, low birth weight and behaviour problems.

# Norwegian Psychiatric Association

The Norwegian Psychiatric Association (NPA), of which most psychiatrists and residents are members, is part of the Norwegian Medical Association. The NPA is concerned with professional conditions and professional development, and the general conditions and structure of the mental health services. It has special sections on preventive psychiatry, biological psychiatry, psychotherapy, forensic psychiatry, old age psychiatry, emergency psychiatry, private practice, quality issues, basic problems in science and psychiatry, and a section on resident education and specialist approval. The association and its sections work in close collaboration with the Norwegian Medical Association, the health authorities and other professional organisations, especially the Psychologists' Association.

The board meets 8–10 times a year, and the sections 2–6 times.

The NPA takes part in public and political processes in developing and changing mental health services. The restructuring and decentralising of the psychiatric services, together with legislative changes in leadership – reducing the administrative and clinical influence of psychiatrists and putting psychologists forward to equal leadership positions – have greatly influenced the role and function of psychiatrists in Norway. There is also an extensive discussion of quality issues, indicators, diagnostic guidelines and treatments, treatment program¬mes, and quality assurance.

# Conclusions

There is great pressure on the emergency wards in the large cities, mainly due to a combination of the reduction in hospital capacity, increasing drug misuse and drug-related psychopathology, and a failure to provide enough housing and services for long-term patients in the community. Although

Norway has more resources at its disposal than most other countries, we are struggling with long waiting lists and unacceptably long waiting times. Hence the government recently has introduced an absolute 'maximum allowed period' for different diagnostic and functional categories; priority is always accorded to the more serious disorders.

The NPA is an active partner in formulating priorities in psychiatry, quality-improvement work and developing quality indicators. There is – and will probably always be – a gap between the expectations of the public and the services that can be provided. The government is determined to give most to those most in need, but in so doing faces the dilemma of how to help those patients with the greatest potential for improvement.

The main ideological basis of modern Norwegian psychiatry rests on a humanistic, biopsychosocial model of understanding and treating psychiatric illness, with the expressed goal of developing better, more specialised and more differentiated hospital treatment, combined with accessible, low-threshold community-based services.

# Poland

Jacek Bomba

Modern mental healthcare in Poland has its foundations in the 19th century, when the country was subject to three different organisational and legal systems – of the Austrian, Prussian and Russian Empires. These differences prevailed even after the First World War. Professionals lobbying for a mental health act had no success. The Second World War left mental healthcare with significant losses among its professional groups. More than half of all Polish psychiatrists lost their lives; some of them were exterminated as Jews, some as prisoners of the Soviets. The Nazi occupation in Poland had dramatic consequences for people with a mental disturbance, as Action T4 turned into genocide on the Polish territory. The majority of psychiatric in-patients were killed. After the Second World War, the mental health system had to be rebuilt, almost from scratch. Major political changes in the country across the second part of the 20th century and revolutionary changes in mental healthcare around the world influenced psychiatric services. The purpose of this paper is to describe mental healthcare in Poland today.

## Mental health policy and legislation

The national mental health policy emphasises promotion, prevention, treatment and rehabilitation; it was initially formulated in 1995 as the National Mental Health Programme. This was followed by the development of regional mental health programmes, specifying particular tasks in each of Poland's voivodships (provinces). However, their realisation is far from satisfactory.

The Mental Health Act enacted in 1994 regulates:

- the promotion of mental health
- the prevention of mental disorders and discrimination
- the provision of accessible mental healthcare services in the community
- the protection of the civil rights of people with mental disorders.

The Act also regulates involuntary treatment. Other acts concern the prevention of alcohol and drug misuse, rehabilitation and employment of people with disabilities; the Penal Code and the Civil and Care Codes also have a bearing on people with mental illness.

The treatment of severe mental disorders is largely free of charge (in-patient treatment, community care, consultations, psychotherapy, rehabilitation and a significant part of medication). Policy regarding the provision of therapeutic drugs is based on a parliamentary act that divides drugs into two groups: 'basic' compounds and 'additional' compounds. The latter include new drugs. The Minister of Health decides which drugs will be supplied free of charge, or at low or reduced prices for persons with specific disorders.

## Mental health service delivery

Mental healthcare is included within the primary care system, although most of it is undertaken within the mental health out-patient clinic system, which is well developed and easily accessible. Primary care physicians are trained in psychiatry, including family psychiatry. However, systemic changes in healthcare financing have disrupted services. Nonetheless, deinstitutionalisation has been continued, and the numbers of day centres, psychiatric units in general hospitals and mobile community teams are increasing. In spite of this, the majority of psychiatric beds are still in psychiatric hospitals (5.2 per 10 000 population) rather than general hospitals (1.2 per 10 000). The overall number of mental health professionals is not satisfactory (Fig. 1); in addition, they are unevenly distributed across the country.

Mental healthcare, as one aspect of general healthcare, is financed by the National Health Fund (NHF), an obligatory, tax-based health insurance system. The NHF, in cooperation with the regional governments, is responsible for satisfactory provision of services. In-patient treatment is financed by the NHF, as is the majority of out-patient care (82% of such care for adults in 2004–05, 94% for children in 2005; Institute of Psychiatry and Neurology, 2006).

In addition, consultation and psychotherapy facilities within the social care system have an important role in the provision of mental healthcare, as do programmes appointed by local authorities and within the educational system (for children, adolescents and their families).

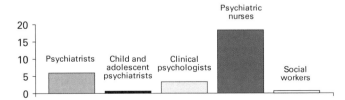

Number of professionals per 100 000 population

**Fig. 1** Numbers of mental health professionals (Institute of Psychiatry and Neurology, 2006).

# Psychiatric training

## Undergraduate

Undergraduate training in psychiatry is based upon a national curriculum. However, medical schools have developed their own programmes, often more extended than the national curriculum. Many specific subjects are taught within elective courses. For example, the programme at the Jagiellonian University Collegium Medicum, Krakow, in addition to a basic course in psychiatry covering child and adolescent psychiatry, general psychiatry and old age psychiatry, also includes medical psychology and basic psychotherapy (which are obligatory), as well as psychoanalysis and sexology (elective).

## Postgraduate

Since 1999, postgraduate training in psychiatry has been a 5-year residency programme based on standards developed by the Section of Psychiatry of the European Union of Medical Specialists. The rotation scheme is dominated by general psychiatry in in-patient settings; however, out-patient services, community psychiatry and psychotherapy centres are also obligatory. Child and adolescent psychiatry, intellectual disabilities, old age psychiatry and forensic psychiatry, although obligatory, are not given adequate amounts of time (Table 1). The theoretical part of training is organised as a series of courses that training centres are obliged to deliver.

## Psychiatric subspecialties

In 1999, postgraduate training in child and adolescent psychiatry was organised as an additional 2 years of residency-based programme for psychiatrists. The number of trainees then significantly decreased, endangering the future of mental healthcare for children and adolescents. To prevent this, a 5-year training programme for physicians was introduced.

## Allied professions

Psychiatric nurses have a two-stage undergraduate university training in general nursing (3 years to become a licensed nurse and a further 3 years to obtain an MSc). Postgraduate training in psychiatric nursing follows a national curriculum and comprises 300 hours of theory and 560 hours on rotations.

Psychologists have a 5-year undergraduate training that is based on a national curriculum, although the final programme is designed by the universities. Postgraduate training in clinical psychology was suspended in the late 1990s because of major legal changes to the profession; it was reintroduced in 2004. It comprises a 5-year rotation-based training scheme that follows a national curriculum.

Table 1 Postgraduate training in psychiatry (numbers of hours)

| | 1st year | 2nd year | 3rd year | 4th year | 5th year |
|---|---|---|---|---|---|
| *Mandatory practical training* | | | | | |
| In-patient unit, short stay | 8 | | | | |
| In-patient unit | 3 | 4 | 3 | 4 | |
| Child and adolescent psychiatry service | | 4 | | | |
| Neurology | | 3 | | | |
| Neurotic disorders service | | | 6 | | |
| Community psychiatry service | | | 2 | | |
| Out-patient service | | | | 5 | |
| Consultation–liaison psychiatry | | | | 2 | |
| Substance dependency service | | | | | 3 |
| Facultative | | | | | 8 |
| *Theoretical courses* | | | | | |
| Foundations of psychiatry | 80 | | | | |
| Health promotion | 25 | | | | |
| Psychotherapeutic relations | | | 40 | | |
| Foundations of child and adolescent psychiatry | | | 40 | | |
| Introduction to family therapy | | | | 40 | |
| Clinical practice of psychotherapy | | | | 40 | |
| Forensic psychiatry | | | | 35 | 40 |
| Balint Seminar (recommended) | 20 | 20 | 20 | 20 | 20 |

The regulation of postgraduate training in psychotherapy is presently being discussed. Until now, the Polish Psychiatric Association, Polish Psychological Association and several other psychotherapeutic societies have provided training and certification procedures (the two named organisations being the main ones; only their certificates are recognised by the NHF).

# Research

The majority of research in the mental health field is conducted at the governmental Institute of Psychiatry and Neurology and research centres in medical schools across the country. Research projects can be supported by grants from the Ministry of Science and Higher Education, and by international sources. Several research groups participate in collaborative projects run by the World Health Organization and the European Union. These are mainly studies of the genetics of mental disorders, the epidemiology of mental disorders, economics, health promotion and combating stigma. Affective disorders, schizophrenia, cognitive disorders, child and adolescent mental health problems, and old age mental disorders are approached from different perspectives.

A long-term prospective study of people diagnosed with schizophrenia, being carried out in Kraków, deserves special mention (Cechnicki, 1998).

The effectiveness of psychotherapy has been extensively studied. The problem has been approached by tracking changes in symptoms and personality traits in response to psychotherapy in the treatment of patients with neuroses (Aleksandrowicz, 1991); additionally, symptoms, defence mechanisms and quality of life have been looked at in the integrated treatment of patients suffering schizophrenic and affective disorders (Bomba & Cichocki, 2005; Zieba *et al*, 1997).

Methods of rehabilitation and community care and their effectiveness are yet another group of problems researchers are concerned with (Meder & Cechnicki, 2002).

Eating disorders, which have significantly increased in incidence in recent decades, have also been given special attention (Józefik & Pilecki, 2004).

For the last 50 years, starting with the group of Auschwitz concentration camp survivors, the consequences of trauma have been studied (Kepinski, 1970). Also studied have been Holocaust survivors (Orwid *et al*, 2002) and prisoners of the former political Soviet and communist regime (Heitzman & Rutkowski, 2002); second- and third-generation survivors have been studied consecutively. Methods of treatment for the various forms of post-traumatic stress disorder will form the next important research topic.

Results of studies are published in both international and Polish journals. The major Polish psychiatric journals are Psychiatria Polska (in Polish, with English, French, German and Russian abstracts) and Archives of Psychiatry and Psychotherapy (in English).

## Human rights issues

From the late 1940s to the 1980s, as the Polish Psychiatric Association watching group noted (Bomba *et al*, 1993), there was no abuse of psychiatry for political reasons. Since 1994 the Mental Health Act has provided for the prevention of abuse of the right to personal freedom in psychiatric practice. Professionals are obliged to offer treatment, if needed, after obtaining informed consent. The major human rights issue remains deprivation of privacy in psychiatric wards due to chronic unsatisfactory funding (Buda *et al*, 1998).

## References

Aleksandrowicz, J. (1991) Psychotherapiefgorschung in Polen. [Psychotherapy research in Poland.] In *Psychotherapie in der Medizin [Psychotherapy in medicine]* (ed. E. Brahler). Westd Verl.

Bomba, J. & Cichocki, Ł. (2005) Czy neuroscience wyjasnia efekty psychoterapii schizofrenii? [Does neuroscience explain the effects of psychotherapy in schizophrenia?] *Psychoterapia*, **2**, 5–11.

Bomba, J., Szymusik, A. & Piotrowski, A. (1993) Psychiatry in Eastern Europe. *American Journal of Psychiatry*, **150**, 988–989.

Buda, B., Gondios, A. & Demetrovics, Z. (eds) *(1998) Costs of Rights in Psychiatry.* CLPI.

Cechnicki, A. (1998) Analiza wpływu wybranych czynników na wyniki leczenia w obszarze społecznym. Krakowskie prospektywne badania przebiegu schizofrenii. [Selected factors impact on social area results of schizophrenia treatment. The Krakow prospective follow-up study.] *Badania Nad Schizofrenia*, **1**, 37–48.

Heitzman, J. & Rutkowski, K. (2002) Mental disturbances in former political prisoners persecuted in Poland in the years 1944–1956. *Dialog. Zeszyty Polsko–Niemieckiego Towarzystwa Zdrowia Psychicznego, Hefte dre Deutsch–Polnishen Gesellschaft fur Seeliche Gesundheit*, **11**, 206–211.

Institute of Psychiatry and Neurology (2006) *Zakłady psychiatrycznej oraz neurologicznej opieki zdrowotnej. Rocznik statystyczny 2005.* [Psychiatric and neurological health care services. Statistical yearly 2005.] Institute of Psychiatry and Neurology.

Józefik, B. & Pilecki, M. (2004) Therapeutic implications of the individual, familial and cultural context of eating disorders in Poland. *World Psychiatry*, **3 (suppl. 1)**, 293.

Kepinski, A. (1970) The so-called 'KZ-syndrom' – an attempt at a synthesis. *Przeglad Lekarski*, **26**, 18–23. Reprinted in *Przeglad Lekarski*, Krakow, 141–156 (ed. J. Z. Ryn, 2002).

Meder, J. & Cechnicki, A. (2002) Rehabilitation of the mentally ill in Poland. In *Images in Psychiatry. Poland* (eds A. Bilikiewicz & J. Rybakowski), pp. 142–157. WPA, PTP, Via Medica.

Orwid, M., Domagalska-Kurdziel, E., Kaminska, M., *et al* (2002) The Holocaust in Polish publications. In *Images in Psychiatry. Poland* (eds A. Bilikiewicz & J. Rybakowski), pp. 83–114. WPA, PTP, Via Medica.

Zieba, A., Dudek, D. & Jawor, M. (1997) Cognitive style in depressed patients over three-year follow-up. *European Journal of Psychiatry*, **11**, 244–250.

# Portugal

## João Marques-Teixeira and Elisabete Fradique

Portugal is in the south-west of Europe; its territory includes the Azores and Madeira islands, giving it an area of 91 900 km². The total resident population of Portugal was 10 579 000 in 2006. The population density was 115 per km². The birth rate has been declining, from 20.0 per 1000 population in 1970 to 10.4 in 2004. Life expectancy at birth in 2006 was 75 for males and 82 years for females. Healthy life expectancy at birth in 2003 was 67 and 72 years, respectively. The infant mortality rate decreased from 10.8 per 1000 in 1991 to 3.5 per 1000 in 2005. The median age of the population has been steadily rising.

Portugal has been a constitutional democratic republic since 1974. The main institutions of state are: President of the Republic, Parliament and government. First two are directly elected by the population. Since 2005, the Socialist Party has formed a government with an absolute majority of seats in Parliament.

Gross national income per capita is $19 960 (sums here and below are in international dollars, purchasing power parity, 2006). Total expenditure on health per capita is $2080. The health budget represents 9.2% of gross domestic product.

## Mental health policy

A mental health policy has been present since 1995, with advocacy, promotion, prevention, treatment and rehabilitation as aims. A substance misuse policy has been present since 1999, and an alcohol policy since 2000.

Ministerial Order 10 464 (9 April 2008) set out the current national goals for mental health:

- permanent monitoring of the mental health status of the Portuguese population
- creation of programmes promoting the well-being, mental health, prevention, treatment and rehabilitation of people with mental illness

- organisation of mental health services for adults, children and adolescents
- articulation of psychiatric care with primary healthcare through an integrated continuous care network
- participation of both users and care providers in the rehabilitation and the social integration of patients with serious mental illnesses.

Mental health is one of the priority areas of the National Health Plan 2004–10. Special concerns are depression and alcohol misuse and dependence.

# Mental health service delivery and resources

Decree Law 2118 of 1963 approved the principles of mental healthcare provision, and mental health centres were created in 1964. In the early 1970s, the need to integrate mental health services with the general healthcare system became obvious. Thus, in 1984, the General Directorate for Primary Healthcare was created, with a Division of Mental Health Services. Decree Law 127 of 1992 integrated these mental health centres into general hospitals, but this served to reveal problems within healthcare in relation to an over-dependence on the regional health authorities. After recommendations from the United Nations and the World Health Organization regarding an emphasis on community services, it was necessary to change the organisation of mental healthcare, to shift the focus to rehabilitation and social inclusion. Decree Law 36 of 1998 regulated the organisation of services in this sector and created a clear referral system alongside a community care network.

The following points summarise the current principles for the organisation of services, although these are still awaiting nationwide implementation:

- the referral model is that of community care
- local (or regional) mental health services are the base of the care system, together with primary care units and hospitals
- teams are multidisciplinary, and each serves a population of approximately 80 000
- primary care units are the basis for ambulatory services; in-patient and emergency care are both provided at hospitals
- social rehabilitation is carried out in conjunction with the state health sector, social security and employment departments
- psychiatric hospitals provide residential services and specialist in-patient care for patients who have no family or social support.

Portugal has 923 general psychiatrists (401 women, 522 men), 508 child and adolescent psychiatrists (242 women, 266 men), about 1000 psychiatric nurses, 160 social workers and 200 psychologists, organised in a mixed system where public (free) and private practice (supported either by the patients or by insurance companies) work together. Some private institutions and enterprises have service agreements with the public system.

The majority of psychiatrists have their practice in both the public and the private domains. In private practice they are not obliged to have any type of service agreement with insurance companies or the public system.

In addition, psychiatric care is provided within the prison service and in the military forces.

Adult public psychiatric care is provided by 30 local healthcare services, predominantly located in general hospitals. There are also one psychiatric hospital and three psychiatric centres (two in Lisbon and one in Coimbra).

## Psychiatric training

Undergraduate psychiatric training is structured around two disciplines directly connected to psychiatry (general psychiatry and psychiatric practice) and two disciplines indirectly connected to psychiatry (basic psychology and medical psychology).

Postgraduate psychiatric training was recently modified. It is now focused not only on mental pathology but also on the influence of medical and surgical pathology on mental health and the influence of mental health on physical illness. We believe this will contribute to the humanisation of care and to the reinforcement of psychiatry's medical identity. The training is centred on diversity of professional experience. After 12 months of basic medical training, the trainee will have 60 months of training specifically in psychiatry. Of these, 48 months cover in- and out-patient care, day care facilities, drug addiction services, liaison psychiatry, old age psychiatry and forensic psychiatry. Three months are dedicated to neurology and another three to child and adolescent psychiatry. The last 6 months of training are on an optional area. Throughout, trainees must be integrated within a psychiatric emergency team.

## Psychiatric subspecialties and allied professions

Child and adolescent psychiatry is organised as an autonomous specialty.

A new and first subspecialty of psychiatry – forensic psychiatry – is currently being developed by the College of Psychiatry of the Portuguese Medical Association (PMA).

Concerning allied professions, the public system offers professional careers to psychiatric nurses, psychologists, occupational therapists and social workers.

Psychotherapeutic training and certification are undertaken by the different psychotherapy societies.

## Research and publications

Almost all research in psychiatry is undertaken within academia, with a few excellent exceptions coming from private research institutes. The main areas of research are focused on basic matters, on clinical domains and on mental health policies and services. There is no national policy or specific funding for this specialty. A few groups are involved in international research networks.

The first national Portuguese morbidity study is currently being conducted.

There are three well established and regularly published Portuguese journals of psychiatry and mental health (Saúde Mental, Acta Psiquiátrica and Psiquiatria Clínica) and a few internet-based facilities for exchange of scientific and clinical material.

## Workforce issues

The PMA, through its Colleges of Psychiatry and Child and Adolescent Psychiatry, defines and supervises good psychiatric practice in both the public and the private domains. This is done through an ethical committee (elected every 3 years). The elaboration of the training programme and the nomination of three of the five examiners for the final examination of trainees (the one that credits them with the title of specialist) are also responsibilities of the PMA.

Several meetings of all psychiatrists have been held under the auspices of the PMA in order to help it better represent their professional interests.

Non-governmental organisations (NGOs) are involved with mental health and some of them have government support; they are active in areas such as suicide prevention, family support and anti-stigma programmes.

The pharmaceutical industry gives financial support to help general practitioners attend psychiatric training courses and offers information and supportive programmes on mental health and psychiatry for patients and their families.

## Human rights issues

Several anti-stigma campaigns, mostly promoted by NGOs, have been implemented. Patients' rights are guaranteed by legislation, especially that concerning persons who are thought to need compulsory treatment (ambulatory or in hospital). Legislation has now begun to be applied to employment facilities for those with mental illness.

## Future developments

Despite a profusion of legislation in recent years, the landscape of psychiatric care in Portugal remains almost unchanged. Apart from a few areas where community care exists and works, the reforms required for the better rehabilitation and social inclusion of chronic psychiatric patients remain the same as they were 20 years ago.

Palha & Marques-Teixeira (2009) conducted a national survey of rehabilitation facilities and practices for chronic psychiatric patients, and concluded that the present scenario is very far from patients' needs. Pita Barros & de Almeida Simoes (2007) similarly concluded that 'in Portugal we are still far from offering to all the population access to essential mental healthcare'. The main reason for this is the distance between mental health practice and the contents of the laws and guidelines.

Pressure from the profession will transform the current legislation into real psychiatric practice. However, some of these measures are already conceptually and practically out of date. Before implementation, their adjustment to the cultural, financial and traditional characteristics of Portugal is mandatory, as will be some adjustment to account for the experience of other countries that have already evaluated their outcome.

Finally, a national research policy is being demanded by Portuguese psychiatrists in the hope that, in the near future, the results of the reforms can be clearly evaluated.

# Sources

Palha, F. & Marques-Teixeira, J. (2009) *Serviços de Reabilitação na Esquizofrenia em Portugal: situação actual e persprctiva dos profissionais.* [Rehabilitation Services for Schizophrenia in Portugal: Current and Prospective Situation of the Professionals.] Vale e Vale Editores.

Pita Barros, P. & de Almeida Simões, J. (2007) Health system review – Portugal. *Health Systems in Transition,* **9(5).**

World Health Organization (2005) Portugal. In *International Mental Health Atlas.* WHO.

World Health Organization (2009) *Statistics 2008, Portugal.* WHO.

# Romania

## Nicoleta Tataru

Romania is now in a period of transition from communism to democracy. Geographically, Romania, like other Eastern European countries, is on the border between the Western world and the Middle East and Asia; until December 1989 it was behind the 'Iron Curtain'.

It covers 237 500 km$^2$, divided into 42 districts. In 2002 it had a population estimated to be 21 795 000. The unemployment rate was 10.5%. Fourteen per cent of the general population were over the age of 65. The infant death rate was 17.3 per 1000 and life expectancy at birth was 67.6 years for males and 71.1 years for females. The gross domestic product per capita (GDP) expressed in purchasing power parity (PPP) is US$6041, and total health expenditure is 2.60% of GDP. The proportion of the national budget spent on the health system is 4%, and around 2% of the total health budget is for mental health. There are 189 physicians per 100 000 population.

## Mental health services

Nationally, there are 908 psychiatrists (4.16 per 100 000 population), of whom 260 are child psychiatrists (1.19 per 100 000 population). They all work in the public health sector, although some also work in private ambulatory clinics. There are also psychologists and social workers in the mental healthcare system.

Most psychiatric services are provided by hospitals and out-patient clinics attached to the Ministry of Health. There are 38 psychiatric hospitals and many psychiatric departments in the general hospitals (a total of 17 079 beds) as well as day hospitals (1222 beds) to care for patients with both acute and chronic mental illnesses; in addition there are 166 beds for patients with drug dependency. There are also 65 mental health centres for adults and children with mental illness. There are no private psychiatric hospitals.

The special needs of people with mental illness have not always been recognised and respected by the generic health services. However, a mental health law was passed in Romania only in August 2002 (Monitorul oficial al Romaniei, XIV, 589). This was the first step towards reform of the mental health services and care system. In chapter 4 of the law, the forms of specific mental health services existing in Romania are listed, along with care standards for people with mental disorders. Only recently has Romania tried to add community mental healthcare services to the traditional system of active psychiatric hospital care. This started by radically reducing the number of beds, but unfortunately without ensuring adequate community care programmes and services. Many long-stay psychiatric wards were transferred to the social services. In the district of Bihor alone, 178 psychiatric beds out of 900 were transferred from Nucet Psychiatric Hospital (accountable to the Ministry of Health) to the social services (accountable to the Department of Labour and Social Protection).

Stigma remains an obstacle in ensuring access to care for patients who are mentally ill. Stigma leads to the development of negative attitudes (including those of professionals), poor quality of treatment services and inadequate funding at both national and local level.

Standards need to be raised in basic mental healthcare, and in relation to patients' basic needs and quality of life (accommodation, food, sheltered housing, sheltered workplaces and community involvement).

## In-patient services

People with acute or chronic mental disorders are treated in:
- psychiatric hospitals (for those with acute mental disorders)
- day hospitals
- long-stay accommodation
- psychiatric wards in general hospitals (when psychiatric hospitals are not locally available)
- the consultation–liaison psychiatry department in Bucharest University General Hospital
- psychiatric departments in geriatric hospitals
- sheltered homes (for patients with schizophrenia) founded by non-governmental organisations (NGOs).

These kinds of services are available in most but not all districts.

## Out-patient units

In Romania out-patient services are available in only a few districts because there is still a severe lack of resources. The following types of service are usually available:
- out-patient or community assessment units
- day care centres
- primary care
- community mental health centres (which serve as a link between patients and their families, general practitioners and hospitals for acutely or chronically mentally ill people) (Tataru, 1997)

- community and social support services (organised by NGOs and churches in almost all districts).

Day programmes contribute to reducing stigma and dis¬crimination against people with mental disorders by reducing their isolation and increasing the patients' abilities to face daily life.

### Home care

In 2003, a programme began of follow-up home care for all patients, including elderly people with mental disorders and dementia. The programme consists of medical treatment and domiciliary services, such as home-helps and meals-on-wheels, and other help to enable patients to remain at home. There is also some financial support from the Department of Labour and Social Protection to compensate the families or carers of people who are chronically ill and those with handicaps (including those with dementia) who are treated at home.

## Mental health programmes

A national mental health programme has been developed in recent years for the treatment of schizophrenia and depression, to provide free medication for patients from the onset of their illness, and also medication for in-patients in forensic psychiatric units. The national programme for elderly people with a mental illness is lacking financial support at present.

## Education

In 1989 Romania had six schools of medicine; now there are 10. Medical education in psychiatry begins with a half-year programme during the last year of undergraduate study, which comprises theoretical and practical courses, seminars and training in psychiatric hospitals or psychiatric departments in general hospitals. These studies include basic knowledge of child and adolescent psychiatry. The curriculum is based around the nosographic criteria of ICD–10 and the classical clinical presentation of mental disorders. The main goal is to give doctors the capacity to recognise, diagnose and care for people with mental health problems.

The educational programme for psychiatrists continues with 5 years of postgraduate medical education, comprising: courses, workshops, mental health examinations, psychiatric interviews, case presentations and training in psychiatric hospitals with a senior consultant psychiatrist or professor of psychiatry. The curriculum for psychiatrists respects the ICD–10 and DSM–IV criteria for the diagnosis of mental disorders. Psychiatry residents are obliged to use the most well known American and English psychiatric books. During these 5 years, the residents can attend a fee-paying training programme or courses and workshops on different forms of psychotherapy, usually run by psychotherapists from Western European countries. The current demand for training in psychotherapies, especially from recent generations of residents, is a consequence of the prohibition of these approaches (on ideological grounds) up to 1990.

Programmes in continuing medical education comprise postgraduate courses lasting 2–3 months and training in university psychiatric hospitals, as well as participation in national and international psychiatric congresses and conferences. There are also more specialist postgraduate training courses for child psychiatrists, geriatric psychiatrists and psychologists.

## Professional associations and publications

Mental health professionals are organised into many scientific associations and societies, most of them founded after 1989. The largest of these is the Romanian Association of Psychiatry, of which nearly all Romanian psychiatrists are members. Others include the Romanian Mental Health League, the Romanian Alzheimer Society, the Romanian Association of Geriatric Psychiatry, the Romanian Association of Free Psychiatrists, the Romanian Association of Neuropsychopharmacology, the Romanian Association of Psychotherapy and the Romanian Association of Toxicology–Dependence. These associations organise annual local and national scientific meetings and conferences and stimulate their members to participate in national and international congresses.

Some European congresses have been organised in Romania: in 2000 the Romanian Association of Geriatric Psychiatry organised the 28th European Congress of Geriatric Psychiatry in Oradea; in 2001 the Romanian Alzheimer Society organised the 10th European Conference on Alzheimer's Disease in Bucharest; and the 2002 meeting of the European College of Neuro-psychopharmacology was held in Bucharest.

The Romanian Association of Psychiatry works in partnership with other European and international psychiatry associations to improve mental healthcare in Romania and is an active member of the World Psychiatric Association (there are 250 paying members). One of its initiatives has been to translate into Romanian many important documents, psychiatric books and diagnostic guidelines (e.g. ICD–10 and DSM–IV). The Romanian Association of Psychiatry publishes the *Romanian Journal of Psychiatry* (four issues a year) and the Romanian League for Mental Health publishes the *Romanian Journal of Mental Health* (three issues a year) and together with the Mental Health League in Moldavia publishes *Psychiatry Today* (three issues a year). There is also the *Romanian Journal of Child and Adolescent Psychiatry*.

## Geriatric psychiatry

Old age psychiatry has become a basic discipline for all sociomedical providers as well as a specialty for some physicians and health workers

(World Health Organization, 1996). In Romania, old age psychiatry has been officially recognised as a subspecialty of psychiatry since 2001. As in other Eastern European countries, geriatric psychiatry is still not well represented. Scientific organisations such as the Romanian Alzheimer Society (established 1996), the Romanian Association of Geriatric Psychiatry (1999), the Romanian Medical Society of Research of Cognitive Disorders and Alzheimer's Disease (2001) try to improve this situation by organising postgraduate courses for young psychiatrists and general practitioners so that better care of the elderly will be provided.

The number of professionals working in the field is still very low, and they are therefore unable to satisfy the need for care of elderly people with mental disorders. A postgraduate 1-year course is run in Bucharest for a diploma in psychogeriatrics for psychiatrists, geriatricians and medical residents (Camus *et al*, 2003). In addition, an annual summer course on geriatric psychiatry is organised in Romania for psychiatrists from all Eastern European countries. These courses are organised as an Eastern European Initiative by the International Psychogeriatric Association, together with the Romanian Association of Geriatric Psychiatry.

General practitioners and community nurses are also involved in the care of the elderly and so an educational programme has been initiated that includes courses for family doctors.

The Romanian Association of Geriatric Psychiatry and the Romanian Alzheimer Society also participate in the pilot studies on Alzheimer's disease and suicide organised by the World Health Organization.

## Mental health services for the elderly

Elderly people with acute and chronic mental disorders, as well as those with dementia, are taken care of both in psychiatric short- and long-stay hospitals and in social services. The latter are not well placed to care for these patients, as there are insufficient staff with professional qualifications in social work or in geriatric psychiatry. Unfortunately there is not a clear picture of all geriatric services, nor are there epidemiological studies in this field. Certainly, as yet there are few psychogeriatric services and even fewer specialist care services for dementia patients.

The extension of outreach services to nursing and residential homes in conjunction with day care centres, day hospitals and residential care could be a valuable alternative to the high degree of institutionalisation of Romanian elderly people, with or without mental disorders.

## Psychiatry and human rights

The protection of human rights and the dignity of persons with mental disorders has a relatively short history in Romania, although in 1652 Matei Basarab, the voivode (governor) of Walachia, in his *Letter to My Son*, wrote promoting the abolition of punishment for individuals with mental disorders and recommended their living in monasteries while they were ill.

Generally, Romania's legislation is in keeping with principles set out by the World Health Organization, United Nations and so on concerning the protection of people with a mental illness. The legislation calls for adequate treatment and respect for the human rights of people with mental disorders.

Standards and practice regarding involuntary commitment in a psychiatric department have been improved since the introduction of the new mental health law in 2002 (see above). Criminal Code 114 relates to forensic psychiatry. Also in 2002, Decree 313 was introduced, which pertained to the prevention of individuals with mental disorders becoming dangerous; this decree has recently been improved.

Involuntary commitment to a psychiatric department or involuntary treatment in an ambulatory setting of individuals with mental disorders is now established; which of the two orders is used depends on the mental state and the degree of danger. There are legal and ethical limits to involuntary commitment; for example, it may not be indefinite (as it was before the 1960s).

There is no legal discrimination against people with mental disorders but they are nevertheless discriminated against in other ways. Since 1990, because of financial problems, few patients have been able to find employment. The tolerance of society has decreased. Since 1990 it has been necessary to create committees to investigate abuse during involuntary commitment. On the other hand, before 1990 some individuals with (and even some without) mental disorders were committed to a psychiatric department to protect them.

## Conclusions

- In Romania, there is a push to re-orientate mental services from being centred on hospitals towards a community care focus.
- People with chronic mental disorders, including dementia, are taken care of both in long-stay psychiatric hospitals and by social services, where the personnel are inadequately trained to care for them.
- Stigma remains an obstacle in ensuring access to care for patients with a mental illness. The battle against stigmatisation needs to be prioritised.
- There is considerable room for improvement in education and training in psychiatry, in research, and in the promotion of mental health and illness prevention.
- It is important for the future development of community services to distinguish between care and treatment.
- The basic quality of care for those who are mentally ill needs to be improved by: developing a community psychiatric network based on

geographical catchment areas; developing a complex rehabilitation programme with more substantial social and financial support; involving the community, carers and users more; and involving the government and local authorities in mental healthcare.

In Romania, as in all former communist countries, there are economic problems and a need for national fundraising to support national psychiatric organisations and services.

# References

Camus, V., Katona, C., De Mendonca Lima, C. A., *et al* (2003) Teaching and training in old age psychiatry: a general survey of the World Psychiatric Association member societies. *International Journal of Geriatric Psychiatry*, **18**, 694–699.

Tataru, N. (1997) Project for the development of an ambulatory and semi-ambulatory centre for the third age. *Dementia and Geriatric Cognitive Disorders*, **8**, 128–131.

World Health Organization, Division on Mental Health and Prevention of Substance Abuse (1996) *Psychiatry of the Elderly – A Consensus Statement*. Geneva: WHO.

# Russian Federation

Valery Krasnov, Isaak Gurovich and Alexey Bobrov

The Russian Federation is a country with an enormous territory, of over 17 million km². Its population is 141.9 million (2010 figure). The population was declining, especially at the end of the 1990s, but in more recent years the tendency has been towards stabilisation. Life expectancy has remained relatively low, although it has increased somewhat over the past few years, to reach 67.5 years in 2008 (61.4 for men and 73.9 for women), up from 65.3 years in 2004 (58.9 for men and 72.3 for women).

The budget for healthcare has remained low compared with that in other countries, both high-income and low- and middle-income ones, and constituted in 2009 about 5.5% of gross national product (GNP). However, it should be mentioned that the federal allocations during the same period had grown from 2.3% to 3.5% of GNP; the rest of the total budget was provided by the state medical insurance system. There are significant differences between different regions in the financial support for local healthcare from municipal budgets. Psychiatric care is financed from the federal budget and is not included in the state medical insurance system.

## Psychiatric care

In general, the psychiatric care system is based on two main types of facility: the territorial psychiatric out-patient clinics, termed 'dispensaries' (in rural areas these are units located by general hospitals), which provide care for the population residing in a specific territory; and the psychiatric hospitals, which generally provide in-patient treatment for the population within a certain catchment area (district, city or region). As a rule, a dispensary district psychiatrist provides care for an adult catchment population of around 25000, whereas child psychiatrists (who usually work in a child territorial polyclinic) provide care for a catchment population of 15000 children and adolescents. These figures, though, will adjusted for territories with a lower population density.

Psychiatric dispensaries may additionally provide specialist services such as psychotherapy, neurology, epileptology, sexology and gerontopsychiatry;

they may also set up day hospitals. So-called 'narcology' services for people with alcohol and drug addiction were established in Soviet times, and until now they have mostly operated separately from regular mental health services.

A specific feature and principal defect of in-patient psychiatric care in Russia is its over-centralisation. The majority of psychiatric hospitals have more than 500 beds and some more than 1500. Nevertheless, over the past few decades the total number of beds has decreased by 25% and this process is continuing gradually. However, the decrease in psychiatric bed numbers has not always been accompanied by an increase in the provision of extramural forms of psychiatric care (Table 1).

The system of psychiatric care has shown contradictory tendencies in its development. On the one hand, taking into account the shortages in state budget allocations, psychiatric care on the basis of local psychiatric dispensaries that are open to the general public and connected to local psychiatric hospitals is expedient. On the other hand, psychiatric patients' stigma and societal prejudices against psychiatry and psychiatric institutions hinder the development of psychiatric dispensaries.

Only about 30–35% of all patients with a mental illness apply for psychiatric assistance in the dispensary. However, recently the number of patients asking for an initial psychiatric consultation has started to increase. The prevalence of mental disorders registered in psychiatric institutions has reached 2978.7 per 100 000 population (Table 2). At the same time, the problem of mental disorders in primary care is becoming more and more serious, such that, at present, some 25–30% of primary care patients need a psychiatric consultation. The need has arisen to reform and develop out-patient psychiatric care.

**Table 1** Extent of psychiatric care resources

| Mental health resource, *n* | 1999 | 2008 |
|---|---|---|
| Psychiatric dispensaries | 164 | 145 |
| Dispensary departments in psychiatric hospitals | 122 | 123 |
| Narcological dispensaries (for people with alcohol and drug addiction) | 171 | 144 |
| Dispensary units in general hospitals (in rural areas) | 2322 | 2078 |
| Psychotherapeutic units in general out-patient clinics | 1118 | 1107 |
| Psychiatric hospitals | 278 | 257 |
| Narcological hospitals | 13 | 12 |
| In-patient departments in psychiatric dispensaries | 107 | 88 |
| Total psychiatric beds (in psychiatric plus general hospitals) | 170 440 | 155 834 |
| Total beds in general hospitals (included in total above) | 14 015 | 13 890 |
| Total beds in narcological hospitals | 28 700 | 26 550 |
| Total places in day hospitals | 13 645 | 17 289 |

**Table 2** Patient populations

| Patient population, *n* | 1999 | 2008 |
|---|---|---|
| Persons with mental disorders (without substance misuse) | 3 813 500 | 4 226 899 |
| Persons with alcohol misuse | 2 230 050 | 2 728 010 |
| Persons with drug addiction | 209 080 | 358 120 |

National data from state psychiatric and narcological dispensaries and psychotherapeutic units.

The suicide rate in Russia is one of the highest in the world, although in recent years it has decreased slightly, from 38.7 per 100 000 in 1999 to 27.1 in 2008. The figure for men is six times higher than that for women, which may be related to greater alcohol consumption among men. Alcohol consumption in Russia is approximately 14–15 litres per capita (Nemtsov, 2009). The prevalence of alcoholism, including alcohol psychoses, has been more or less stable over the past decade, but with a slight tendency to increase, up to 1922.4 per 100 000 population in 2008; the male:female ratio was 5:1 (Koshkin, 2009; see also Table 2). Addiction to other substances has also apparently increased in recent years. The prevalence rate was 252.2 per 100 000 in 2008 (Koshkina, 2009). Opioid dependence accounted for 87.5% of this group.

Over the past few years, the total number of people with a mental illness who are registered disabled has increased by 20%, and in 2008 reached 1 020 002 (in 1999 it was 826 036). This increase has arisen not merely through personal deterioration in health but also because social adaptation has become more difficult.

In the past decade, a significant number of psychologists, psychotherapists, specialists in social work and social workers have been incorporated into the staff of psychiatric institutions, which has created a basis for transition from a largely medical to a biopsychosocial model of mental healthcare and a team approach to its provision (Table 3).

In some regions mental health services have begun to give greater emphasis to care in the community, where a system of psychosocial rehabilitation is

**Table 3** Numbers of specialists providing psychiatric care

| Specialists | 1999 | 2008 |
|---|---|---|
| Psychiatrists (including psychotherapists) | 15 860 | 16 184 |
| Psychotherapists (included in total above) | 3 248 | 3 438 |
| Narcologists (specialists providing care for people with alcohol or other substance misuse) | 4 470 | 5 329 |
| Specialists in social work (with higher education) | 70 | 772 |
| Social workers | 840 | 1 857 |
| Clinical psychologists (in psychiatric and narcological institutions) | 1 407 | 3 652 |

organised, hostels and other types of protected housing are set up, interaction with social services is developed, assertive treatment departments (teams) are set up, and 'hospital at home', employment, psychoeducation and psychosocial work with families are provided (Gurovich & Neufeldt, 2007). Non-governmental organisations (NGOs) are becoming more involved in mental health assistance, although not yet sufficiently so.

# Legislation and patients' rights

The Law on Psychiatric Care, adopted in 1992, works successfully enough at both federal and regional levels, and generally provides for patients' rights. However, social care services and guarantees regarding the provision of mental healthcare have not been implemented sufficiently.

Although there have been some notable omissions and errors in routine clinical practice in recent years (like the nationally well known Rakevich and Arap cases), these have not involved a deliberate violation of patients' rights. In some cases, especially connected with hospitalisation, mental health specialists do not pay enough attention to accounting for their actions to patients and relatives. It is not a matter of violation of the legislation, but rather a question of professional ethics. All such cases or conflicts in psychiatric care are discussed at meetings of the Russian Society of Psychiatrists and in professional journals.

# Research

Because of the urgent need for reform in mental healthcare, Russian psychiatrists consider applied clinical/organisational studies to be the main scientific task in their work. Epidemiology, the formation and trials of new models, new approaches to treatment and rehabilitation on the basis of multiprofessional teamwork, with the involvement of NGOs, are the priority for most researchers and research groups.

The detection and treatment of depressive and anxiety disorders at primary level is also one of the important directions for research, alongside investigating optimal forms of multidisciplinary work and joint research with doctors, cardiologists, neurologists and other specialists (Smoulevich *et al*, 2005; Krasnov, 2008).

Socially oriented studies have been supported by a special federal programme. Studying the mental health of populations living for a long time under the strain of an emergency situation and then under reconstruction and reconciliation processes, as has been the case in the Chechen Republic (Idrissov & Krasnov, 2009), is supporting the development of appropriate mental healthcare in specific regions.

Recently, new branches of research and practical psychiatry have emerged in Russia, such as ecological psychiatry and ethnocultural aspects of mental health (Krasnov & Gurovich, 2007).

# Education in psychiatry

Postgraduate education for clinical practice (after 6 years of formal medical education) comprises an additional 2-year course termed 'ordinature' and then 500 hours of specialisation in forensic psychiatry, narcology or psychotherapy (psychotherapy is possible only after at least 3 years of practical work in psychiatry). There are also courses on psychogeriatrics, child psychiatry, psychosomatics and the organisation of psychiatric services. All doctors have to validate their professional status in certificate confirmation courses, once every 5 years.

There is also a variety of training schemes for clinical psychologists and social workers.

# References

Gurovich, I. Ya. & Neufeldt, A. H. (eds) *(2007) Current Trends and New Service Models in Mental Healthcare*. Medpractica-M. (In Russian.)

Idrissov, K. A. & Krasnov, V. N. (2009) Mental health of the population of the Chechen Republic: a dynamic population 2002–2008 study. *Zhurnal nevrologii i psikhiatrii*, **109**, 76–81. (In Russian.)

Koshkin, A. V. (2009) *Prevalence of alcoholism in Russia in 2008*. First Russian National Congress on Narcology, November 24–27. Proceedings, Moscow (ed. N. N. Ivanets), pp. 237–238. NNC Narkologii. (In Russian.)

Koshkina, E. A. (2009) *Substance abuses in modern Russia*. First Russian National Congress on Narcology, November 24–27. Proceedings, Moscow (ed. N. N. Ivanets), pp. 236–237. NNC Narkologii. (In Russian.)

Krasnov, V. N. (ed.) *(2008) Improvement of Early Diagnostics of Mental Disorders (on the Basis of Interrelationship with Primary Care Specialists)*. Medpracitca-M. (In Russian.)

Krasnov, V. N. & Gurovich, I. Y. (2007) Russian culture and psychiatry. In *Culture and Mental Health* (eds K. Bhui & D. Bhugra), pp. 109–121. London: Hodder Arnold.

Nemtsov, A. V. (2009) *Alcohol History of Russia: Newest Period*. Librokom. (In Russian.)

Smoulevich, A. B., Syrkin, A. L., Drobijev, M. Y., *et al* (2005) *Psychocardiology*. Mental Informational Agency. (In Russian.)

# Serbia

Dusica Lecic Tosevski, Saveta Draganic Gajic
and Milica Pejovic Milovancevic

Serbia is located on the Balkan peninsula, which served for centuries as a vulnerable crossroads between the East and the West. At the beginning of the 1990s, some of the republics of the former Yugoslavia, including Serbia, were involved in disastrous civil conflicts. In 2006 Serbia became a sovereign republic. At the 2002 census, its population was 7 498 000.

The country has been exposed to many severe stressors, such as civil war in neighbouring countries, United Nations economic sanctions, which lasted for 3.5 years, and 11 weeks of NATO bombing in 1999. As a consequence, Serbia has experienced the destruction of infrastructure, large numbers of refugees and internally displaced people (currently there are half a million of them in Serbia), social instability, economic difficulties and deterioration of its healthcare system. In addition, a serious problem is the brain drain, since around 300 000 people, mostly young intellectuals, have left the country in recent years (Lecic Tosevski & Draganic Gajic, 2005).

After 2000, the country underwent economic liberalisation, and experienced relatively fast economic growth: gross domestic product per capita rose from US$1.160 in 2000 to US$6.782 in 2008, according to the International Monetary Fund (2008). The country is now passing through social transition and harmonisation with the European Union (EU). At present, the main problems are the high unemployment rate (18.8% in 2008 and currently rising due to the economic crisis) and the large trade deficit (US$11 billion). The major source of finance for public health is the national Health Insurance Fund, to which is allocated 6.1% of gross domestic product.

## Mental disorders

The events outlined above caused a steady rise in mental and behavioural disorders. The prevalence of mental disorders increased by 13.5% between 1999 and 2002 and they now represent the second largest public health problem, after cardiovascular disease. The incidence rates of stress-related disorders, depression, psychosomatic illnesses, substance misuse and suicide are still high, as are rates of delinquency and violence among young people (Lecic Tosevski *et al*, 2007). Furthermore, the burnout syndrome is pronounced in many physicians, who have shared adversities with their patients and experienced secondary traumatisation (Lecic Tosevski *et al*, 2006). An international multicentre study carried out 7 years after major trauma has shown that the prevalence of chronic post-traumatic stress disorder (PTSD) is still very high (current, 18.8%; lifetime, 32.3%), as is that of major depressive episode (current, 26.2%; recurrent, 14.4%) (Priebe *et al*, 2009).

## Mental health policy and legislation

In 2000, when the international community decided to take a proactive attitude rather than intervening only during crises, nine countries entered the Stability Pact for South-Eastern Europe (SEE): Albania, Bosnia and Herzegovina, Bulgaria, Croatia, the Former Yugoslav Republic of Macedonia, Moldova, Montenegro, Romania and Serbia. The mental health project 'Enhancing social cohesion through strengthening community mental health services' (Mental Health Project for SEE, www.seemhp.ba/index. php) brought together experts from the region with the aim of harmonising national mental health policies and legislation. The renewal of collaboration was also important for conflict resolution and reconciliation.

The National Committee for Mental Health was established in January 2003 by the Serbian Ministry of Health. As a coordinating body of the SEE Mental Health Project, the Committee prepared a national policy and action plan, and drafted a law on the protection of rights of persons with mental disorders. Both documents were reviewed by distinguished international experts. The National Strategy for Development of Mental Healthcare was approved by the government in January 2007 (Ministry of Health of the Republic of Serbia, 2007). A national programme for substance misuse has also been prepared and approved.

## Mental health services

The oldest psychiatric institution in the Balkans was established in Belgrade (capital of Serbia) in 1861 (the 'Home for Insane People'), with 25 beds. Nowadays, there are 46 in-patient psychiatric institutions in Serbia (specialist hospitals, psychiatric institutes and clinics, clinics for child and adolescent psychiatry, and psychiatric departments in general hospitals) and 71 out-patient services in municipal health centres. The entire mental health sector has 6247 beds, approximately half of which are in large psychiatric hospitals. Admissions in 2002 totalled 5833. The number of psychiatrists (neuropsychiatrists) in the country is 947, but some of them are involved in the treatment only of patients with neurological problems and do not deal with persons with a mental disturbance. A third of them work in the capital, Belgrade. About 5% of psychiatrists are engaged in child and adolescent psychiatry (Lecic Tosevski *et al*, 2005; Lecic Tosevski & Pejuskovic, 2005).

Healthcare in Serbia is free of charge and is provided through a wide network of public healthcare institutions, controlled by the Ministry of Health. The private provision of healthcare services, although limited, is on the rise, particularly in certain specialties, such as drug addiction.

Mental healthcare is well integrated with the primary healthcare system, at least in larger cities, which have mental health and developmental counselling units within municipal health centres. The first community mental healthcare centre was opened in 2005 in the southern part of Serbia. However, the widening of the network of community centres is rather difficult because of the economic crisis. There are other problems in mental healthcare, such as a lack of residential homes, as well as the poor condition of some of the large psychiatric hospitals. There are five of these in Serbia, and some patients have been hospitalised in them for many years, since they have no relatives, or the community would not accept them. Many patients with chronic mental disabilities are accommodated in social care homes, which are in need of deinstitutionalisation.

Non-governmental organisations are also involved with mental healthcare. Their role was invaluable during years of conflict since they supported local experts in preventive programmes for refugees and internally displaced persons, ex-detainees and torture victims. Non-governmental and paraprofessional groups have an increasing role within the mental health system, through various psychosocial programmes for deinstitutionalisation, destigmatisation, domestic violence, human rights and so on.

Until recently, prevention was not financed by the state and was carried out by enthusiastic professionals. Fortunately, the government has recently recognised its importance and is now supporting programmes for the prevention of suicide and violence among children and young people, as well as the prevention of substance misuse and alcoholism.

## Training

The specialties of psychiatry and neurology were separated in 1993, and child psychiatry was established as a separate specialisation. The duration of training for adult and child psychiatry is 4 years. Both curricula are developed according to European standards and are accredited (Pejovic Milovancevic *et al*, 2009).

Postgraduate psychiatry training is well developed – there are subspecialties in psychoanalytical psychotherapy, forensic psychiatry, clinical pharmacology and so on. Psychotherapy has a long tradition and many psychotherapists were trained abroad, primarily in England and France, in various approaches – psychoanalytical, group analysis, systemic, cognitive–behavioural, and so on. Continuing medical education has become obligatory for all mental health professionals.

# Research

Professionals from Serbia are publishing in leading psychiatric journals, books and textbooks. Serbia was included in two multicentre studies, supported by the EU, which have been carried out in the Balkans – STOP and CONNECT (Priebe *et al*, 2002, 2004). It is hoped that the results of these studies will represent an empirical basis for adequate programmes for people with PTSD.

The Belgrade Institute of Mental Health is a partner in the exciting EU project 'Copy number variations conferring risk of psychiatric disorders in children'. The aim of the project is to identify genetic variants that confer an enhanced risk of major mental disorders on children and adolescents.

# Professional associations

There are several psychiatric associations in Serbia, including the Serbian Psychiatric Association, the Serbian Association of Psychiatric Institutions, the Association for Child and Adolescent Psychiatry and Allied Professions of Serbia, and the Serbian Psychotherapeutic Association. These associations collaborate closely with international organisations such as the World Psychiatric Association, the European Psychiatric Association and the European Association of Psychiatry. Collaboration with the World Health Organization (WHO) is also flourishing and the Serbian Institute of Mental Health was recently nominated to be the WHO Collaborating Centre for Workforce Development.

# Human rights issues

The human rights of all patients in Serbia are protected by the Healthcare Law. The Mental Health Act is expected to be approved shortly. In 2006, the government introduced the concept of 'carer of patient's rights' and now each hospital has a professional with such a duty, usually with a legal background. In addition to this, most institutions have ethical committees and are obliged to apply an ethical code in treatment and research.

# Conclusion

The organisation of mental healthcare in Serbia has many advantages, as well as disadvantages. The main advantages are a balanced territorial coverage of psychiatric departments in general hospitals, well-educated professionals, as well as a relatively low proportion of institutionalised patients at the onset of the mental healthcare reform. Of special importance is a long tradition of psychosocial orientation, with day hospitals in clinics of all larger towns.

However, there is insufficient cooperation between primary, secondary and tertiary healthcare. This is exacerbated by a lack of catchment areas and patients' legal right to choose their own doctor (often by affinity or reputation of doctors), as well as lack of skills of general practitioners in mental healthcare. Stigma in relation to mental illness is prevalent among the public, which hinders early recognition and treatment. Furthermore, there is a lack of cooperation between the psychiatric and the social welfare institutions, a lack of community mental healthcare centres and other out-patient psychiatric services in the community (rehabilitation and professional orientation services), as well as insufficient information systems for registering and monitoring mental disorders.

The ongoing psychiatric reform certainly represents a challenge and opportunity for mental health professionals. The process of reform is not easy, especially in a country facing social transition, so it is expected that the implementation of the national strategy and action plan will take time.

# References

International Monetary Fund (2008) *World Economic Outlook (WEO): Financial Stress, Downturns, and Recoveries*. Available at http://www.imf.org/external/pubs/ft/weo/2008/02/weodata/index.aspx (accessed October 2009).

Lecic Tosevski, D. & Draganic Gajic, S. (2005) The Serbian experience. In *Disaster and Mental Health* (eds J. J. Lopez-Ibor, G. Christodoulou & M. Maj, *et al*), pp. 247–255. Wiley.

Lecic Tosevski, D. & Pejuskovic, B. (2005) Mental health care in Belgrade – challenges and solutions. *European Psychiatry*, **20**, 266–269.

Lecic Tosevski, D., Curcic, V., Grbesa, G., *et al* (2005) Mental health care in Serbia – challenges and solutions. *Psychiatry Today*, **37**, 17–25.

Lecic Tosevski, D., Pejovic Milovancevic, M., Pejuskovic, B., *et al* (2006) Burnout syndrome of general practitioners in postwar period. *Epidemiologia e Psichiatria Sociale*, **15**, 307–310.

Lecic Tosevski, D., Pejovic Milovancevic, M. & Popovic Deusic, S. (2007) Reform of mental health care in Serbia: ten steps plus one. *World Psychiatry*, **6**, 51–55.

Ministry of Health of the Republic of Serbia (2007) *Strategy for the Development of Mental Health Care*. Available at http://www.imh.org.rs (accessed October 2009).

Pejovic Milovancevic, M., Lecic Tosevski, D., Popovic Deusic, S., *et al* (2009) Mental health care of children and adolescents in Serbia: past steps and future directions. *Epidemiologia e Psichiatria Sociale*, **18**, 262–265.

Priebe, S., Gavrilovic, J., Schützwohl, M., *et al* (2002) Rationale and method of the STOP study – study on the treatment behaviour and outcomes of treatment in people with posttraumatic stress following conflicts in ex-Yugoslavia. *Psychiatry Today*, **34**, 133–160.

Priebe, S., Jankovic Gavrilovic, J., Schützwohl, M., *et al* (2004) A study of long-term clinical and social outcomes after war experiences in ex-Yugoslavia – methods of the 'CONNECT' project. *Psychiatry Today*, **36**, 111–122.

Priebe, S., Bogic, M., Ajdukovic, D., *et al* (2010) Mental disorders following war in the Balkans – a study in five countries. *Archives of General Psychiatry*, **67**, 518–528.

# Slovak Republic

## Jozef Dragašek and Alexander Nawka

The Slovak Republic is a landlocked country in central Europe with a population of over 5 million. The Czech Republic and Austria lie to the west, Poland to the north, Ukraine to the east and Hungary to the south. The largest city is the capital, Bratislava; the second largest city is Košice. Slovakia is a member of the European Union, the United Nations, the Organisation for Economic Cooperation and Development (OECD) and the World Trade Organization, among other international organisations. The majority of the inhabitants of Slovakia are ethnically Slovak (85.8%). Hungarians are the largest ethnic minority (9.5%). With a gross domestic product (GDP) of €63.3 billion in 2009, Slovakia is classified as a middle-income country. In that year total health expenditure represented 6.7% of GDP (Pažitný, 2008), 34% of which went on pharmaceuticals, the highest share among all OECD countries (World Health Organization, 2010).

## Prevalence of mental disorders

Two epidemiological studies have recently been conducted to assess the prevalence of depressive and anxiety disorders in Slovakia – the EPID (Heretik et al, 2003) and EPIA (Novotný et al, 2006) surveys. According to the EPID survey, the 6-month prevalence rate of depression is 41% (13% major depression, 5% minor depression and 23% depressive symptoms only); and according to the EPIA survey, the 6-month prevalence of generalised anxiety disorder is 4%.

The overall rates for first lifetime contact with mental health out-patient services for all mental disorders has been reported to be 1724.4 per 100000 inhabitants (NCZI, 2009). Almost 27% of treated mental disorders were classified as neurotic disorders; organic disorders were the second most commonly treated conditions in the out-patient setting (20.5%), followed by affective disorders (17.5%) and substance use disorders (12.7%) in 2008 (NCZI, 2009).

## Policy and legislation

Slovakia has no laws specific to mental healthcare and there is no monitoring of the quality of care. Several independent bodies monitor human rights in general and some non-governmental organisations address the human rights of those with mental illness (Bražinová *et al*, 2008).

Slovakia ratified the main human rights instruments in 1992, shortly before the division of Czechoslovakia and the establishment of the Slovak Republic. Mental healthcare falls under the general system of healthcare and is regulated by general healthcare legislation, which reflects much of the international thinking about human rights. An anti-discrimination act, adopted in 2004, bans discrimination on the grounds of health status. The government adopted the Charter of Patients' Rights in 2001 and this has since been promoted through various non-governmental activities. The Charter defines all the rights and entitlements of patients within healthcare delivery as they are stipulated in other legally binding documents. The Slovak Public Defender of Rights, for instance, monitors the legality of official decisions that affect individuals and the Slovak National Centre for Human Rights is an independent human rights monitoring centre that provides information and assistance.

The act on healthcare specifies forms of out-patient and in-patient care (Bražinová *et al*, 2008). It has improved the protocols for informed consent, the right to information, choice of provider, access to documentation, right to dignity, confidentiality and refusal of care. The Healthcare Surveillance Authority was established in 2005; it supervises public health insurance and the overall delivery of healthcare services.

## Personnel

The professionals involved in mental healthcare may be classified as follows:
- medical doctors – psychiatrists, child and adolescent psychiatrists
- nurses – general nurses with secondary education, nurses with a bachelor's degree and nurses with a specialisation ('nursing in psychiatry')
- other health professionals with a degree – psychologists, social workers, physiotherapists, 'pedagogues' in health establishments, etc.
- health workers without a degree.

In 2004 the Slovak Republic had 32 psychiatric nurses, 10 psychiatrists, 3 psychologists and 1 social worker per 100 000 inhabitants (UZIS, 2006). The shortage of nurses, social workers and case managers sometimes results in patients having no one to coordinate comprehensive care packages for them.

## Service delivery

Nationally, there are 26 psychiatric wards in general hospitals (including the psychiatric departments in university hospitals), with a total of 1744 beds. These beds are used for short-term acute hospitalisations. The length of stay is limited by the health insurance companies to around 21 days (NCZI, 2009). The comparatively large number of beds can be explained by the tradition of in-patient care in central Europe and because hospital psychiatric services sometimes have to compensate for the lack of social care and community services. Community-based services, such as case management, rehabilitation centres, sheltered housing and employment schemes, are few in number (Table 1) and in fact only one region (Michalovce) has a system of community-based mental healthcare (Nawka *et al*, 2008).

## Training in psychiatry and in allied professions

On the basis that well-trained mental healthcare personnel are at the foundation of quality care, the Slovak Republic has made important reforms in the post-communist period (Vevera *et al*, 2008). The structure of the system where most psychiatric patients are treated in general hospitals is, however, mirrored in the training requirements.

Slovakia has three medical faculties that provide comprehensive courses in psychiatry: the Faculty of Medicine, Comenius University, in Bratislava; the Jesenius Faculty of Medicine, Comenius University, in Martin; and the Faculty of Medicine, University of P. J. Šafárik, in Košice. Postgraduate training is directed by the Ministry of Health and executed mainly by the Slovak Medical University and other accredited institutions. The postgraduate curriculum is in accordance with the Charter of the Union Européenne des Médecins Spécialistes (UEMS; European Union of Medical Specialists) for training in psychiatry; it includes a variety of psychiatric in-patient and out-patient services. There are also 2-year certified courses for specialisation in geriatric psychiatry, psychiatric sexology and substance misuse. Two of three existing medical faculties, in Bratislava and Košice, are able to grant PhDs in psychiatry.

Psychology as an independent bachelor and masters degree programme is delivered by faculties of philosophy. There are also three public faculties

**Table 1** Mental health services in Slovakia (2006) (population 5.44 million)

| Facility/service | *n* |
| --- | --- |
| Psychiatric out-patient clinics | 201 |
| Psychology out-patient clinics | 179 |
| Day clinics | 14 |
| Case management services | 1 |
| Rehabilitation centres | 60 places |
| Sheltered workshops | 12 places |
| Sheltered living services | 1 (8 beds total) |
| Psychiatric departments in general hospitals | 26 (1744 beds total) |
| Psychiatric hospitals | 5 (1392 beds total) |
| Mental hospitals | 4 (630 beds total) |

and one private faculty for healthcare and nursing and one medical university focusing mainly on training, as well as 24 secondary medical schools.

## Research and publications

Research in Slovakia is mostly carried out at universities and institutions attached to the Academy of Sciences. The most important are psychiatric departments within medical schools (Bratislava, Košice and Martin) and the Slovak Medical University. Unfortunately, mental health research in Slovakia is fragmented and largely ad hoc in nature, financed from different resources (Veselý & Ocvár, 2008). Most scientific research is in biological psychiatry (e.g. electrophysiology in schizophrenia and addiction), epidemiology (depressive and anxiety disorders, suicide), quality of life and psychopathology.

There are only two professional Slovak mental health journals in which researchers can publish their results, and neither is indexed in the ISI Web of Knowledge. Research findings are often published in conference brochures.

## Plans for future

In recent years, Slovakia has achieved important results in the organisation of its mental health services, but there is still a lot to do in order to achieve sustainability. Developments will focus on the following areas (Nawka *et al*, 2008).

### Prevention

Primary, secondary and especially tertiary prevention had been largely neglected. There is now, though, promotion of social integration and employment of individuals with mental illness in their community. Special focus should be placed on the mental health needs of children, adolescents and the elderly.

### Adequate resources

A system with adequate resources must be created to support better quality of care and more consumer-driven services. This should actually reduce overall spending on mental health.

### Community-based care

Most chronic beds in psychiatric hospitals should be eliminated or transformed to social health beds. Specialised secure departments for the compulsory long-term treatment of non-voluntary patients are planned in psychiatric hospitals.

## Integration

Mental healthcare is due to be better integrated into general health and social services, as care shifts away from psychiatric hospitals to psychiatric departments in general hospitals.

## Local participation

Local government must be involved in health promotion, and in the treatment, rehabilitation and integration of patients into the community and labour market.

## Training

New curricula will be needed for the transformation to community mental healthcare, which will require both traditional and new categories of personnel: social workers, case managers, primary care physicians, self-help group workers, patient advocates and advocacy experts.

# References

Bražinová, A., Baudiš, P., Háva, P., *et al* (2008) Mental health policies and legislation. In *Mental Health Care Reform in the Czech and Slovak Republics, 1989 to the Present* (eds R. M. Scheffler & M. Potucek), pp. 81–112. Charles University Press.

Heretik, A., Sr, Heretik, A., Jr, Novotný, V., *et al* (2003) *EPID – Epidemiológia depresií na Slovensku.* [Epidemiology of Depression in Slovakia.] Psychoprof.

Nawka, P., Dragomirecká, E., Dzúrová, D., *et al* (2008) Organizational structures. In *Mental Health Care Reform in the Czech and Slovak Republics, 1989 to the Present* (eds R. M. Scheffler & M. Potucek), pp. 113–141. Charles University Press.

NCZI (Národné Centrum Zdravotníckych Informácií; National Health Information Centre) (2009) *Zdravotnícka Rocenka Za Rok 2008.* [Health Yearbook Year 2008.] NCZI.

Novotný, V., Heretik, A., Sr, Heretik, A., Jr, *et al* (2006) *EPIA – Epidemiológia Vybraných Uzkostných Porúch na Slovensku.* [Epidemiology of Selected Anxiety Disorders in Slovakia.] Psychoprof.

Pažitný, P. (2008) *Stanovisko HPI k Rozpoctu Zdravotníctva na Roky 2009–2011.* [Health System Budget 2009–2911 from the Standpoint of the Health Policy Institute.] Available at http://www.hpi.sk/hpi/sk/view/2213/stanovisko-hpi-k-rozpoctu-zdravotnictva-na-roky-2009-2011.html (accessed August 2010).

UZIS (Ústav Zdravotnických Informací a Statistiky; Institute of Health Information and Statistics) (2006) *Trendy Vývoje Zdravotnických Dat v SR a CR v Letech 1994–2004.* [Trends in Evolution of Health Data in the SR and CR, 1994–2004.] UZIS.

Veselý, A. & Ocvár, L. (2008) Research and evaluation. In *Mental Health Care Reform in the Czech and Slovak Republics, 1989 to the Present* (eds R. M. Scheffler & M. Potucek), pp. 225–250. Charles University Press.

Vevera, J., Bražinová, A., Nemec, J., *et al* (2008) Human resources and training. In *Mental Health Care Reform in the Czech and Slovak Republics, 1989 to the Present* (eds R. M. Scheffler & M. Potucek), pp. 197–223. Charles University Press.

World Health Organization (2010) *Slovakia. Country cooperation strategy at a glance.* Available at http://www.who.int/countryfocus/cooperation_strategy/ccsbrief_svk_en.pdf

# Slovenia

Slavko Ziherl and Blanka Kores Plesnicar

Slovenia, with an area of 20 000 km² and a population of 2 million, is one of the smallest members of the European Union. It gained its independence from Yugoslavia in 1991. The country has a gross domestic product (GDP) of US$27 300 per capita. (Largely because of its historical links with Western Europe, Slovenia has a higher GPD compared with other countries in transition in Central Europe.) The health budget represents 8.4% of GDP. Slovenia has a low birth rate and an ageing population. It is divided into 210 municipalities; however, the reorganisation of government into several separate regions with more administrative and economic autonomy is in progress. The prevalence of mental illness is comparable to that in other European countries, although there are high levels of alcoholism and suicide.

## Mental health policy and legislation

Slovenia is a democratic country with a parliamentary form of government. The government must generally endorse all healthcare reforms before they are implemented. The Law of Healthcare and Health Insurance presents the basis for compulsory and voluntary health insurance and also allows for the privatisation of healthcare. The Health Insurance Institute of Slovenia is a public non-profit institution, which is overseen by the state and is bound by the Law on Compulsory Health Insurance. Ministries, government agencies and offices have an administrative and regulatory function and are also responsible for the development of health policy, preventive programmes and health promotion. The state is also the owner and director of public health institutions, such as hospitals and clinics.

Currently the National Programme for Mental Health is in the process of being passed in parliament, as is the new Law on Mental Health. Until now, the provisions of the Non-contentious Procedure Act from 1999 have been used, but these are not in accordance with the constitution. The new Law on Mental Health establishes a network of implementers of mental health programmes and services, defines the rights of people in the network (including the right to a representative or lawyer), establishes the conditions and manner of the appointment of representatives, coordinators of supervisory proceedings and coordinators of services, and regulates the procedure for voluntary or involuntary admission to a psychiatric hospital or social welfare institution. It also contains an innovation, the supervision of patients with psychiatric disturbances in their local community. This would mainly hold true for patients with severe psychiatric disturbances.

## Mental health service delivery

The healthcare system and mental health service delivery are both defined by the Law on Medical Services. Mental health institutions are part of the public health network; there are no private psychiatric hospitals or centres for long-term care in the country. Only community care is private, with the majority of providers having contracts with the Health Insurance Institute. Access to psychiatric services is available to everyone and it is paid for by the Health Insurance Institute with funds from compulsory health insurance.

Real deinstitutionalisation of psychiatry has never been achieved in Slovenia. There are four general psychiatric hospitals, one psychiatric clinic and one department of a university clinical centre. This provision amounts to 0.85 beds/1000 inhabitants, which includes beds occupied by patients under compulsory and forensic care. There are 5.4 psychiatrists per 100 000 inhabitants and 5.8 psychiatric nurses per 100 000 inhabitants, who are mainly employed in psychiatric hospitals. Within the Psychiatric Clinic and the University Clinical Centre there are two departments of child and adolescent psychiatry, while another department of child psychiatry is located at the Children's Hospital. In Slovenia there are 24 specialists in child and adolescent psychiatry.

Adults with special needs or those with severe and chronic mental disorders are treated in five institutions, which are partly financed by health insurance funds and partly from social welfare.

Community psychiatric treatment is provided by psychiatrists who are otherwise employed in psychiatric hospitals, by those in health centres and by private psychiatrists who have contracts with the Health Insurance Institute. There are community care facilities for patients with mental disorders, but a broader system of community mental health has not yet been developed. Psychiatric hospitals and clinics provide professional support and education for those employed in non-government organisations, which are active in rehabilitation, the integration of patients into society, counselling and other forms of assistance, and also play an active role in anti-stigma programmes. Within their framework there are 44 residential groups, 22 day centres and 14 information offices.

Slovenia also has specific programmes for the mental health of minorities, refugees, the elderly and children. Educational programmes are run for general practitioners, and teachers, school counsellors and others for the recognition of suicidal tendencies.

# Psychiatric training

In Slovenia there are two medical faculties. Medical studies last 6 years. One faculty is linked to the Psychiatric Clinic in Ljubljana, the other to the Psychiatric Department of the University Clinical Centre in Maribor. After completion of studies and a 1-year internship it is possible to specialise in psychiatry.

The Medical Chamber of Slovenia is responsible for specialisation, licensing, issuing a code of medical ethics and supervising clinical practice. Membership of the Medical Chamber is compulsory for all professionals. A call for applications for specialisation in all fields is made by the Medical Chamber twice a year, according to national needs. Annually there are on average advertisements for 15 vacant positions for specialisation in psychiatry, but the positions remain unfilled because of the severe shortage of doctors throughout the country. Training for specialisation in psychiatry lasts 5 years, as does training in child and adolescent psychiatry. Both specialisations have a common 2-year programme, after which they differ.

# Psychiatric subspecialties and allied professions

Psychotherapy is only partly included in the specialisation programme (4 months); a longer period of psychotherapy training is not compulsory. The specialisation in clinical psychology lasts 4 years, and is advertised by the Ministry of Health. There is no special specialisation for psychiatric nurses, but only additional education, which is run by the two university psychiatric institutions with the assistance of the Nursing Chamber of Slovenia.

# Main areas of research

Slovenian psychiatry is rather underdeveloped in the area of research. Only one professional psychiatric journal is published, and this does not have an impact factor. There is no research institute in the field of psychiatry in the country; hence research is left to interested and highly motivated professionals.

The Institute of Public Health of the Republic of Slovenia has carried out research in the field of suicide. Slovenia has one of the highest suicide rates in the world, with 22.7 suicides per 100 000 inhabitants per year. The suicide rate has, though, declined since 1992, when it was 28.9 per 100 000 population. There is a higher suicide rate among men (38.2 per 100 000 population) than among women (9.19 per 100 000 population). Most alarming is the extremely high suicide rate in the over-65 age group, of 48.45 per 100 000, with the rate in males reaching 94.85/100 000 population. This places Slovenia foremost globally for suicides among the elderly.

Other research is being carried out in the field of pharmacogenetics, in collaboration with faculty institutions, and into cognitive functions in some severe physical illnesses.

## Workforce issues, resources

There is still too little employment in the field of psychiatry. There is a shortage of doctors in Slovenia and despite increased enrolment in the medical faculties no increase in the number of doctors or psychiatrists can be expected until 2015. The employment of psychologists, psychiatric nurses, occupational therapists and social workers is dependent on the budget of each institution. Perhaps part of the problem will be solved by increased privatisation in health, especially in community care. Private psychiatrists can choose between patients, as they have long waiting lists; this places a heavy burden of patient management onto hospital psychiatrists, who run a 24-hour emergency service. The new national health programme envisages larger work obligations for private psychiatrists.

## Human rights issues

Slovenia has a human rights ombudsman, whose office intensively oversees human rights, especially in psychiatric hospitals and prisons. In parliament, a new law on patients' rights was approved in April this year. This introduces more ombudsmen for patients' rights throughout the country (previously there had been only one). Also in parliament, a new Mental Health Act is awaiting approval. This will introduce a national plan on mental healthcare, and reform psychiatric services towards a more community-oriented approach.

## Sources

Statistical Office of the Republic of Slovenia (2007) *Slovene Regions in Figures*. Statistical Office of the Republic of Slovenia.

Švab, V., Groleger, U. & Ziherl, S. (2006) The development of psychiatric reform in Slovenia. *World Psychiatry*, **5**, 56–58.

Ziherl, S. (1997) Psychiatric training in Slovenia. *European Archives of Psychiatry and Clinical Neuroscience*, **247 (suppl.)**, S38–S40.

# Spain

## Juan J. López-Ibor and Blanca Reneses

Spain covers an area of some 506 000 km² and has a population of just over 41 million. It is a high-income country (according to World Bank criteria) and devotes 7.5% of its gross domestic product to health.

## Organisation of healthcare

Spain's National Health System has universal coverage and is financed through the general budget of the state, although the system is organised territorially. Healthcare has two levels: primary care, which is the gate into the system, and specialised care, which is managed independently of primary care, although some regions are considering unifying the two. Psychiatric care is part of specialised care.

Around 6% of the population have additional health insurance and can be treated privately, which gives them greater choice in their healthcare. The private insurance companies set limits on the length of psychiatric hospital stays and the number of out-patient consultations per year that can be reimbursed.

## Mental health policy and service organisation

The budget, planning and provision of health services are taken care of by each of the 17 *comunidades autónomas* (regions), which are responsible for their own mental health policies under the framework of the 1986 General Health Law and the 1995 Decree for Psychiatric Reform. The Law on the Cohesion and Quality of Healthcare reinforces the uniformity and standards of the care provided in each *comunidad autónoma*.

Each of the *comunidades autónomas* has a mental health plan, framed as part of a general health plan. Social reintegration is a key feature of mental health policy. The details of each region's policy are set out in its plan. There is a specific national plan for drug misuse, which is drawn up by the Ministry of Internal Affairs, since it includes actions pertaining to the control of the traffic in illicit drugs.

For mental health services there is also a general (i.e. national) decree that covers clinical diagnosis and follow-up, pharmacological therapy, individual, group and family psychotherapies and hospitalisation; hypnosis and psychoanalysis are excluded. The cost of all psychotropic drugs is covered by the National Health System.

All *comunidades autónomas* share the following organisational principles for their mental health services (Reneses, 2003).

- Care is based on the principles of community psychiatry.
- Services are sectorised. Each sector (district) has from 50 000 to 200 000 inhabitants. Mental health services in each sector consist of a multidisciplinary team of psychiatrists, psychologists, nurses, occupational therapists and social workers. Each sector has one or more mental health centres and one or more admission units for acute processes, as well as day hospitals and psychosocial rehabilitation centres.
- People experiencing acute psychiatric episodes are preferably hospitalised in general hospitals. Traditional mental hospitals have been progressively transformed to fit their services to the needs of the population in areas such as rehabilitation, units for sub-acute processes and units for residential care.
- There are specific programmes for the care of children and adolescents in general mental health services or in independent centres. These programmes include out-patient care, day hospitals and admission units, although only some regions have specialist mental health units for minors (in the others they are admitted to general paediatric units).
- The net of social services is tightly coordinated with the healthcare one in different forms in the different *comunidades autónomas*. In some of them out-patient rehabilitation services are provided by the social services.
- Residential non-hospital care is perceived to be less and less sufficient and is usually provided by social services.
- Specific programmes of psychotherapy, the treatment of alcohol-related problems and rehabilitation are present in all regions but have different degrees of development.

There are some further differences in the way the *comunidades autónomas* organise their services:

- Some of them have an independent net for the care of people who misuse drugs.
- Some have non-hospital admission units for the long-stay care of people with sub-acute and chronic processes.
- The number of resources, both structural and human, varies among the *comunidades autónomas*, as a result of the differing budget allocations for mental health.

# Mental healthcare resources

The territorial organisation of health services means that there is no easily accessible national source of information on resources. However, the National

Health System publishes online statistics on hospitals (*Establecimientos Sanitarios con Regimen de Internado*; ESCRI) and these provide the following information. The number of psychiatrists providing out-patient care in public health services varies from 7.2 psychiatrists per 100000 population in Asturias to 1.6 in Extremadura; the average is around 4 psychiatrists per 100000. Across the regions, the number of beds in units for acute care in public hospitals is between 7.2 and 12.0 per 100000 population. The total number of beds, public and private, is 50.4 per 100000 inhabitants, of which 12.6 are in services for acute processes and 38.6 are for long-stay patients. For acute cases, 60.2% of beds are located in general hospitals.

The number of hospital discharges with a main psychiatric diagnosis per 100000 inhabitants in the year 2002 was 279 (Instituto Nacional de Estadística, 2002).

## Information systems

The national minimum data-set (CMBD) facilitates the collection of basic healthcare data. It covers the whole of public hospital care and collects data on all hospital discharges, and includes information on mental health. The Questionnaire on Hospital Morbidity (Instituto Nacional de Estadística, 2002) and the ESCRI provide statistical information on the structure, activity and finances of all public and private hospitals.

The specific information systems for mental health are decentralised, each *comunidad autónoma* having its own system. At least five *comunidades autónomas* have information systems based on cumulative case records; the rest have systems based on group activity (Ministerio de Sanidad y Consumo, 2003). There is no specific national information system for mental health.

## Patients' rights

The national civil and penal codes have been modified to protect the rights of psychiatric patients and improve conditions of detention for offenders with a mental illness. As a part of these reforms, prison hospitals were closed and special units within the National Health System were opened.

The latest civil legislation relating to mental illness was enacted in 2000; this regulates all involuntary admissions and treatments, which can be carried out only after judicial authorisation and with supervision.

## Training and education

### Training of specialists

The training of psychiatrists, clinical psychologists and psychiatric nurses is regulated at state level; services have to be authorised to undertake training (Ministerio de Sanidad y Consumo, 1996). There is no specialisation in child psychiatry or in geriatric psychiatry. A limited number of residency posts are offered, again organised at state level. There is a state examination common to all medical disciplines. (In the case of psychologists and nurses, the examination is specific to each specialty.) The attainment of a residency post depends on the results obtained in the selective examinations.

The training of psychiatrists takes 4 years and includes: psychiatric in-patient and community care, liaison psychiatry, child psychiatry, day-hospital care, neurology and internal medicine (Ministerio de Sanidad y Consumo, 1996).

The training of clinical psychologists takes 3 years and includes hospital and community care, care of children and adolescents, and psychosocial rehabilitation.

Training in psychotherapy is in preparation. At present it is not carried out in a systematic way nationally, although some hospitals do provide their own.

## Undergraduate training

Two mental health disciplines generally feature in the curricula of medical schools: medical psychology in the preclinical, basic curriculum; and psychiatry during the clinical period. Some medical faculties have a third discipline, psychopathology, which is otherwise taught as part of either the medical psychology or the psychiatry curriculum. Several non-compulsory disciplines are also included, among them drug dependence and eating disorders.

# Mental health professions

Professional practice is regulated at national level by the 2003 Law for the Regulation of Healthcare Professions. The specialty of child psychiatry does not exist, officially, and this has impeded the organisation of psychiatric care for children and adolescents.

The practice of psychotherapy is not regulated in Spain. Normally training in psychotherapy is carried out by psychiatrists and clinical psychologists in the private sector.

Clinical practice is not allowed to psychologists not qualified as clinical psychologists.

# Psychiatric associations

The two best-established national associations are the Sociedad Española de Psiquiatría (SEP), a scientific medical association of psychiatrists, and the Asociación Española de Neuropsiquiatría (AEN), whose membership consists of all mental health professionals. In the past it also included a significant number of neurologists and neurosurgeons. The SEP holds a national congress every year jointly with the Sociedad Española de Psiquiatría Biológica (SEPB), which is a smaller, mainly research society.

The AEN also organises annual congresses. There are various regional associations, most of which are linked to the SEP or to the AEN.

Other national scientific associations cover more specific fields, such as child psychiatry, psychogeriatrics, psychiatric epidemiology, alcoholism and drug addiction and forensic psychiatry.

## Scientific journals

The oldest Spanish psychiatric journal still published is *Archivos de Neurobiologia*. *Actas Españolas de Psiquiatría* is the most widely distributed psychiatric journal in the Spanish-speaking world and is among those with the highest impact factor of all non-English psychiatric journals. Another widely distributed journal is the *Revista Española de Psiquiatría Biológica*.

## References

Instituto Nacional de Estadística (2002) *Encuesta de Morbilidad Hospitalaria*. Available at: http://www.ine.es/inebase/menu3_soc.htm

Ministerio de Sanidad y Consumo (1996) *Guía de Formación de Especialistas [Guide to the Formation of Specialties] (3rd edn)*. Madrid.

Ministerio de Sanidad y Consumo (2003) *Informe de Situación de Salud Mental*. [Information on the Mental Health Situation.] Madrid: Observatorio del Sistema Nacional de Salud. See http://www.msc.es/Diseno/informacionProfesional/profesional_observatorioSNS.htm

Reneses, B. (2003) Planificación de los Servicios Psiquiátricos en España. [Planning *of psychiatric services in Spain.] In Tratado de Psiquiatría [Textbook of Psychiatry]* (eds M. Gelder, J. J. López-Ibor & N. Andreasen), Vol. III. Barcelona: Ars Médica.

## Further reading

López-Ibor, J. J., Leal, C. & Carbonell, C. (2004) *Images of Spanish Psychiatry*. Madrid: Editorial Glosa.

# Sweden

Helena Silfverhielm and Claes Göran Stefansson

With an area of 450000 km², Sweden is one of the largest countries in Western Europe. It is 1500 km from north to south. It has nearly 9 million inhabitants (20 per km²). It is a constitutional, hereditary monarchy with a parliamentary government. Sweden is highly dependent on international trade to maintain its high productivity and good living standards. Many public services are provided by Sweden's 289 municipalities and 21 county councils. Municipal responsibilities include schools, child care and care of the elderly, as well as social support for people with a chronic mental illness. The county councils are mainly responsible for healthcare, including psychiatric care, and public transport at the regional level. Sweden is characterised by an even distribution of incomes and wealth. This is partly a result of the comparatively large role of the public sector.

## The healthcare system

Sweden's healthcare system is governed through the three levels of government – central, county and municipality. Central government is responsible for legislation within the healthcare system, higher education (universities), research funding, the health insurance system, and general and directed subsidies to the counties and municipalities to help them carry out different public service measures. The 21 counties are responsible for specialised healthcare activities, which include hospitals and primary healthcare (general practitioners) and the medical professionals working there. The 290 municipalities are responsible for social services for elderly persons and those with a disability, including a mental disability. This includes not only social support but also medical nursing.

The public healthcare system is financed by taxes raised at all three levels of government. A minor part of healthcare is carried out on a private basis (mostly short-term treatment). Private care is most common in the big cities and is rare in rural regions. The management of the care and social services provided for people with mental disorders is handled by the counties and the municipalities.

In 2001 the total expenditure on medical care in Sweden was a19.1 billion, which represented 8.0% of gross domestic product (GDP). After allowing for income from patient fees and so on, the net cost to government was a12.1 billion.

Mental healthcare has achieved political prioritisation over the past 20 years, on the one hand through a national action plan for the development of healthcare and on the other by the introduction of a national mental health coordinator, combined with directed subsidies from the government for the development of mental healthcare.

## Mental health services

Net expenditure on psychiatric care is a1.4 billion per year. The psychiatric treatment prevalence of adult persons is about 2–3% of the total population per year. In the bigger cities the treatment prevalence is higher (e.g. 4–5% in Stockholm).

Psychiatric care is divided between four different types of organisation: general psychiatry (for those aged 18 years or more); child and adolescent psychiatry; forensic psychiatry; and psychiatry of persons with drug misuse.

### Hospital beds

In 1967 the mental hospitals were transferred from the state to the counties. At that time there were in total some 35 000 psychiatric beds (4 beds/1000 inhabitants), of which about 70% were in mental hospitals. Thereafter they began to close, and since the mid-1990s Sweden has had no beds in mental hospitals. Today there are about 4000 psychiatric beds (0.5 beds/1000 inhabitants), all of them in psychiatric wards in general hospitals (except 350 in forensic high-security hospitals).

### In-patient care

The number of in-patients continues to decline. The proportion of beds occupied by persons under compulsory and forensic care was higher in 2005 than previously (Table 1). The reduction in bed numbers has been made possible through the out-patient care centres and the commitment of the municipalities to the psychiatric reforms of 1995 (see below). But there has been a re-institutionalisation. The beds in the former psychiatric hospitals have now to a certain degree been replaced by nursing homes and supported housing managed by the municipalities.

## Social services

The social services are responsible for the care of people with a disability, which includes people with a long-term mental illness. Expenditure on

**Table 1** Number of in-patients in Sweden, based on data from a single-day census

| Form of care | 1991 Men | 1991 Women | 1994 Men | 1994 Women | 1997 Men | 1997 Women | 2005 Men | 2005 Women |
|---|---|---|---|---|---|---|---|---|
| Voluntary | 4270 | 4659 | 3218 | 3396 | 1884 | 2141 | 2228 (total) | |
| Compulsory | 1003 | 919 | 557 | 551 | 522 | 409 | 394 | 461 |
| Forensic | 731 | 106 | 677 | 58 | 699 | 71 | 809 | 126 |
| Total | 6004 | 5684 | 4452 | 4005 | 3105 | 2671 | 4022 (total) | |

Source: National Board of Health and Welfare, Sweden (2005).

social services was a13.2 billion in 2000, or 5.7% of GDP. Unfortunately it is impossible to separate costs for mental healthcare within social services from other costs. In 2002 there were some 8000 people with mental disabilities in 850 sheltered homes for whom the social services were responsible.

The social services also have responsibility for long-term care and economic support for persons with substance misuse disorders. In the year 2000 some 21 000 people aged 21 years or more were in receipt of such services, at a total cost of a 406 million.

# Development of psychiatric care

## Community Mental Healthcare Reform, 1995

An evaluation of the sectorised organisation of psychiatric care showed, among other things, that patients with a long-term mental illness, for example those with schizophrenia, in a number of respects were not receiving satisfactory care. Their needs for medical treatment were mostly being met, but other needs (e.g. social support) were not. The responsibility for interventions regarding these needs was given to the social service agencies, with the Swedish Social Services Act of 1982. However, a parliamentary commission of 1992, the Committee on Psychiatric Care, concluded that social services were still largely inadequate and were not being provided in a satisfactory manner. Therefore, the mandate upon municipal social services was clarified through the Community Mental Healthcare Reform, which came into effect on 1 January 1995. The reform is directed towards individuals with severe and long-standing mental illness.

The aim of the reform was to take back into the local community people undergoing long-term treatment in psychiatric hospitals and nursing homes and to force social service agencies and psychiatric units to cooperate in their care for these people. The reform also clarified that social services had the primary responsibility to support anyone with a chronic mental illness in the community with housing, daily activities and rehabilitation.

Today there are about 45 000 people with a chronic mental illness (0.7% of the total adult population) yearly in the care of social services or psychiatric care organisations. This is about a quarter of all patients in psychiatric treatment.

## Legislation concerning psychiatry

The Swedish Disability Act 1994 aims to provide support and services for people with disabilities of various kinds, including psychiatric disorders. The law states a number of specific forms of assistance that these people can receive, including counselling and support, personal assistance, housing with special services, contact persons and companions. The Act is 'complementary' in that it cannot entail any curtailment of assistance to which the individual is entitled under other legislation. Moreover, it is civil rights legislation, and decisions can therefore be appealed against in the administrative courts. As of 2002, 2700 persons with a mental disability were in receipt of benefits under the Disability Act.

The Healthcare Act 1982 regulates the treatment of persons in need of medical or psychiatric treatment, whether by nurses in sheltered homes within social services or by specialised psychiatric care in these homes or in clinics.

The Social Services Act 2001 obliges the municipal social services to conduct outreach activities among persons with psychiatric disabilities. Social services are also obliged to plan their assistance programmes for these people in collaboration with the psychiatric care organisation and other social bodies and organisations.

The Municipal Financial Responsibility Act 1995 makes it incumbent upon the municipalities to pay for the care of patients who, after three consecutive months of in-patient treatment by a psychiatrist, have been deemed as fully medically treated within the psychiatric in-patient system but who are still being cared for in hospital because they cannot be transferred into community-based independent living or sheltered housing. One of the aims of this municipal financial responsibility is to stimulate the development of new forms of housing within the community for people with a mental disability who have been in long-term institutional care.

## Problem areas

There are three groups for whom care provision in Sweden is at present problematic:
- patients with a chronic mental illness
- those aged 18–25 years
- those with a dual diagnosis of personality disorders and substance misuse.

## Patients with a chronic mental illness

These persons belong mainly to the diagnostic categories of the psychoses and most (75–80%) have schizophrenic disorders. The Community Mental Healthcare Reform has meant that about 80% of these people live in the community, with support mostly from social services. The predominant problem is the degree of cooperation between social services and the psychiatric care organisations, which both have some responsibility for people with schizophrenia. Central government is trying to force the counties (psychiatric care) and the municipalities (social services) to create a joint organisation for the care and social support of these people. This has been legally possible since 1 July 2003.

## Younger patients

The treatment prevalence of persons within psychiatric care has increased notably in recent years, mostly in out-patient services. In Stockholm county (in which one in five of the Swedish population resides) this number increased by 33% between 1997 and 2001 (from 45 000 persons to 60 000, or from 3.5% of the adult population to 4.5%). The increase is, however, most marked for people aged 18–25 years. Substance misuse is common in this group. A large part of psychiatric out-patient resources are directed to this problem but there has been no systematic effort to provide services directed to the psychiatric problems of 'young adult' persons. One solution would be to merge child psychiatry with adult psychiatry services. These care organisations at present mostly operate entirely independently.

## People with personality disorders and substance misuse (dual diagnosis)

This category of psychiatric disorder has come to public prominence recently because of a few high-profile cases, notably one which involved the murder of Sweden's foreign minister, Anna Lind. Investigations showed that these persons often have a long history of treatment, have had early contact with social services and from a young age have engaged in criminal behaviour. A government inquiry has been launched to investigate how medical/psychiatric treatment and social services can be better coordinated for these people.

# Suicide

Sweden has traditionally had a reputation as a country with a high suicide rate, but after marked increases in the 1960s and 1970s the rate steadily fell after 1979 (Table 2). The suicide rate for 2000, 19.0 per 100 000 population aged 15 years and over, was the lowest since the current classificatory system was introduced in 1969, and Sweden is now part of the middle group among European countries. Furthermore, the age differences in

**Table 2** Numbers of suicides and suicide rates per 100 000 (men and women, aged 15 years and over), by age-group, for selected years 1980–2002

| Year | 15–24 years | | 25–44 years | | 45–64 years | | 65+ years | | Total | |
|---|---|---|---|---|---|---|---|---|---|---|
| | *n* | Rate | *n* | Rate | *n* | Rate | *n* | Rate | *n* | Rate |
| 1980 | 174 | 15.4 | 805 | 34.4 | 790 | 42.3 | 468 | 34.4 | 2237 | 33.4 |
| 1985 | 158 | 13.5 | 749 | 31.1 | 664 | 36.6 | 495 | 34.0 | 2066 | 30.2 |
| 1990 | 153 | 13.1 | 638 | 26.2 | 676 | 35.2 | 513 | 33.6 | 1980 | 28.1 |
| 1995 | 131 | 12.1 | 568 | 23.4 | 663 | 31.3 | 444 | 28.8 | 1806 | 25.2 |
| 2000 | 106 | 10.3 | 416 | 17.1 | 483 | 21.4 | 375 | 24.5 | 1380 | 19.0 |
| 2001 | 110 | 10.6 | 445 | 18.3 | 601 | 26.3 | 390 | 25.5 | 1546 | 21.2 |
| 2002 | 146 | 13.9 | 418 | 17.2 | 586 | 25.3 | 335 | 21.8 | 1485 | 20.3 |

Source: Swedish National Centre for Suicide Research and Prevention of Mental Ill-Health, 2005.

suicide fatalities are, from an international perspective, relatively small. In line with the general decrease, suicide rates for both men and women fell in the 20 years up to 2001, when certain suicide rates increased from the rather low levels in 2000. Public health specialists became concerned that this increase could announce a change in trend towards rising suicide rates. Figures for 2002 published by the National Board of Health and Welfare indicate a decrease in the female suicide rate in 2001/02, accompanied by a marginal increase in the male rate.

The reduced suicide rate has not been as evident among younger groups, however; in parallel, in international comparisons, the oldest age-group has a relatively low suicide rate.

## Recruitment trends

According to statistics from the National Board of Health and Welfare, in 2002 there were 1700 doctors with a specialist qualification in psychiatry. Of these, 1400 were actively engaged in healthcare. The number of new psychiatrists who had received their training in Sweden increased over the period 1996–99 but the number fell thereafter (Fig. 1).

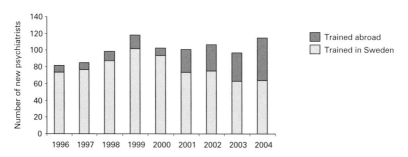

**Fig. 1** Total number of specialty licences in psychiatry distributed to doctors trained in Sweden or abroad, 1996–2004. Source: National Board of Health and Welfare, NPS database.

The number of psychiatrists employed in the public healthcare system care is forecast to rise to 2010. Thereafter the number will be stabilised at around 1500, and then fall again so that by 2020 it is expected to be at the same level as in 2001 (Fig. 2).

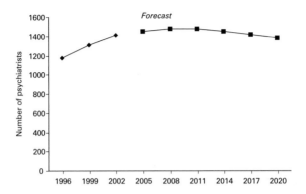

**Fig. 2** Total number of psychiatrists in the healthcare system, 1996–2002 and forecast for 2005–20. Source: National Board of Health and Welfare, NPS database.

According to a 2004 nationwide inquiry by the National Board of Health and Welfare directed at the county councils, there was some optimism regarding their ability to recruit new professionals, not only psychiatrists but also nurses and psychologists.

# Switzerland

## Dan Georgescu

Switzerland – officially the Swiss Confederation – is a federal republic situated in central Europe. It covers an area of 41 287 km² and has a population of just over 7 600 000. Switzerland consists of 26 federated states, of which 20 are called cantons and 6 are called half-cantons. German, French and Italian are Switzerland's major and official languages.

Switzerland has the second highest per capita level of healthcare spending as a proportion of gross domestic product (11.3%). Although there are no exact data available, based on international comparisons, one may assume that at least 10–12% of total healthcare costs are attributable to mental health problems. A characteristic of Swiss society and therefore of Swiss psychiatry is the federal and liberal tradition. Although there is hardly any central state coordination of mental health policy, there is to some degree a homogeneous level of care services throughout the whole country. The cohabitation of the public and private sectors reflects the liberal tradition. Swiss modern psychiatry goes back to the second half of the 19th century, when the first psychiatric hospitals and chairs and a professional association of psychiatrists were founded.

## Mental health policy and legislation

On a political level, there is no national mental health policy, common strategy or binding principles to ensure the uniform national delivery of psychiatric care. The national strategy for mental health, developed in 2004 by the Federal Department for Health, is actually only a guide to help the cantons and the federal government design concrete projects.

Even with respect to involuntary admission, there is no uniform legal framework at a national level, but only basic federal legislation (article 397 of the Code of Civil Law), with corresponding supplementary laws on preventive custody at the cantonal level. With respect to compulsory treatment there is only a guideline entitled *Compulsory Measures in Medicine of the Swiss Academy for Medical Sciences*. Further legal documents relevant to psychiatry are, at the national level, those regarding the right of self-determination, bodily injury and a duty to take care, as well as, at the cantonal level, health laws and patient decrees. There are several decisions of the Federal Tribunal determining the duty to obtain informed consent.

An important milestone of Swiss health law, the federal health law of 2006 regarding the academic medical professions, regulates the training, specialty-related and personal licensing conditions and the professional duties of physicians. This law strongly influences not only the universities but also private practice, as well as the law-makers at canton level.

# Mental health services

## Funding

In Switzerland, the cantons are in charge of the organisation of mental health services. The cantonal healthcare concepts differ to a certain extent as far as the services offered and the health delivery structures are concerned. However, in recent years a certain degree of convergence has occurred, although the federal structure has favoured a fragmentation of the funding agencies and the healthcare providers.

Services provided by the psychiatric hospitals are reimbursed mainly by health insurance companies – mandatory insurance being imposed since 1996 by the Law on Sickness Insurance for all Swiss residents – and by the cantons. Private funding, additional private insurance and the municipalities contribute to the funding to a much more moderate extent. Out-patient treatment is covered mainly by health insurance, followed by self-payment for such treatment.

Consultations in private practice are reimbursed also for those patients who have only basic (mandatory) health insurance, provided that the psychiatrist is recognised by the cantonal authority. Those with additional, private health insurance have a choice of hospital, even if this is situated in another canton or if it is a private one.

Besides psychiatrists there are also many psychologists practising in the private sector, their bills being reimbursed only for patients with additional insurance.

Traditionally, the Swiss greatly value the ability to make their own choice in matters related to healthcare, but in the last decade political pressure has come from both the state and the insurance companies to limit the number both of doctors in private practice and of reimbursed sessions of psychotherapy, as well as to introduce a system of managed care, including gatekeepers. This pressure, aimed at reducing healthcare costs, has stirred up some controversies and confrontations in Switzerland.

## Service delivery

At present there are 1.06 psychiatric beds (forensic and addiction psychiatry beds not included) per 1000 inhabitants; there has been a continuous reduction in recent years in the number of beds in hospitals, in favour of community-based settings. Under the slogan 'ambulant before hospital', out-patient care and day hospital care have been extended to assume a major role in prevention, crisis intervention and rehabilitation. Despite the expansion of community-based services in recent years, there are differences in the availability of psychiatric services – as well as private practices – between urban and rural areas.

Mental health services are delivered by the state as well as by the private sector. The cantonal governments are responsible for the organisation of psychiatric care in the state sector. The state sector includes a wide range of well equipped services with a high degree of specialisation. In addition to general adult psychiatry and child and adolescent psychiatry, the psychiatric institutions also have substance dependence, old age, psychosomatic medicine and liaison psychiatry services, as well as forensic psychiatry services.

The private sector consists of eight private psychiatric institutions and psychiatrists working in private practice. The private institutions offer in-patient as well as out-patient facilities for a range of mental disorders, with the exception of severe psychotic illness and hostile, agitated or self-harming behaviours.

It should be emphasised that mental healthcare in Switzerland involves cooperation between psychiatric services (both state and private) and adjacent sectors, such as public health, disability services, social services, youth welfare services and senior services, as well as justice and police.

# Workforce issues and professional organisations

Relative to its population, Switzerland has the highest number of psychiatrists in the world: 30 per 100 000 inhabitants, according to the World Health Organization (WHO). At present, Switzerland has, according to the Federal Department of Health, 2603 adult psychiatry specialists, of whom 2016 are in private practice, the rest being employed in public institutions. For child and adolescent psychiatry the numbers are 1257 (overall) and 439 (in private practice). However, the overall number of psychiatrists is actually significantly higher, given that many psychiatrists with foreign diplomas, working mainly in state hospitals, are not included in these statistics. Thirty-nine per cent of adult psychiatrists and 47% of child and adolescent psychiatrists are female.

The Swiss Society of Psychiatry and Psychotherapy (SSPP) – which includes among others the cantonal psychiatric societies and the affiliated subspecialty organisations – has 1884 members; the Swiss Society of Child and Adolescent Psychiatry and Psychotherapy (SSCAPP) has 592 members.

In 2002, the SSPP and SSCAPP co-founded an umbrella organisation, the Foederatio Medicorum Psychiatricorum et Psychotherapeuticorum (FMPP), to promote the common interests of the two psychiatric associations. *The Bulletin Psy & Psy* is the common organ of the SSPP and the SSCAPP, informing its readers about issues of professional politics. The joint website is www.psychiatrie.ch.

# Training

## Undergraduate training

Undergraduate medical education in Switzerland lasts 6 years. There are six medical schools, in Basel, Berne, Geneva, Lausanne, Zurich and Fribourg, though the last offers only the pre-clinical, basic curriculum. All medical schools are subsidised by their home cantons. At the undergraduate level there are three disciplines concerned with mental health: psychosocial medicine, adult psychiatry and child and adolescent psychiatry.

## Postgraduate training in psychiatry

Responsibility for the education of medical specialists lies with the Swiss Medical Association (Foederatio Medicorum Helveticorum, FMH) and the medical professional associations, on behalf of the Federal Department of Home Affairs. The professional associations develop the training programmes, which are afterwards examined and put into force by the FMH, whereas the diplomas are issued by the Federal Department. Devising the psychiatric training curriculum and its periodic review, organising and administering the specialty board examinations as well as visits to the training centres are the responsibility of the Standing Committee on Psychiatric Training and Education of the SSPP. The Committee includes representatives of the universities, of the training directors, of psychiatrists in private practice, of trainees, and so on.

The recently revised competence-based training programme is due to become effective in 2009. It stipulates a 6-year residency, of which 1 year is to be spent in a somatic specialty and 5 in psychiatry. Both in-patient and out-patient settings need to be part of the residency experience, and a rotation between different institutions is required.

Training in psychiatry and psychotherapy is decentralised and not a matter only for university centres. Around 150 psychiatric institutions of varying size are recognised by the FMH as places of residency, each with an *a priori* specified period of recognised training, in a hospital or ambulant setting, and psychiatric subspecialty.

Theoretical psychiatric education is offered within the framework of the eight regional networks for postgraduate education. Together with psychiatric training in the narrow sense, trainees are taught the basics of health economics, the legal foundation and ethical aspects of psychiatric practice. Training in psychotherapy, which accounts for a considerable part of the postgraduate programme, is provided by SSPP-recognised private institutes of psychotherapy in German-speaking Switzerland, as well as by the universities in the French-speaking part. The current residency programme stipulates 3 years of training in one of the recognised models (psychoanalytic, cognitive–behavioural or systemic). Traditionally, efforts have been made to ensure the Swiss curricula have a well balanced biological and psychosocial content.

## Psychiatric subspecialties

Child and adolescent psychiatry developed at the beginning of the 20th century out of adult psychiatry and paediatrics. In Switzerland, the development started early, in comparison with other European countries, with the establishment of care structures specific to this age group. Child and adolescent psychiatry became a separate psychiatric discipline in 1953. It has its own chairs in all medical schools, 30 postgraduate training centres as well as more than 17 cantonal services with out-patient as well as in-patient or day hospital structures. Although Switzerland boasts a higher incidence of child and adolescent psychiatrists than its neighbours, the supply of such services is insufficient, in particular outside the densely populated cities.

The first subspecialty of adult psychiatry to be officially recognised by the Medical Chamber was old age psychiatry (2005), followed by consultation–liaison psychiatry (2008). For old age psychiatry, several university chairs have already been established; there are 37 training centres and about 100 certified old age psychiatrists. At present, there are ongoing efforts to establish two further psychiatric subspecialties (forensic psychiatry and addiction psychiatry).

## Research and scientific journals

Swiss research in psychiatry has always been valued nationally and internationally. Research is done at all the universities, mostly of a clinical nature or on basic science. Currently, there is a tendency to form collaborative research groups connecting several neurosciences.

The only Swiss psychiatric journal still published is *Swiss Archives of Neurology and Psychiatry* (founded 1917, eight issues a year, published in German, French and English). Swiss authors are frequently present on the editorial boards of widely distributed scientific journals in English, German, French and Italian.

## Sources

Bundesamt für Gesundheit (BAG) (*2009*) *Psychische Gesundheit* [Mental health]. At http://www.bag.admin.ch/themen/medizin/00683/01916/index.html?lang=de (accessed May 2009).

Foederatio Medicorum Helveticorum (FMH) *(2001) Facharzt für Psychiatrie und Psychotherapie: Weiterbildungsprogramm* [Psychiatry and Psychotherapy: Programme of Specialist Education.]. At http://www.fmh.ch/de/data/pdf/psychiatrie_version_internet_d.pdf (accessed May 2009).

Joint Conference of Swiss Medical Faculties (SMIFK) *(2002) Swiss Catalogue of Learning Objectives for Undergraduate Medical Training*. At http://sclo.smifk.ch (accessed May 2009).

Schweizerische Gesundheitsdirektorenkonferenz (GDK) *(2008) Leitfaden zur Psychiatrieplanung* [Guideline for psychiatry planning]. At http://www.gdk-cds.ch/fileadmin/pdf/Themen/Gesundheitsversorgung/Versorgungsplanung/Psychiatrieplanung/GDK-Psychiatrieplanung15-d__def_.pdf (accessed May 2009).

# Ukraine

## Semyon Gluzman and Stanislav Kostyuchenko

Ukraine, at 603 700 km$^2$, has the second largest landmass in Europe. It has a population of about 47.4 million. Ukraine is a lower-middle-income country with a gross national income per capita of US$1260 (World Bank, 2002).

## Healthcare

The health and well-being of the Ukrainian population, as in other former Soviet countries, are generally very poor. Life expectancy at birth is 69.7 years (64.4 years for men and 75.3 years for women). Overwhelmingly the most important reason for this is the combination of poverty, poor diet and living conditions, and lifestyle factors such as tobacco and alcohol use. Cardiovascular disease and trauma (accidents and poisonings) are the two most common causes of death, followed by cancer (UNDP & UNICEF, 2002).

Healthcare expenditure amounts to 3.5% of gross domestic product. In-patient care accounts for two-thirds of total healthcare expenditure. The number of physicians per 100 000 is 229; hospital bed provision is 903.2 per 100 000 (1998 figure), much in line with the average of 812.0 per 100 000 across Europe.

During the past 10–15 years government programmes have sought to strengthen primary healthcare on the basis of family medical practice, to develop a system of health insurance, and to create the conditions for private medical practice. A key feature of the current situation in Ukraine is the low level of remuneration for doctors and other healthcare staff (International Labour Office, 2001).

## Mental health services

In-patient psychiatric care is delivered in 89 psychiatric hospitals. Of a total of 44 812 psychiatric beds, only 1468 are in general hospitals. There are also 6535 beds in 40 in-patient drug misuse facilities. The main features of the network of mental health services are their centralised structure, their focus on patients with a psychosis and their relative separation from other medical services.

## Mental health legislation

The Law on Mental Healthcare was adopted by the Ukrainian Parliament in February 2000. It defines the legal and organisational principles for the provision of psychiatric care to citizens. The Law also defines forms of mental healthcare and the legal basis for psychiatric assessment, as well as for out-patient and in-patient treatment. For the first time, the Law set up a system for the provision of involuntary psychiatric care. Also, the responsibilities of state authorities with respect to the protection of the rights and legitimate interests of persons with mental disorders are defined in the Law. Further, it sets out the rights and obligations of the persons responsible for the provision of psychiatric care.

## Training

The graduate 6-year study programme in a medical university includes an obligatory 54 hours of training in medical psychology and 108 hours of training in psychiatry. Internship to become a specialist in psychiatry lasts 2 years. The programme includes some training in child psychiatry, the treatment of substance misuse, psychotherapy and neurology, but most of the training is in adult psychiatry.

After 3 years of work as a physician after graduation from medical university it is possible to receive training in the following specialties: psychiatry, child psychiatry, the treatment of substance misuse (in Ukraine and other post-Soviet countries this is a separate specialty named narcology), psychotherapy and sexology. This training takes 4–5 months.

Every psychiatrist should receive at least 1 month of professional training once every 5 years.

## Resources

The state network of mental health services employs 3477 psychiatrists (7.33 per 100000 population); of this total, 1783 work in out-patient facilities, 238 are psychotherapists, 94 are forensic psychiatrists and 1317 are narcologists (2.78 per 100000). Other mental health professionals, such as nurses, psychologists, occupational specialists and social workers, are not included in the official statistics. Also, there are private mental health and substance misuse services, primarily in large cities, but again statistics are unavailable.

# Research

There are wide networks of scientific institutions and departments of psychiatry at medical universities. However, few papers reporting Ukrainian research in the field of mental health appear in the world literature.

In 2002 the Ukrainian Psychiatric Association, in collaboration with Division of Epidemiology of the Department of Psychiatry at the State University of New York at Stony Brook and Kiev's International Institute of Sociology, conducted the first epidemiological survey of mental health and substance use disorders. This found that close to one-third of the population experienced at least one psychiatric illness in their lifetime, 17.6% had experienced an episode in the past year and 10.6% had a current disorder. There was no gender difference in the overall prevalence rates. In men, the most common diagnoses were alcohol disorders (26.5% lifetime) and mood disorders (9.7% lifetime); in women, they were mood disorders (20.8% lifetime) and anxiety disorders (7.9% lifetime). The rates of treatment seeking were very low. The person to whom respondents talked most often about their symptoms was their general medical provider. For lifetime mood disorders, 16.6% talked to a professional; for anxiety disorders, the figure was 21.1%. The rates were higher in those with more severe forms of these disorders. Thus, for the subgroup of respondents with mood disorder who acknowledged suicidal thoughts, the percentage who talked to a professional was 25.1%.

# The Ukrainian Psychiatric Association

The Ukrainian Psychiatric Association (UPA) is a non-governmental, non-profit organisation working in the field of psychiatry and professional training. It was founded in 1990. The UPA has become a leader among the similar organisations in Eastern Europe and Central Asia. It is an information centre for psychiatrists, psychiatric nurses, psychologists, lawyers and politicians working in the field of mental health and health system reform.

Since its inception, the UPA has considerably widened its network: there are now 31 UPA branches and more than 800 members. A priority for the UPA is to diminish the 'information isolation' of Ukrainian medical specialists.

In 1990 the UPA founded its special Experts' Commission for rendering social and legal assistance to mental health service users and their relatives. It provides assistance on a daily basis to all those who appeal to it. People appeal to the Commission with requests to protect their rights. The experts working on it represent the interests of people with psychiatric illnesses in the courts and provide juridical and social assistance to them. Their activities are wide in scope: specialist consulting; legal assistance (including representation in court); the assistance of forensic psychiatrists (including support in courts); the provision of consultations by forensic psychologists;

psychological help; and the attendance of a social worker. The Commission has registered an increase in the number of cases pertaining to human rights and psychiatry abuses. This serves to confirm, unfortunately, the inadequacy of government assistance. The UPA's Expert Commission regularly informs the mass media, legal and law-enforcement authorities in relation to the human rights of people with a mental illness in Ukraine. The UPA more generally fulfils an important societal service, through its independent expert groups, in carrying out regular monitoring of human rights abuses in the field of psychiatry. The UPA provides assistance and consultations without charge. Since its establishment in 1990, the UPA has been actively engaged in overcoming the stigmatisation of psychiatric patients in Ukraine.

The UPA publishes two periodicals, in Ukrainian, the *Review of Contemporary Psychiatry* and the *UPA Bulletin*. These are distributed not only to psychiatrists in Ukraine and other ex-Soviet countries but also to psychiatric patients and their relatives. Moreover, the UPA has assisted in starting other journals, such as *Social, Psychological and Medical Aspects of Cruelty* and *Social Policy and Social Work*.

The research activities of the UPA have included the implementation of programmes in the following fields:

- sociological – 'monitoring of human rights observance', 'public opinion on mental health and psychiatric illness'
- economic – 'provision of a basic economic rationale of psychiatric system reorganisation'
- epidemiological – 'mental health of children', 'Chernobyl disaster victims', 'alcoholism and mental disorders in Ukraine'
- historical – 'history of psychiatry in pre-revolutionary and Soviet periods'.

In addition, a special project has been launched on the adaptation of ICD–10 in Ukraine, in cooperation with American psychiatrists.

# Conclusion

The outline above reflects only one aspect of the situation, the formal one, as described by many international experts from the World Bank and other agencies.

The situation has another side, however, and it is a sad one. As in all post-Communist states, our psychiatric service is archaic (it does not correspond to the political, legal and economic realities of the country), ineffective and costly. The principles of evidence-based medicine are ignored within the system of psychiatric services. The collection of medical statistics, for example, is archaic and not of the best quality. Epidemiological studies (in the Western sense of the term) have not been carried out in this country. Financial institutions have never sought to examine the cost-effectiveness of the existing mental health system, responsibility for which is dispersed across at least seven government ministries and departments.

The Ministry of Healthcare of Ukraine formally admits the use of out-of-date, exotic and harmful methods of treatment (ranging from the well known sulfazine of Soviet punitive psychiatry to unmotivated psychosurgical intervention and inadequate application of electroconvulsive therapy).

Only recently has there emerged some hope that the system will be improved. For the first time in this country a competent and determined person has been appointed to the post of the Chief Psychiatrist. Hope is also inspired by the establishment of a national service users' association, the activism of the officers of the Department of Mental Health and Substance Dependence, and the World Health Organization's collaboration with various partners in this country.

## References and further reading

Adams, R. E., Bromet, E. J., Panina, N., *et al* (2002) Stress and well-being in mothers of young children 11 years after the Chernobyl nuclear power plant accident. *Psychological Medicine*, **32**, 143–156.

Bromet, E. J., Gluzman, S. F., Paniotto, V. I., *et al* (2005) Epidemiology of psychiatric and alcohol disorders in Ukraine: Findings from the Ukraine World Mental Health survey. *Social Psychiatry and Psychiatric Epidemiology*, **40**, 681–690.

Bromet, E. J., Goldgaber, D., Carlson, G., *et al* (2000) Children's well-being 11 years after the Chernobyl catastrophe. *Archives of General Psychiatry*, **57**, 563–571.

Drabick, D. A., Gadow, K. D., Carlson, G. A., *et al* (2004) ODD and ADHD symptoms in Ukrainian children: external validators and comorbidity. *Journal of the American Academy of Child and Adolescent Psychiatry*, **43**, 735–743.

International Labour Office (2001) *Healthcare in Central and Eastern Europe: Reform, Privatization and Employment in Four Countries. A report to the International Labour Office.* Geneva: ILO.

UNDP & UNICEF (2002) *The Human Consequences of the Chernobyl Nuclear Accident: A Strategy for Recovery.* http://www.undp.org/dpa/publications/chernobyl.pdf

Webb, C. P., Bromet, E. J., Gluzman, S., *et al* (2005) Epidemiology of heavy alcohol use in Ukraine: findings from the world mental health survey. *Alcohol and Alcoholism*, **40**, 327–335.

WHO World Mental Health Survey Consortium (2004) Prevalence, severity, and unmet need for treatment of mental disorders in the World Health Organization World Mental Health Surveys. *JAMA*, **291**, 2581–2590.

World Bank (2002) *World Development Report*. Washington, DC: World Bank.

# United Kingdom

Vicky Banks, Geoff Searle and Rachel Jenkins

The National Health Service (NHS) serves the UK through four devolved organisations for England, Scotland, Wales and Northern Ireland. It is one of the largest public healthcare systems in the world, universal and free at the point of delivery. Its key challenge is to maintain this approach within tight financial constraints, while embracing new technologies, treatments and styles of service delivery, as well as meeting the health needs of an ageing population.

The population of the UK was 61 792 000 in mid-2009. Children aged under 16 represented approximately one in five of the total population, around the same proportion as those of retirement age (over 65). In mid-2009 the average age of the population was 39.5 years, up from 37.3 in 1999. Population growth is greatest in the over-85s, who currently number around 1.4 million, a figure which is estimated to reach 3.5 million by 2034, which will represent 5% of the population.

## Mental health in the UK

Mental illness contributes 22.8% of the total burden of disability-adjusted life years (DALYs) in the UK (World Health Organization, 2008). One in six adults has a mental health problem at any one time (World Health Organization, 2004).

Half of those with a long-term mental illness have it by the age of 14 (Kim-Cohen *et al*, 2003) and three-quarters by their mid-20s (Kessler & Wang, 2007). The most deprived communities in the UK have the poorest mental health and physical health (McManus *et al*, 2009). People with severe mental illness die on average 20 years earlier than the general population. Mental health problems cost England approximately £105 billion each year, including costs of lost productivity and the wider impacts on well-being (Centre for Mental Health, 2010), and represent the largest single cost to the NHS, accounting for 11% of the secondary care budget (Department of Health, 2009).

Further key statistics are presented in Box 1.

---

**Box 1** Mental illness in England: some illustrative figures

- 10% of children and young people have a mental disorder. Of 5- to 16-year-olds, 6% have conduct disorder (Green *et al*, 2005), 4% an emotional disorder (Green *et al*, 2005) and 18% subthreshold conduct disorder (Colman *et al*, 2009)
- 17.6% of adults in England have at least one common mental disorder and a similar proportion have symptoms which do not fulfil full diagnostic criteria for common mental disorder (McManus *et al*, 2009)
- Postnatal depression affects 13% of women following childbirth (O'Hara & Swain, 1996)
- In any one year, 0.4% of the population suffer from a psychosis (McManus *et al*, 2009) and a further 5% from subthreshold psychosis (Van Os *et al*, 2009)
- 5.4% of men and 3.4% of women have a personality disorder (Singleton *et al*, 2001); 0.3% of adults have antisocial personality disorder (McManus *et al*, 2009)
- 24% of adults have hazardous patterns of drinking, 6% have alcohol dependence (Singleton *et al*, 2001), 21% tobacco dependence (McManus *et al*, 2009) and 3% dependence on illegal drugs (Singleton *et al*, 2001)
- 25% of older people have depressive symptoms which require intervention: 11% have mild depression and 2% severe depression (Godfrey *et al*, 2005); the risk increases with age – 40% of over-85s are affected
- 20–25% of people with dementia have major depression, whereas 20–30% have minor or subthreshold depression (Amore *et al*, 2007)
- Dementia affects 5% of people aged over 65 and 20% of those aged over 80 (Knapp & Prince, 2007)
- In care homes, 40% of residents have depression, 50–80% dementia and 30% anxiety (Godfrey *et al*, 2005)
- A third of people who care for an older person with dementia have depression (Milne *et al*, 2001).

---

# Mental health service policy development and delivery

When it was created in 1948, the NHS took over a large number of old mental asylums. The movement towards community care for people with severe mental illness started in the 1950s with the advent of phenothiazines and the exploration of rehabilitation methods in community settings. The movement received government policy endorsement in the 1970s. Research from the 1960s through to the 1980s demonstrated the damaging effects of institutionalisation and the improved health and social outcomes which accompanied deinstitutionalisation. A major Department of Health drive to close the large asylums started in the 1980s, accompanied by expansion of district community teams and the development of comprehensive local care systems. The Care Programme Approach (CPA) was introduced in 1990 to ensure systematic assessment of needs, individual tailored care plans, regular review and assignment of a key worker. Mental health was prioritised in the 1992 white paper The Health of the Nation, which set outcome targets to reduce morbidity from mental illness and suicide. This was followed by frameworks for intersectoral working (Building Bridges, 1995) and for local comprehensive care (The Spectrum of Care, 1996). A national psychiatric morbidity survey programme was started in 1993 (see http://www.mentalhealthsurveys.co.uk).

The Mental Health National Service Framework (NSF) was established in 1999; it sets standards of care for suicide prevention, access to services, mental health promotion, and carer support and involvement, with prescribed models of service delivery in both primary and secondary care. In 2000, the NHS Plan aimed to strengthen community care and reduce the use of acute in-patient beds; this was followed by major investment, which led to an additional 700 mental health teams, 1300 consultant psychiatrists, 2700 clinical psychologists and 10000 mental health nurses, who were deployed in highly specialised teams (community mental health teams, crisis resolution and home treatment teams, assertive outreach teams and early intervention teams); these were able to reduce admissions, but their operation was often rather fragmented.

The past few years have seen more highly structured care delivery, using care pathways. Consultant psychiatrists use their expertise at the beginning of the care pathways, assess complex cases, review those in crisis and advise team members and primary care staff (Royal College of Psychiatrists, 2010a). Psychological treatments have been expanded with a tiered programme of brief psychotherapeutic interventions (particularly cognitive–behavioural therapy) provided by the Improving Access to Psychological Therapies (IAPT) programme (Department of Health, 2008).

Service users and their carers have been increasingly involved in service development, supported by a number of voluntary organisations. An important focus has been the 'personalisation' of care, which has been led by a new national body, Health Watch, which has pilot projects already established in a number of services.

Both public and private mental health services are regularly inspected, most recently by the Care Quality Commission (CQC) (see http://www.cqc.org.uk), which also monitors the use of the Mental Health Act, and protects the rights and interests of detained patients.

A recent national patient satisfaction survey showed that 77% of community patients rate their care as good, very good or excellent. The suicide rate in England has fallen steadily since 1990, alongside implementation of a national suicide prevention strategy (National Mental Health Development Unit, 2009) and the World Health Organization has declared that England has the best services in Europe (see Appleby, 2007).

The past few decades have seen continuous organisational change in the NHS, ranging from the separation of the purchase and provision of services in the late 1980s to several moves to achieve greater autonomy for local health providers. The 2010 white paper *Equity and Excellence: Liberating the NHS* sets out plans to form new purchasing organisations run by family physicians ('GP consortia'), while the new mental health strategy, 'No Health Without Mental Health' (with a supporting paper, *Delivering Better*

**425**

*Mental Health Outcomes*; HM Government, 2011*a*,*b*), adopts a life course approach, as advocated by the 'Foresight' report on mental capital and well-being (Cooper *et al*, 2008), and aims to create parity of esteem between physical and mental health. These have been followed by a statement on public mental health from the Royal College of Psychiatrists (2010*b*).

Many of the developments described above relate to England but similar challenges face the devolved administrations in the other countries of the UK, which are evolving their own tailored responses.

## Mental health legislation

There have been a number of recent changes in mental health legislation. The essential principles of the Mental Health Act 1983 remain unchanged, but the Mental Health Act 2007 (England and Wales) introduced community treatment orders (CTOs), changes in professional roles and additional safeguards for patients receiving electroconvulsive therapy.

The Mental Capacity Act 2005, followed by Deprivation of Liberty Safeguards 2007 (DoLS), provides a legal framework for those who lack capacity, with key principles, procedures and safeguards in line with human rights legislation.

There is a similar Mental Health (Care and Treatment) (Scotland) Act 2003 and new legislation for Northern Ireland covering capacity and mental health is due in 2011.

## Undergraduate training

In the UK there are 31 undergraduate medical schools which train doctors on behalf of the NHS (50% of these undergraduates will go on to become family physicians). Medicine is usually a first degree course, that is, entered directly from school, although some medical schools offer graduate entry and some offer an intercalated second degree. Training is guided by the UK General Medical Council (GMC) (see GMC, 2003). Learning has become both more learner led and more research based (including problem-based learning), with clinical experience earlier in training.

Psychiatry undergraduate training lasts 6–12 weeks but, in order to achieve parity with physical health, this should be increased to reflect the prevalence of mental health problems in the community.

## Postgraduate training in psychiatry

Training in psychiatry follows a 6-year programme: 3 years in core training; then, after passing their professional examinations, trainees re-apply for higher training and a further 3 years as a (sub)specialty trainee. Successful completion leads to the Certificate of Completion of Training (CCT) in psychiatry. Recruitment into psychiatry is at a low level, with many unfilled posts in core training across the UK.

The education of the trainee is actively managed within a structured framework of competencies, which are continuously assessed through workplace-based assessments (WPBAs) – which are now web based. Progress through training is managed by an annual review of competency progression (ARCP), which is informed by an electronic portfolio of experience, hosted by the Royal College of Psychiatrists. Core trainees must pass the MRCPsych examination (which comprises three written papers and a clinical examination) to progress to advanced training. The curricula for the new training programmes are approved and quality assured by the GMC, which recently took over responsibility for postgraduate education.

There are 21 deaneries responsible for the delivery of postgraduate medical education in England, Scotland, Northern Ireland and Wales. In 2006–07, deaneries introduced 'specialty schools', which, together with the Royal College of Psychiatrists, lead national recruitment and training, maintain standards and support innovation and diversity in psychiatry education, and work closely with the College's Psychiatric Trainees' Committee.

## Research and academic psychiatry

Research in mental health is undertaken by universities, NHS trusts and charities. There has been a growing trend to involve users and carers in research design and conduct, and all research with human participants has to receive prior ethical approval. There are a variety of UK funding sources, including the Department of Health, the Medical Research Council, the Economic and Social Research Council, the Wellcome Trust, and smaller foundations, as well as international sources such as the European Union. Many UK researchers have strong links to researchers in other countries, and participate in international studies. Universities run master's degree courses and PhD training programmes, and some funders offer PhD scholarships. A number of high-impact mental health research journals are based in the UK. The UK Department of Health also funds the regular production of 'good practice' guidelines by the National Institute for Health and Clinical Excellence, based on systematic reviews of the research evidence.

## Conclusions

In the UK the delivery of mental healthcare is under constant change, against a backdrop of regular reform of the NHS. Recent changes in legislation and organisation offer opportunities to improve the mental health of the UK. To deliver these changes strong consultant leadership, increased recruitment to psychiatry, and a drive for equity for physical and mental healthcare in the UK are needed.

# References

Amore, M., Taqariello, P., Laterza, C., *et al* (2007) Subtypes of depression in dementia. *Archives of Gerontology and Geriatrics*, **44**, 23–33.

Appleby, L. (2007) *Mental Health Ten Years On: Progress on Mental Health Care Reform*. Department of Health.

Centre for Mental Health (2010) *The Economic and Social Costs of Mental Health Problems in 2009/10*. Centre for Mental Health. Available at http://www.centreformentalhealth.org.uk/pdfs/Economic_and_social_costs_2010.pdf (last accessed March 2011).

Colman, I., Murray, J., Abbott, R. A., *et al* (2009) Outcomes of conduct problems in adolescence: 40 year follow-up of a national cohort. *BMJ*, **338**, a2981.

Cooper, C., Field, J., Goswami, U., *et al* (2008) *Mental Capital and WellBeing Final Project Report*. Government Office for Science.

Department of Health (2008) *Improving Access to Psychological Therapies Implementation Plan: National Guidelines for Regional Delivery*. DH.

Department of Health (2009) *Departmental Report 2009: The Health and Personal Social Services Programmes*. DH. Available at http://www.official-documents.gov.uk/document/cm75/7593/7593.pdf (last accessed March 2011).

GMC (2003) *Tomorrow's Doctors*. General Medical Council.

Godfrey, M., Townsend, J., Surr, C., *et al* (2005) *Prevention and Service Provision: Mental Health Problems in Later Life*. Institute of Health Sciences and Public Health Research, Leeds University, and Division of Dementia Studies, Bradford University.

Green, H., McGinnity, A., Meltzer, H., *et al* (2005) *Mental Health of Children and Young People in Great Britain, 2004*. Office for National Statistics.

HM Government (2011a) *No Health Without Mental Health: A Cross Government Mental Health Outcomes Strategy for People of All Ages*. Department of Health.

HM Government (2011b) *No Health Without Mental Health: Delivering Better Mental Health Outcomes for People of All Ages*. Department of Health.

Kessler, R. & Wang, P. (2007) The descriptive epidemiology of commonly occurring mental disorders in the United States. *Annual Review of Public Health*, **29**, 115–129.

Kim-Cohen, J., Caspi, A., Moffitt, T., *et al* (2003) Prior juvenile diagnoses in adults with mental disorder. *Archives of General Psychiatry*, **60**, 709–717.

Knapp, M. & Prince, M. (2007) *Dementia UK: A Report into the Prevalence and Cost of Dementia*. Alzheimer's Society.

McManus, S., Meltzer, H., Brugha, T., *et al* (2009) *Adult Psychiatric Morbidity in England, 2007: Results of a Household Survey*. NHS Information Centre for Health and Social Care.

Milne, A., Hatzidimitriadou, E., Chryssatholoplou, C., *et al* (2001) *Caring in Later Life: Reviewing the Role of Older Carers*. Help the Aged.

National Mental Health Development Unit (2009) *National Suicide Prevention Strategy for England: Annual Report on Progress 2008*. NMHDU.

O'Hara, M. W. & Swain, A. M. (1996) Rates and risk of postpartum depression – a meta analysis. *International Review of Psychiatry*, **8**, 37–54.

Royal College of Psychiatrists (2010a) *Looking Ahead: Future Development of UK Mental Health Services: Recommendations from a Royal College of Psychiatrists' Enquiry*. Occasional Paper OP75. Royal College of Psychiatrists.

Royal College of Psychiatrists (2010b) *No Health Without Public Mental Health: The Case for Action*. Position Statement PS4. Royal College of Psychiatrists.

Singleton, N., Bumpstead, R., O'Brien, M., *et al* (2001) *Psychiatric Morbidity Among Adults Living in Private Households, 2000*. TSO.

Van Os, J., Linscott, R. J., Myin-Germeys, P., *et al* (2009) A systematic review and meta analysis of the psychosis continuum: evidence for a psychosis–proneness–persistence impairment model of psychotic disorder. *Psychological Medicine*, **39**, 179–195.

World Health Organization (2004) *Projections of Mortality and Global Burden of Disease 2004–2030*. WHO.

World Health Organization (2008) *Global Burden of Disease Report*. WHO.

# North America

# Bermuda

## David Price

Bermuda comprises a group of small islands in the Atlantic Ocean, situated approximately 1000 km east of the USA. It is a self-governing crown dependency of the UK. It is the third richest country in the world, with average wages per head of US$41 495 in 2000. Its economy is based on a flourishing offshore insurance industry and tourism.

## Psychiatric services

Bermuda's healthcare comprises both private and public initiatives. Employees are required to obtain health insurance for themselves and their dependants. For those who are not insured, the government provides through the public system.

The island has two hospitals, King Edward VII Memorial Hospital, a general medical hospital, and a separate psychiatric unit, St Brendan's Hospital. The latter provides mental healthcare for the majority of the islanders and receives a budget of over US$28 million per year.

## Human resources

St Brendan's Hospital employs three adult and one child and adolescent psychiatrist. Each adult psychiatrist takes on the responsibility for providing one specialist area of service. The majority of staff in the hospital are Bermudian, although, given the global shortage of suitably qualified mental health staff, Bermuda recruits actively for doctors, nurses and allied staff in jurisdictions such as the UK, Canada, Australia and the USA. The cultural diversity of the staff produces an interesting mix of perspectives and ideas about healthcare policy.

## Overview of services

Since the early 1980s, mental health policy within Bermuda has focused on making services more accessible, more community oriented and less stigmatised.

The closure of two long-stay wards in the 1980s provided the momentum for the development of community mental health teams. Teams are multidisciplinary; individual members case manage up to 50 patients. Bermuda's small size facilitates assertive outreach.

There is a housing shortage for people with severe mental illness. The high cost of real estate due to the expansion of the business sector makes accommodation costs prohibitive for those on a low income and finding cheaper accommodation, such as at the island's Salvation Hostel, can be difficult. Many individuals with severe mental health problems live with their families, despite the high level of burden this frequently places on carers.

There are 25 acute hospital beds, including 5 on a psychiatric intensive care unit. Shortage of beds is unusual and this reduces the pressure to discharge patients before recovery is complete. A small rehabilitation unit offers a comprehensive package of psychosocial interventions for patients with complex needs; it has a philosophy of engagement for up to 2 years.

Two learning disability wards remain within the hospital but a government initiative aims to provide one new group home each year and a community learning disability service.

## Consumers of mental health services

The population of Bermuda is some 65 000, approximately 60% Black and 40% White. The population is relatively wealthy and well educated.

Despite the turnover of expatriates employed in the business sector, the population is relatively static and this allows for an accurate and up-to-date case register of clients who use the service.

## Education and research

St Brendan's Hospital is currently accredited for training by the Royal College of Psychiatrists. This is important to the hospital, as it helps to maintain standards of care and benchmarks training against UK standards and practice.

A recent community survey commissioned by the hospital board highlighted the need to improve the awareness of mental health issues in Bermuda; a campaign to reduce stigma and provide education is under way.

The relative stability and small size of the population of Bermuda facilitate genetic and epidemiological studies into mental illness. In particular, there appears to be a strong line of schizophrenia and bipolar affective disorder among the St Davids islanders. Collaborative research projects are currently being explored. One study is currently looking at the effect of cannabis on the presentation of psychosis.

# Mental Health Act

The Mental Health Act is largely based on the English Act. There is an assessment order and a longer treatment order that lasts for up to 1 year. Two consultant psychiatrists make a recommendation to either a nearest relative or a mental welfare officer. Appeals are allowed and there is a tribunal which hears cases, presided over by a lawyer.

# Canada

Nady el-Guebaly

The delivery of healthcare in Canada is shaped by a number of variables – geography, legislation, federal structure, location and culture.

## A vast geography

At 10 million km$^2$, Canada is the second largest country in the world but it is sparsely populated – it has only 32 million inhabitants. Canada would cover the whole of Europe and part of Asia but two-thirds of the population live within 300 km of the US border.

## A federally monitored Health Act

Since 1967, the country has embarked on the ambitious provision of 'medically necessary' healthcare to all its citizens based on five tenets – universality, comprehensiveness, accessibility, portability of coverage and non-profit public administration. These equally apply to mental and addiction disorders. Currently, the main problem is long waiting lists interfering with accessibility.

## The dynamics of provincial jurisdiction

Each of the governments of the ten provinces and three territories has the responsibility and control of healthcare within its own boundaries. The national congruence of service delivery remains remarkable.

## Location

Canada's contiguity with the USA shapes the public debate concerning healthcare. On the one hand, national pride is readily expressed at the high standards of North American care delivery, while training and publishing in the USA are highly valued; on the other hand, there is widespread public concern about the excesses of US-based managed care and the significant portion of that population without insurance. This results in a determined effort to learn from both US and European influences to create a uniquely Canadian blend (Rae-Grant, 2001).

# A cultural mosaic

Canada is a welcoming land of opportunity to a steady stream of immigrants and with a birth rate of 1.5 children per couple the country will continue to depend on migration for its sustenance. With two official languages, English and French, and many unofficial cultures, multiculturalism rather than a 'melting pot' policy is one of the prized social characteristics. The healthcare workforce reflects society's mosaic. The first inhabitants of this country, the First Nations, have not fared well so far and this is reflected in higher morbidity and mortality risks.

Canadians in general highly value their healthcare system, known as medicare (which is publicly financed but privately run) and public polls suggest that medicare is considered an essential ingredient of Canadian identity. There are concerns, however, about the capacity to sustain it (Romanow, 2002).

# Mental health policies and statistics

The Canadian Community Health Survey (CCHS) in 2002 reported that some 20% of Canadians personally experience some form of mental illness during their lifetime (Health Canada, 2002). Eighty-six per cent of hospital admissions for mental illness are to general hospital. Seven major mental illnesses (excluding addiction) account for 3.8% of all general hospital admissions. Between 1950 and 1975, 35 000 beds for patients with mental illness were eliminated from psychiatric hospitals but only 5000 were added to general wards. In 2001–2002, while psychiatric hospitals accounted for only 13% of all admissions for mental illness, the average length of stay in psychiatric hospitals was 162 days, compared with 25 days for general hospitals. These average lengths of stay were down 35% from 1994–1995. The widespread policy of deinstitutionalisation did not, however, induce an appropriate increase in community-based services. Provincial Mental Health Acts have increasingly upheld patients' rights, and involuntary hospitalisation is currently limited to the presence of 'immediate danger to self or others'.

Canada's suicide rate is relatively high. Suicide accounts for 24% of all deaths among 15- to 24-year-olds and 16% among 25- to 44-year-olds. Suicide rates among the First Nations population are three to six times the national average. In 1998, the direct and indirect costs related to mental health problems were estimated to be arguably the highest of all conditions, representing some 14% of the national corporate net operating profits.

# Human resource planning for psychiatry

Physician resource planning is a puzzling task. Canadian psychiatry has been involved in human resource planning for some 40 years and in the process doubled the number of psychiatrists per population between 1972 and 1997 (el-Guebaly, 1999). Severe shortages remain in all geographical areas and all subspecialties. Since the 1990s, a target psychiatrist: population ratio of 1:8400 has been achieved and surpassed in many urban areas. Some 4000 psychiatrists, 10% of whom are child psychiatrists, address the needs of the population of 32 million, with an average working week of 46 hours. Only the USA and The Netherlands have comparable ratios. The patients seen display a DSM–IV Axis I diagnosis (American Psychiatric Association, 1994) in 86% of cases and half will have more than one diagnosis.

There are on average 600 residents in training programmes and of the graduates of medical school 6–7% choose psychiatry. While statistics about the supply of physicians abound, less is known about the drivers of demand for their services – demographics, prevalence of illness, standard of living or accessibility or cost. Family physicians are the most commonly consulted professionals for mental health problems, followed by psychiatrists and psychologists. Of late, a shared-care model of delivery with family physicians and, on a more limited basis, with paediatricians has been implemented (Kates *et al*, 1997). Interdisciplinary teams staff most publicly funded mental health services, but national figures about other professions specialising in mental health are not readily available.

International medical graduates have accounted for about a quarter of the supply of physicians in Canada, this portion doubling in the provinces of Newfoundland and Saskatchewan. The current shortage of physicians and the fact that their average age is 49 years have spurred a renewed effort to streamline the entry of prospective immigrants through the Medical Council of Canada, provincial licensing colleges and medical schools.

# Educating physicians in psychiatry: a lifelong process

## Undergraduate courses

The 16 medical schools generally have a 4-year medical curriculum, although a few offer a 3-year course. The Canadian Psychiatric Association, founded in 1951, supports the organisation of Coordinators of Undergraduate Psychiatric Education (CUPE) to provide a forum for identifying the core knowledge, attitudes and skills required for graduation. Graduating students are evaluated by the Medical Council of Canada Licensing Examination, where about 20% of the questions are on psychiatry. A multiple-choice format as well as observed structured patient interviews are used to test the students. Broad topics taught in the pre-clinical years include interviewing skills, the doctor–patient relationship, detection of psychopathology and diagnosis, as well as specific subjects such as violence and mental health legislation.

Currently most schools have autonomous courses in psychiatry somewhat complementary to the neurosciences. The clinical clerkship rotation in the final years varies between 6 and 8 weeks. Medical students, particularly female students, have of late regarded psychiatry as a much more attractive specialty than in the past (Leverette *et al*, 1996).

## Evolving postgraduate education

The accreditation of postgraduate training is the purview of the Royal College of Physicians and Surgeons of Canada (RCPSC), which has the task of certifying specialists from all disciplines. With the incorporation of the internship year under the direction of the chosen specialty, training in psychiatry is, in fact, a 5-year process, not uncommonly complemented by a 6th year of academic fellowship.

Training requirements and objectives reflect a balance between biological and psychotherapeutic approaches, as well as the promotion of evidence-based clinical practice guidelines (Cameron *et al*, 1999; Paris, 2000). The 'social contract' required of medical specialties is also a concern of the Royal College. The 'Can MEDS 2000' project identified a cluster of seven competencies to be achieved in training: medical decision maker, communicator, collaborator, manager, health advocate, scholar and professional (Societal Needs Working Group, 1996). It remains uncertain as to how well these requirements are being met.

Other training challenges have included the provincial budget reductions to the hospital sector, which have resulted in a shift to 'community-based care' training and increased involvement in multidisciplinary teams. This shift has also resulted in the increased involvement of family physicians in the care of people with a mental illness and 'shared care' programmes, where psychiatrists and trainees provide consultations in family physicians' offices.

A perennial organisational issue has been the accommodation of subspecialty training. Canadian psychiatry, compared with US psychiatry, has been very conservative in recognising subspecialties and currently identifies only three – child, geriatric and forensic psychiatry. The Royal College recommends a 2-year subspecialty programme, one within the 5-year complement and one additional to it, but the debate continues. Members of other subspecialty practices such as addiction or administration have sought credentialing from US organisations to remedy the lack, so far, of such an avenue in Canada.

Pressure to incorporate new knowledge and skills in the training programme has somewhat eased with the concept of lifelong education.

# Continuing professional development and maintenance of certification

Education does not end with graduation from a training programme. Indeed, graduation certifies the acquisition of necessary skills to embark upon a journey of lifelong learning. It is of interest that several of the less popular topics among training residents are in high demand in continuing education activities.

'Top down' lectures are of limited value and have been partly replaced by needs-based activities, including reading, meeting with colleagues, quality assurance and brief traineeships. The Royal College Maintenance of Competence programme rates continuing medical education programmes, including their funding source, particularly from industry; there is also a random audit of learning diaries. An annual report of these activities for a total of 400 credits over a 5-year period is required to maintain specialty certification (Royal College of Physicians and Surgeons of Canada, 1999).

# The challenges of psychiatric research

Following the Second World War, Canada made a far-reaching decision not to create national research institutes like those in the USA but to create instead a Medical Research Council and develop research capacity within the 16 medical schools. This initiative has had mixed results and over the past 5 years the Canadian Institutes of Health Research have channelled research funds from governments while fostering the creation of multidisciplinary, inter-provincial research teams to implement a consensual research agenda.

Compared with the burden on society placed by mental illness and addiction disorders, research into these has been persistently underfunded, at about 4% of the total government expenditure on health research. Indeed, this funding shortage would have been worse were it not for the ability of Canadian researchers to access US funds. This has also led to the pharmaceutical industry assuming a prime role in funding pharmacological clinical trials, which range from the truly innovative to post-marketing surveys.

In the 1950s, the McGill University group, headed by Dr Lehman, was credited for introducing several neuroleptics and tricyclics to North America. Currently the Canadian College of Neuropsychopharmacology monitors a thriving network of trials in schizophrenia, mood and anxiety disorders and more recently pharmacological trials on the early manifestations of mental illness.

In the field of epidemiology, Dr Leighton's Stirling County Study of Psychiatric Disorders has now developed into a multi-sited group of collaborators, which has resulted in achievements such as Dr Bland's Edmonton city-wide surveys, Dr Offord's Ontario Child Health Study, and Dr Arboleda-Florez's forensic work.

Several diagnosis-specific clinical investigations have had a significant effect on practice. These studies have looked at: linkage and association in schizophrenia (Drs Bassett and Maziade), sex differences (Dr Seaman), eating disorders (Dr Garfinkel), personality disorders (Drs Paris and Livesley), affective disorders (Dr Kennedy), anxiety disorders (Dr Stein), addiction (Drs Negrete and el-Guebaly) and psychotherapy (Drs Azim, McKenzie and Leszcs).

# Conclusion

Psychiatry in Canada is a vibrant specialty within an evolving universal healthcare system. A recently formed coalition of 12 non-governmental organisations, including the Canadian Psychiatric Association, has urged government to identify specific mental health goals, a policy framework embracing both mental illness and mental health promotion, adequate resources to sustain the plan and an annual public reporting mechanism (Canadian Alliance on Mental Illness and Mental Health, 2000).

At the same time, the practice of psychiatry is increasing in complexity, with such cumulative demands on practitioners as lifelong learning, as well as the expectations of increasingly informed consumers. Hospitals downsizing and the pressure to discharge patients early without a significant increase in community resources have increased workload stress. Programmes addressing physicians' stress and impairment are increasingly popular. Expanding telehealth programmes appear to provide some relief to poorly resourced communities. While fee-for-service was the main form of remuneration for physicians, alternative forms of sessional payments are becoming popular. The motto 'the only constant is change' describes well Canada's current healthcare and psychiatric practice.

# References

American Psychiatric Association (1994) *Diagnostic and Statistical Manual of Mental Disorders (4th edn) (DSM–IV)*. Washington, DC: APA.

Cameron, P., Leszcz, M., Bebchuck, W., et al (1999) The practice and roles of the psychotherapies: a discussion paper. *Canadian Journal of Psychiatry*, **44** (suppl. 1), 18S–31S.

Canadian Alliance on Mental Illness and Mental Health (2000) *A Call for Action: Building Consensus for a National Action Plan on Mental Illness and Mental Health*. Ottawa: CAMIMH.

el-Guebaly, N. (1999) Thirty-five years of psychiatrist workforce planning: what do we have to show for it? *Bulletin of the Canadian Psychiatric Association*, **31**, 101–104.

Health Canada (2002) *A Report on Mental Illness in Canada*. Ottawa: Health Canada.

Kates, N., Craven, M., Bishop, J., et al (1997) Shared mental health care in Canada. *Canadian Journal of Psychiatry*, **42(8) (insert)**.

Leverette, J., Massabki, A. & Peterson, H. (1996) Factors affecting medical students' selection of Canadian psychiatric residency programs: Part II – some contemporary issues. *Canadian Journal of Psychiatry*, **41**, 582–586.

Paris, J. (2000) Canadian psychiatry across 5 decades: from clinical inference to evidence-based practice. *Canadian Journal of Psychiatry*, **45**, 34–39.

Rae-Grant, Q. (2001) *Psychiatry in Canada: 50 Years 1951–2001*. Ottawa: Canadian Psychiatric Association.

Romanow, R. (2002) *Building on Values: The Future of Health Care in Canada – Final Report*. Ottawa: Commission on the Future of Health Care in Canada.

Royal College of Physicians and Surgeons of Canada (1999) *Maintenance of Certification: Information Guide for Fellows*. Ottawa: RCPSC.

Societal Needs Working Group (1996) Can MEDS 2000 project. Skills for the new millennium. *Annals of the Royal College of Physicians and Surgeons of Canada*, **29**, 207–216.

# Jamaica

Frederick W. Hickling

The intense historical relationship linking Jamaica and Britain to 300 years of the transatlantic slave trade and 200 years of colonialism has left 2.7 million souls living in Jamaica, 80% of African origin, 15% of mixed Creole background and 5% of Asian Indian, Chinese and European ancestry. With a per capita gross domestic product of US$4104 in 2007, one-third of the population is impoverished, the majority struggling for economic survival. The prevailing religion is Protestant, although the presence of African retentions such as Obeah and Pocomania are still widely and profoundly experienced, and the powerful Rastafarian movement emerged as a countercultural religious force after 1930. The paradox and contradictions of five centuries of Jamaican resistance to slavery and colonial oppression have spawned a tiny, resilient, creative, multicultural island people, who have achieved a worldwide philosophical, political and religious impact, phenomenal sporting prowess, astonishing musical and performing creativity, and a criminal underworld that has stunned by its propensity for violence.

## Policy and service

Hickling & Sorel (2005) discuss mental health policy and legislation in Jamaica and the English-speaking Caribbean, and the development of the Lunatic Asylum in Kingston.

Mental health legislation originated from colonial Britain in 1872, cementing the draconian policy of police arrest for lunacy and incarceration in the oppressive lunatic asylums that has dogged the history of mental healthcare in the UK, with successive attempts at legislative reform in that country in the 20th century. Jamaica broke with this British tradition in 1974 by virtually abandoning the custodial approach to the treatment of mental illness, and by the creation of a nationwide system of care that marginalised police involvement in the management of people with a mental illness, and placed their treatment squarely in the purview of the medical and nursing professions. As a result, a community mental health system has now evolved that is situated firmly in the primary healthcare system of the country, with seminal links to public sector medical and nursing professionals.

A network of over 300 clinics in the island of 4400 square miles provides a full range of mental health services, delivered primarily by community mental health nurses (called mental health officers), supervised by 30 psychiatrists. More than 40 000 patients are treated annually. Treatment is provided free of charge, with the full range of internationally available psychotropic medications and psychiatric treatments. The community mental health service provides a mobile community follow-up service that keeps track of the hundreds of patients who have problems with medication adherence, and provides emergency services, crisis intervention and acute hospitalisation when necessary.

More than 60% of those patients requiring hospital admission for acute mental illness are admitted to the medical wards of the 13 general hospitals island-wide (Hickling *et al*, 2000). The generally trained medical and nursing practitioners who work in these hospitals provide care for those admitted for psychiatric treatment, side by side with those with diabetes and heart disease, under the supervision of the community psychiatrist and mental health officers assigned to those hospitals. A Cochrane review (Hickling *et al*, 2007) found that this remarkable therapeutic reality is unique to Jamaica.

The remaining 40% or so of patients requiring hospital admission are admitted to specialised psychiatric units in three major hospitals serving the two major urban centres of Kingston and Montego Bay. The average length of hospital stay for acutely ill patients is about 14 days. The Mental Health Law of 1997 provides the legal statute that allows patients to be admitted and detained involuntarily for up to 14 days. The majority of all admissions are voluntary, and no facility outside of prison exists where a patient can be detained involuntarily for a longer period. Community treatment orders and legal sections that can determine the involuntary incarceration of a patient for up to 6 months at a time, as exist in countries such as England, do not exist under Jamaica's mental health legislation.

After 37 years of measured deinstitutionalisation, the Bellevue Mental Hospital is now a 700-bed institution with 100 acute beds serving a catchment area of 90 000 persons in the city of Kingston, with custodial facilities for more than 600 indigent patients over the age of 65.

Although the island's mental health service accounts for 5% of the health budget, which in turn is 6.5% of the national budget, vibrant private treatment facilities in psychology and psychiatry now exist island-wide.

## Training

The Jamaican mental health success story is due in no small measure to the effect of the medical, psychiatric and nursing training at the University of the West Indies (UWI), Mona. The UWI, which was established in 1948 as a school of the University of London, has trained nearly 6000 medical practitioners since its inception. In addition, its School of Nursing (UWISON) has provided the undergraduate and postgraduate training for many thousands of nurses in Jamaica. Psychiatric training was introduced for all nurses and medical students in 1965, thus providing a comprehensive primary and secondary medical care programme provisioned by 3000 medical and 5000 nursing practitioners, which buttresses the psychiatric service in the island. Psychiatric residents and medical students receive apprenticeship and academic tutoring in the 20-bed open ward unit run on therapeutic community principles at the University Hospital of the West Indies. The accident and emergency department and the in- and out-patient services of the University Hospital reinforce the broad, eclectic secondary care training experience, with practical primary care training being provided in the government-run community mental health services.

Recent postgraduate training programmes for clinical psychologists (Hickling & Matthies, 2004) now provide the basis for the development of psychological assessment and psychotherapy services.

A robust child and adolescent service has emerged around the country in tandem with the adult mental health services, and the UWI is now implementing a training programme in child and adolescent psychiatry to provide the specialists to further develop these services. Similar training programmes in substance misuse and forensic psychiatry are being developed at the UWI. UWISON also conducts a robust nurse practitioner and mental health officer training programme.

# Specialist services and research

In 2005, the UWI launched the Caribbean Institute of Mental Health and Substance Abuse (CARIMENSA) for delivering primary prevention in mental health across the country and the region. Aimed at developing programmes to reduce national problems such as violence, substance misuse, teenage pregnancy, HIV/AIDS and other chronic diseases, this Institute, situated in the Faculty of Medical Sciences, has developed a novel cultural therapy programme (Hickling, 2004), which incorporates innovative ethnographic group methods with creative arts therapies for risk reduction for people of all ages, classes and ethnicities. A 3-year 'Dream-a-World' cultural therapy pilot programme (Hickling, 2006) was initiated with a cohort of 9-year-old inner-city primary school children who were exhibiting behavioural and academic problems. The preliminary results of this programme indicated significantly higher scores on the government grade-6 achievement test for the study group compared with a control group, as well as a reduction in behavioural problems, more significantly in boys. In 2008, CARIMENSA implemented a novel MSc in cultural therapy at the UWI, to train cultural therapists in primary prevention processes for the nation.

The UWI has had a seminal influence on mental health research in Jamaica. The institutional public policy at the beginning of the new millennium of

**443**

appointing Caribbean psychiatrists with a high-output research record to lead mental health at the university certainly paid dividends in terms of mental health research output (Hickling *et al*, 2008). This strategy has resulted in considerable increases in overall psychiatric research output (Gibson *et al*, 2007).

Collaboration with the Pan American Health Organization has highlighted Caribbean mental health research (Hickling, 2005) in the areas of epidemiology, public policy, treatment outcomes and service evaluation.

Recent quantitative (Gibson *et al*, 2008) and qualitative (Arthur *et al*, 2008) studies have demonstrated a profound reduction in stigma regarding mental illness in the island, related to a 'psychological deinstitutionalisation' process over the past 40 years, described by Whitley & Hickling (2007). The establishment of the CARIMENSA Press in 2005 has triggered the launch of a Mental Health Observatory and the publication of five books on Caribbean psychology and psychiatry.

## Conclusion

Detailed information on the mental health profile of Jamaica can be found in the World Health Organization's mental health atlas (2005) and in the book edited by Hickling & Sorel (2005). The revolutionary transformation of the mental health landscape in Jamaica highlights the practical possibilities for efficient liberalisation of mental health practices worldwide, but especially in low- and middle-income countries. This transformation into an affordable, humane, modern and efficient system integrated into primary healthcare services, for all Jamaicans, is largely unrecognised at home and abroad and the comprehension of many people seems stuck at the image of the custodial 'snake pit' lunatic asylum that existed in the early 1960s. Old myths and legends are hard to eradicate, and no doubt this image will persist until the deinstitutionalisation process of the Bellevue Mental Hospital, started in 1972, is completed.

## References

Arthur, C., Hickling, F. W., Gibson, R. C., *et al* (2008) The stigma of mental illness in Jamaica. In *Perspectives in Caribbean Psychology* (eds F. W. Hickling, B. K. Matthies, K. Morgan, *et al*). CARIMENSA Press.

Gibson, R. C., Morgan, K. A. D., Abel, W. D., *et al* (2007) Changing the research culture at the Section of Psychiatry, the University of the West Indies, Mona. *West Indian Medical Journal*, **56**, 171–177.

Gibson, R. C., Abel, W. D., White, S., *et al* (2008) Internalizing stigma associated with mental illness: findings from a general population survey in Jamaica. *Revista Panamericana de Salud Pública/Pan American Journal of Public Health*, **23**, 26–32.

Hickling, F. W. (2004) Popular theatre as psychotherapy. *International Journal of Postcolonial Studies – Interventions*, **6**, 45–56.

Hickling, F. W. (2005) The epidemiology of common mental disorders in the English-speaking Caribbean. *Pan American Journal of Public Health*, **18**, 256–261.

Hickling, F. W. (ed.) *(2006) Dream a World: CARIMENSA and the Development of Cultural Therapy in Jamaica.* CARIMENSA Press.

Hickling, F. W. & Matthies, B. (2004) The establishment of a clinical psychology postgraduate program at the University of the West Indies, Mona. *Caribbean Journal of Education*, **25**, 25–36.

Hickling, F. W. & Sorel, E. (eds) *(2005) Images of Psychiatry – the Caribbean.* Department of Community Health and Psychiatry, University of the West Indies Mona, and World Psychiatric Association.

Hickling, F. W., McCallum, M., Nooks, L., *et al* (2000) Treatment of first contact schizophrenia in open medical wards in Jamaica. *Psychiatric Services*, **51**, 659–663.

Hickling, F. W., Abel, W., Garner, P., *et al* (2007) Open general medical wards versus specialist psychiatric units for acute psychoses. *Cochrane Database of Systematic Reviews*, **issue 3**, CD003290.

Hickling, F. W., Gibson, R. C. & Abel, W. D. (2008) Public policy and mental health research at the University of the West Indies, 1995–2005. *Journal of Education and Development in the Caribbean*, **10**, 87–96.

Whitley, R. & Hickling, F. W. (2007) Open papers, open minds? Media representations of psychiatric de-institutionalisation in Jamaica. *Transcultural Psychiatry*, **44**, 659–671.

World Health Organization (2005) Jamaica. In *Project Atlas: Resources for Mental Health*, pp. 254–256. WHO. Available at http://www.who.int/mental_health/evidence/atlas/ (accessed October 2009).

# Mexico

Shoshana Berenzon, Héctor Sentíes and Elena Medina-Mora

Mexico is a culturally, socially and economically heterogeneous country, with a population of over 100 million. Although it is regarded as a country with a medium–high income according to World Bank criteria, inequality continues to be one of its main problems. In addition to this, the country is going through a difficult period. Large parts of the population face economic insecurity, as a result of which feelings of despair, fear and impotence are common. It is hardly surprising, then, that mental disorders should constitute a major public health problem: depression is the main cause of loss of healthy years of life (6.4% of the population suffer from it), while alcohol misuse is the 9th (2.5%) and schizophrenia the 10th (2.1%) most common health problem (González-Pier *et al*, 2006).

## The Mexican health system

The Mexican health system is divided into three types of service provision.

First, social security provides services for the formal, salaried sector of the economy and covers 47% of the population. This type of security guarantees free access to healthcare and is financed through contributions from both employers and employees.

Second, those not covered by social security (45% of the total Mexican population), who are also the poorest, were long regarded as a residual group, for whom the Health Secretariat provided a poorly defined benefits package. In 2000, the Popular Insurance Scheme was created to provide protection for this vulnerable population. The intention was to expand the coverage of this insurance only gradually. Two kinds of mental health service are included under this scheme: preventive medicine and external consultation services. Beneficiaries of the Popular Insurance Scheme are entitled to receive treatment for the diseases included in the Universal Catalogue of Essential Health Services (CAUSES), which covers all the medical services provided at primary health centres and associated medication. In relation to mental health, CAUSES include: attention deficit disorder, eating disorders, alcohol misuse, depression, psychosis, epilepsy, Parkinson's disease and convulsive crises.

Third, there is a heterogeneous group of private service providers who attend non-insured families who are able to afford them and the population which, despite having some form of social security, is dissatisfied with the quality of services; this group accounts for just 4% of the population (Frenk, 2007).

# Mental health services

## Mental health policy and legislation

The main axes of the legislative and political actions related to mental health, formulated in 1983, were promotion, prevention, treatment and rehabilitation. In order to restructure these policies, consultations were carried out in 2001 with the participation of politicians, government officials, professionals, non-governmental organisations (NGOs) and patients. On the basis of these consultations, the 2001–06 Mental Health Programme of Action proposed an integrated care model. That programme, in addition to psychiatric hospitals, community health centres, day hospitals and intermediate residences, emphasises patients' rights and their social inclusion. Its main components are: strategies to reform existing services, mental health promotion and prevention, improving mental health training programmes for staff, and the encouragement of research work in this field.

The most recent National Health Programme (2007–12) proposes five social policy objectives:

- improve the population's health conditions
- provide efficient health services, guaranteeing quality, warmth and safety for the patient
- reduce health inequalities
- prevent the impoverishment of the population for health reasons
- guarantee that health will contribute to overcoming poverty.

On the basis of these objectives and in order to reinforce and lend continuity to the care model formulated in 2001, a proposal was made to create a national mental health network, comprising specialist units within primary care (UNEMES), organised on the basis of a community model. The aim is for these specialist units to offer out-patient services for timely detection, care and rehabilitation, while offering the necessary services for effective treatment. The aim is for UNEMES to function as the axis around which out-patient and community mental healthcare will function. They must therefore consist of multidisciplinary teams offering integrated care. In addition to their welfare functions, they will be an important space for health prevention and promotion, as well as offering training opportunities for other levels of care.

Although major efforts have been made in Mexico to advance the care of patients with mental disorders, the main challenge at present is to achieve the integration of mental healthcare into general healthcare programmes. This is the only way the gap between care and treatment needs will be bridged.

## Mental health service resources

The Mexican mental health system has 0.667 psychiatric beds for every 10 000 inhabitants. There are 0.51 beds in psychiatric hospitals plus 0.051 beds available at general hospitals for this same population rate. As for human resources, it is estimated that for every 100 000 inhabitants there are 2.8 psychiatrists, 44 psychologists, 0.12 psychiatric nurses, 1.5 neurosurgeons, 1.2 neurologists and 0.20 social workers specialising in psychiatry (World Health Organization, 2005). As Fig. 1 illustrates, Mexico has a significant shortfall in resources compared with other countries on the American continent.

## Organisation of services

There are three types of service at the primary healthcare level: mental healthcare modules integrated into general hospitals; health modules integrated into health centres; and psychiatric units integrated into general hospitals. However, many of these units or modules lack sufficient minimum personnel to be able to cover the demand for treatment; also, they are not uniformly distributed geographically.

At the secondary healthcare level, the Health Secretariat only has eight specialised mental healthcare units designed for out-patients and the provision of specialised psychological medical care. At this level of care, 41% of all institutional psychiatrists and psychologists are concentrated in Mexico City.

Lastly, there are the psychiatric hospitals. Mexico has 31 public institutions, distributed unevenly throughout 23 of the country's 31 states. The units operate on the basis of two main schemes: short and long hospital stays. Although these are their main activities, in recent years they have largely been devoted to specialist out-patient care, because of the high demand for and the limited supply of services of this nature. 'Day hospital management' is a concept that is currently being implemented at certain institutions. The experience has been satisfactory, since this form of management reduces the number of relapses and increases patients' social inclusion (Secretaria de Salud, 2004).

In rural areas there are no local specialist mental healthcare institutions. A visit to the psychiatrist or psychologist may involve a day's travelling as well as considerable expense. Consequently, the rural population often consults traditional doctors and other informal agents.

# Psychiatric training

The teaching of psychiatry in Mexico is relatively recent. The earliest psychiatry hospital residences began in 1948. In 1951 a clinical course was established at the National Autonomous University (Universidad Nacional Autónoma de México, UNAM); it is now a 3-year programme. Since 1971, the UNAM has offered specialist courses in the different areas of psychiatry and provides master's degree and PhD programmes.

In 1994, the UNAM with the National Academy of Medicine and other institutions created the Single Medical Specialisation Programme. This has been taught at all schools of medicine and medical faculties, which ensures that the academic course is standardised.

There is only one specialisation in psychiatric social work, taught at the National Institute of Psychiatry and coordinated by the UNAM. There are two formal courses for psychiatric nursing, one taught at the UNAM National School of Nursing and another at the Instituto Politecnico Nacional (IPN) School of Nursing. Courses are also taught after the basic nursing degree at Mexico's largest psychiatric hospitals and at the National Institutes of Neurology and Psychiatry.

# Mental health research

Mental health research in Mexico faces difficulties due to the shortage of trained professionals and a lack of high-technology equipment. Despite this, various Mexican institutions undertake research in the clinical, neuroscience, epidemiological and social spheres of mental health.

The main clinical areas researched are genetics, clinimetry, neurochemistry, psychopharmacology, immunology, phyto-pharmacology, brain cartography and imaging. The most important fields of research in the field of neuroscience are: neurophysiology, chronobiology, neurobiology, bioelectronics, ethology and comparative psychology. The main lines of research related to the

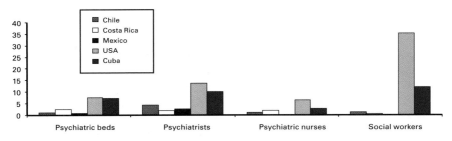

**Fig. 1** Mental healthcare human resources per 100 000 inhabitants (does not include psychologists because the data are not available in Mexico) (World Health Organization, 2005).

epidemiological and social areas are: psychiatric epidemiology, health systems, drug dependence, suicide, violence, mental health in vulnerable groups and evaluation of intervention models.

# Human rights and future challenges

In 1995, an official Mexican regulation for the provision of psychiatric services in medical care hospital units was issued. This regulation focuses on two areas: quality specialised medical care and the preservation of the user's human rights. This regulation fits in with the United Nations' Principles for the Protection of Persons Suffering from Mental Illness and for the Improvement of Mental Health Care (1991). One of the shortcomings of the Mexican regulation is that it fails to mention the rights of children and teenagers with mental illness, and it therefore needs revision.

Important advances have included increasing the budget to treat mental illness and the creation of innovative primary mental healthcare approaches. Nevertheless, the proportion of people suffering from mental diseases who receive treatment remains low. The greatest challenge is to expand coverage and achieve universal mental healthcare services, in order to reach the most neglected groups, but also to develop new, improved, culturally sensitive treatments that can meet the population's needs, fostering help seeking and treatment compliance.

# Sources

Comisión Nacional de Derechos Humanos (1995) *Lineamientos para la Preservación de los Derechos Humanos en los Hospitales Psiquiátricos*. [Guidelines for the Preservation of Human Rights in Psychiatric Hospitals.] Comisión Nacional de Derechos Humanos.

Frenk, J. (2007) Bridging the divide: global lessons from evidence-based health policy in Mexico. *Salud Publica*, **49** (suppl. 1), S14–S22.

González-Pier, E., Gutiérrez-Delgado, C., Stevens, G., *et al* (2006) Priority setting for health interventions in Mexico´s system of social protection in health. *Lancet*, **368**, 1608–1618.

Secretaría de Salud (2004) *Salud México 2004. Información para la rendición de cuentas*. [Health Mexico 2004. Accounting Information.] Secretaría de Salud.

World Health Organization (2005) *Mental Health Atlas: Mexico*. Available at http://www.who.int/mental_health/evidence/atlas/ (last accessed July 2009).

# United States of America

Carol A. Bernstein, Bruce Hershfield and Deborah C. Cohen

The USA has the world's largest economy and the highest per capita spending on healthcare, but it lags behind other countries on a number of key health measures. It ranks 23rd in healthy life expectancy and 32nd in infant mortality (World Health Organization, 2009). In 2000, the World Health Organization ranked the US healthcare system as 1st in responsiveness, 37th in overall performance, and 72nd by overall level of health (among 191 member nations in the study).

## Mental health in the USA

Approximately 25% of US adults have a diagnosable mental disorder in a given year and approximately 6% have a serious mental illness. Mental disorders are the leading cause of disability for people aged 15–44 years (National Institute of Mental Health, 2010).

About 11% of adults experience serious psychological distress, such as anxiety and mood disorders, that result in functional impairment that impedes one or more major life activities. Rates of mental illness are highest for adults aged 18–25 years and lowest for those over 50; rates for women are significantly higher than for men. The most common mental illnesses are anxiety and mood disorders (Substance Abuse and Mental Health Services Administration, 2009).

Some 17% of inmates entering jails and prisons have a serious mental illness (which is nearly three times the rate in the general population) (Steadman et al, 2009). As many as 70% of those in the juvenile justice system have a diagnosable mental disorder and one in five has a mental disorder significant enough to impair functioning (Skowyra & Cocozza, 2006).

Unfortunately, the high rate of mental illness does not correlate with adequate treatment. Fewer than half of adults with a diagnosable mental disorder receive treatment in a given year (Kessler et al, 2005). The number of Americans under care for mental illnesses nearly doubled between 1996 and 2006 (from 19 to 36 million) (Agency for Healthcare Research and Quality, 2009). Among those with serious mental illnesses, adults aged over 50 were more likely to use mental health services (71%) than adults aged 18–25 (40%) (Substance Abuse and Mental Health Services Administration, 2009).

A variety of social, financial and systemic barriers contribute to the lack of psychiatric treatment. Although society's perception of individuals with mental illness has improved, stigma is still significant. A negative attitude to mental illness, which can be expressed as distrust, stereotyping, fear, embarrassment, anger and avoidance, often inhibits people from seeking treatment.

# Service delivery

A range of services and treatments to help people with mental disorders is provided by a variety of caregivers working in public and private settings. There are four major components to these services:

- specialty mental health professionals (psychiatrists, psychologists, psychiatric nurses, psychiatric social workers, etc.)
- general medical practitioners
- social services providers (e.g. school-based counselling, vocational rehabilitation)
- informal volunteers (e.g. self-help groups).

Approximately 15% of adults and 21% of children and adolescents in the USA use these services each year (Surgeon General, 2001). Most care is provided in out-patient settings (public or private clinics or offices). Acute hospital care is usually provided in psychiatric units of general hospitals rather than in free-standing psychiatric hospitals.

Patients frequently seek care exclusively from primary care physicians and clinicians. For example, more than 50% of patients with depression see only primary care physicians or clinicians (Kessler *et al*, 2003).

The roles of consumer self-help, consumer-operated, consumer advocacy, family support and peer support services are expanding. There are also increasing efforts to coordinate not only medical and mental health services, but also other services for those recovering from mental illness, such as education, housing and employment. However, these are generally fragmented and dispersed among a number of organisations, both private and government-based.

# A history of deinstitutionalisation

In 1955 there was one psychiatric bed for every 300 Americans; today there is one for every 3000 (Torrey *et al*, 2010). Beginning in the mid-20th century, large psychiatric hospitals began to close so that care could be provided to patients in less isolated, more inclusive community mental health services – a process referred to as deinstitutionalisation. Although this was successful for some people, community resources have not been available or have been inadequate for many others. People with mental disorders have all too often ended up homeless or as inmates in the criminal justice system.

# New laws providing greater access and coverage

Recently enacted laws are expected to go a long way to improve access to care for those with mental illness. The 2010 Patient Protection and Affordable Care Act will have far-reaching effects on patients, as well as on psychiatrists and other physicians. It will provide comprehensive health insurance coverage, including for the treatment of mental illness and substance misuse, to an estimated 30 million Americans who are currently uninsured.

The Paul Wellstone and Pete Domenici Mental Health Parity and Addiction Equity Act of 2008 specifically expands federal requirements for mental health coverage. Private insurers who cover mental health must provide coverage at least equivalent to that for other medical illnesses. Furthermore, co-payments for mental health services cannot exceed those for general health services, and insurers may not impose special limitations on the number of mental healthcare visits.

# Workforce and resources

There are more than 40000 psychiatrists in the USA. Approximately 137 psychiatry residency programmes accredited by the Accreditation Council of Graduate Medical Education (ACGME) train some 6000 residents each year. There are nearly 9000 advanced practice psychiatric nurses who provide mental health services, including prescribing (under varying state regulations), and more than 90000 psychologists who provide services, generally not including prescribing.

Clinicians providing mental health services do not reflect the ethnic diversity of the US population. Members of the major ethnic/racial minorities in the USA make up about 33% of the population, but only about 25% of physicians, 19% of psychiatrists, 10% of psychologists and 15% of social workers. There is even greater disparity among specific racial/ethnic groups. For example, African Americans make up approximately 13% of the population, but only 3% of psychiatrists and 2% of psychologists, and Latinos make up about 14% of the population but only 5% of psychiatrists and 3% of psychologists (Sribney et al, 2010).

More resources are available in some parts of the country than in others. There are over 3500 'health professional shortage areas' for mental health in the USA, affecting more than 84 million people, 65% of them in non-metropolitan areas. Although the total number of psychiatrists per 100000 population has been relatively stable over the past 20 years, the average age of psychiatrists (half are over 55) has raised concerns that there will soon be too few to meet future demands (Skully & Wilk, 2003).

Key factors in the future are likely to include the changing scope of practice and roles of non-psychiatrists; growth and ageing of the population; mainstreaming of psychotropic drugs; increasing insurance coverage; and changing utilisation patterns in subpopulations (e.g. Latinos) (Vernon et al, 2009).

## Financing mental healthcare

In terms of healthcare expenditure, mental disorders are among the five most costly types of health conditions in the USA (along with cancer, heart disease, asthma and trauma-related disorders) (Agency for Healthcare Research and Quality, 2009). Mental healthcare in the USA is paid for from a combination of public and private sources, including public funding (Medicaid, 18%; Medicare, 22%), private insurance (28%) and out-of-pocket individual/self-pay (25%) (Agency for Healthcare Research and Quality, 2006).

Other sources of federal funding include the Veterans Administration and Department of Defense (through service delivery), the Substance Abuse and Mental Health Services Administration (through block and discretionary grants), and the Health Resources and Service Administration (via federal community health centres).

States have traditionally served as the safety net for people unable to access mental health services and have carried much of the responsibility for low-income individuals with serious mental illness. The recent economic downturn has forced many states to scale back this funding.

## Critical issues

Several critical issues currently affect mental healthcare and will continue to do so in the near future. Access to care is limited by problems in rural areas (travel distance for patients, a scarcity of providers) and also by stigma and too few culturally competent and linguistically diverse providers. Another challenge is the lack of coordination of care – of public and private services, of various specialty services, of general medical and mental health services, and of social services and other institutions (housing, criminal justice, education). Also at issue is growing public concern over the influence of pharmaceutical companies on how physicians practise. The transition to the use of electronic health records is another major adjustment.

Although psychiatry remains an important and fulfilling career in the USA, there will be many challenges for patients and mental healthcare workers for many years to come. However, there will also be many new opportunities to provide better mental health services for all those who need them.

## References

Agency for Healthcare Research and Quality (2006) *Medical Expenditure Panel Survey (Table 4: Total Expenses and Percent Distribution for Selected Conditions by Source of Payment: United States, 2006)*. AHRQ.

Agency for Healthcare Research and Quality (2009) *The Five Most Costly Conditions, 1996 and 2006: Estimates for the U.S. Civilian Noninstitutionalized Population. Statistical Brief No. 248*. AHRQ. Available at http://www.meps.ahrq.gov/mepsweb/data_files/publications/st248/stat248.pdf (accessed July 2010).

Kessler, R. C., Berglund, P., Demler, O., et al (2003) The epidemiology of major depressive disorder: results from the National Comorbidity Survey Replication (NCS-R). *JAMA*, **289**, 3095–3105.

Kessler, R. C., Demler, O., Frank, R. G., et al (2005) Prevalence and treatment of mental disorders, 1990 to 2003. *New England Journal of Medicine*, **352**, 2515–2523.

National Institute of Mental Health (2010) *The Numbers Count: Mental Disorders in America.* NIMH. Available at http://www.nimh.nih.gov/health/publications/the-numbers-count-mental-disorders-in-america.shtml (accessed July 2010).

Skowyra, K. R. & Cocozza, J. J. (2006) *Blueprint for Change: A Comprehensive Model for the Identification and Treatment of Youth with Mental Health Needs in Contact with the Juvenile Justice System.* National Center for Mental Health and Juvenile Justice, Policy Research Associates, Inc. Available at http://www.ncmhjj.com/Blueprint/pdfs/Blueprint.pdf (accessed July 2010).

Skully, J. H. & Wilk, J. E. (2003) Selected characteristics and data of psychiatrists in the United States, 2001–2002. *Academic Psychiatry*, **27**, 247–251.

Sribney, W., Elliott, K., Aguilar-Gaxiola, S., et al (2010) The role of nonmedical human services and alternative medicine. In *Disparities in Psychiatric Care* (eds P. Ruiz & A. Primm), pp. 274–289. Lippincott, Williams & Wilkins.

Steadman, H. J., Osher, F. C., Robbins, P. C., et al (2009) Prevalence of serious mental illness among jail inmates. *Psychiatric Services*, **60**, 761–765.

Substance Abuse and Mental Health Services Administration (2009) *National Survey on Drug Use and Health, 2008.* SAMHSA. Available at http://www.oas.samhsa.gov/NSDUHlatest.htm (accessed July 2010).

Surgeon General (2001) *Mental Health: Culture, Race, and Ethnicity.* US Department of Health and Human Services. Available at http://www.surgeongeneral.gov/library/mentalhealth/cre/ (accessed July 2010).

Torrey, E. F., Kennard, A. D., Eslinger, D., et al (2010) *More Mentally Ill Persons Are in Jails and Prisons Than Hospitals: A Survey of the States.* Treatment Advocacy Center (TAC) and National Sheriffs Association (NSA). Available at http://www.treatmentadvocacycenter.org/storage/tac/documents/final_jails_v_hospitals_study.pdf (accessed July 2010).

Vernon, D. J., Salsberg, E., Erikson, C., et al (2009) Planning the future mental health workforce: with progress on coverage, what role will psychiatrists play? *Academic Psychiatry*, **33**, 187–192.

World Health Organization (2009) *World Health Statistics 2009.* WHO. Available at http://www.who.int/whosis/whostat/2009/en/index.html (accessed July 2010).

# South America

# Brazil

## Marcos Pacheco de Toledo Ferraz and Elisaldo A. Carlini

Brazil is a country with 170 000 000 inhabitants (census for the year 2000), of whom 138 000 000 live in urban areas. The illiteracy rate, that is, people over 15 years of age who cannot write or read even a simple message, is 13.4%. About 25.6% of the population live on a family income less than half the minimum wage (1999 figures). Brazil's gross internal revenue is R$564 800 per capita (1998 figures, about US$1680 today).

The Brazilian population experiences the diseases typically found in underdeveloped countries as well as the pathologies of developed countries. With the exception of obstetrics, most of the morbidities found in hospitals are diseases of the respiratory tract (16.2%) and those of the circulatory system (9.5%), followed by infectious and parasitical diseases (7.4%). Mental and behavioural disorders account for 3.5% of hospital cases (Table 1).

## Psychiatric services and reform

Even though the proportion of psychiatric admissions to hospitals is 3.3% (Table 1), when we analyse the average expenditure on hospital admissions by the Unified Health System (SUS) by specialty, that is, the amount of expenditure divided by the total number of admissions, the amount spent on psychiatry is about four times higher than that on general practice, and

Table 1  Proportion of hospital admissions by specialty, 2000

| Specialty | Proportion of hospital admissions |
|---|---|
| General practice | 34.3% |
| Surgery | 23.0% |
| Obstetrics | 24.1% |
| Paediatrics | 3.3% |
| Psychiatry | 3.3% |
| Psychiatry (day hospital) | 0.2% |

Source: Ministry of Health – System of Information on Hospitals of the SUS (SIH-SUS).

twice as high as that on surgery. The costs of treatment for mental and behavioural disorders, such as schizophrenia, delirious and schizotypal disorders, are far higher than the costs for other disorders (Table 2).

The high costs of schizophrenia are well demonstrated by Leitão (2001), who, by studying patients with the illness in the state of São Paulo, showed that 2.3% permanently resided in hospital and 3.7% had been in hospital for less than 1 year.

The Conference for the Restructuring of Psychiatric Attention, held by the Pan-American Health Organization in November 1990, passed the Declaration of Caracas, which emphasised a policy of hospital bed reductions and highlighted the frequent violations of human rights that took place at psychiatric hospitals in Latin America. This position had already been adopted by the Brazilian Association of Psychiatry (see below).

There are some 10 000 psychiatrists working in Brazil. According to Zago *et al* (2001), the number of specialists is sufficient (5.75/100 000 inhabitants), but they are largely concentrated in the south and south-east of the country.

Until the mid-1980s, public mental health policies strongly favoured admissions to psychiatric hospitals. This approach has since begun to change, slowly but systematically. As a result, there has been a reduction in both the number of hospital beds in psychiatry and the number of admissions. There were 410 003 admissions to psychiatric hospitals in 1997. Data from the Ministry of Health show that this had decreased by 12.8% in 2001, in spite of the population growth during the same period. Admissions to day hospitals doubled, from 10 268 to 22 183.

In April 2001, the Brazilian President passed the Law of Psychiatric Reform after 11 years of discussions in the Congress and wider debates. Law No. 10.216 of 6 April 2001 is explicit with regard to the rights of

**Table 2**   Costs of treatment for mental and behavioural disorders in 2001

| Diagnosis | ICD–10 code | $R |
| --- | --- | --- |
| Dementia | F00–F03 | 16 879 254 |
| Mental and behavioural disorders due to the use of alcohol | F10 | 60 145 522 |
| Mental and behavioural disorders due to the use of psychoactive substances | F11–F19 | 9 061 261 |
| Schizophrenia, delirious and schizotypal disorders | F20–F29 | 264 195 266 |
| Mood (affective) disorders | F30–F39 | 31 783 555 |
| Neurotic and somatoform stress-related disorders | F40–F48 | 1 878 384 |
| Mental retardation | F70–F79 | 47 668 801 |
| Other mental disorders | | 56 932 658 |
| Total | | 488 544 702 |

Source: Ministry of Health – System of Information on Hospitals of the SUS (SIH-SUS).

people with mental disorders, in the area of both psychiatric admission and mental health community services. It clearly defines the issue of self-commitment, that is, admission with the consent of the user, as well as involuntary commitment, which takes place without consent. After extensive discussions, this law determined that the term 'user' should replace the term 'patient'. Involuntary psychiatric admission, which must be reported to the Public Ministry by the direction of the hospital, was subject to much controversy but was eventually adopted.

## Education in psychiatry

Brazil has at present 95 medical colleges from which about 9300 doctors graduate each year. According to Zago *et al* (2001), only 16 of them conduct scientific research.

Scientific research in Brazil began in a modern form after the creation of postgraduate education in 1969. In the area of mental health, there has been a very important increase in the number of indexed Brazilian journals since 1990, while the situation in other areas, such as haematology, rheumatology and oncology, has remained the same. Postgraduate programmes have undergone considerable improvement recently. Nowadays two centres, the University of São Paulo and the Federal University of São Paulo, gain the best ratings in the external evaluation carried out by the Ministry of Education. Other centres – such as the Federal University of Rio Grande do Sul, the Federal University of Rio de Janeiro and the Federal University of São Paulo (Ribeirão Preto campus) – also showed good results in this evaluation.

## Residence in psychiatry

The National Council of Medical Residence (CNRM) was created in September 1977 by means of Decree 80.281. It defines medical residence as a modality of postgraduate education in the form of specialist courses characterised by in-service training aimed at doctors. The programmes comprise two years in psychiatry, with an optional third year. Presently there are 462 residence places in psychiatry in Brazil, most (43.7%) of them in the state of São Paulo.

## Professional bodies

The Brazilian Association of Psychiatry (ABP), founded in 1966, has about 3000 associated psychiatrists. It holds congresses (originally biennial and now annual). The last, the XX Brazilian Congress, was attended by 3100 medical professionals, most of whom were psychiatrists.

In June 1993 the ABP was one of the organisers of the 9th World Congress of Psychiatry, held in Rio de Janeiro, which had approximately 7000 participants. The ABP has published the *Revista Brasileira de Psiquiatria*

(*Brazilian Psychiatry Journal*) since 1979; at first it was called *Revista ABP–APAL*, when it was jointly produced by the ABP and the Latin-American Psychiatry Association (APAL). The ABP's newsletter, *Psiquiatria Hoje* (*Psychiatry Today*), was founded in 1976. Both the journal and the newsletter are distributed to all members.

The Association maintains ongoing educational programmes via the internet at www.pecabp.ecurso.com.br

The Institute of Psychiatry at the Federal University of Rio de Janeiro also publishes a journal of good scientific quality and national circulation, the *Jornal Brasileiro de Psiquiatria* (*Brazilian Journal of Psychiatry*).

# References

Leitão, R. J. C. (2001) *Utilização de Recursos e Custos Diretos da Esquizofrenia para o Setor Público do Estado de São Paulo*. Tese de Mestrado em Epidemiologia da Universidade Federal de São Paulo.

Zago, A. M., *et al* (2001) *Ciência no Brasil*. Texto preparado para a Academia Brasileira de Ciências.

# Chile

Alfredo Pemjean

Chile has approximately 600 psychiatrists for its 15 million people. Although in the capital city, Santiago, the provision (per capita) is twice as high as in the rest of the territory, it is possible to see over the past decade a progressive increase in the number of these specialists in the other main cities. There are no more than 50 child psychiatrists and several cities have no local resource in this subspecialty.

## Training

Ten schools of medicine offer medical undergraduate education. The 7-year curriculum includes courses on medical psychology, psychopathology and general psychiatry.

Physicians may become specialists in psychiatry through a 3-year postgraduate programme of studies, provided by seven universities. All these residence programmes have similar coverage of neurology, in-patient wards and out-patient facilities and community mental health, as well as some adult and child psychiatry, the amount of which depends on the final specialty. Examinations vary across the residence programme: sometimes there are full examinations but, more frequently, there is formal approval after each one of the 6- or 12-month rotations.

Another way to obtain a specialty certificate is by undertaking formal clinical work, in a psychiatric clinical facility, that lasts at least 5 years; accreditation requires attendance at postgraduate courses and passing a formal examination, one week long, in a university centre.

Finally, a national independent organisation, CONACEM, is the authority for specialist certification of physicians; the certificate is necessary for professional work and insurance purposes.

## Professional bodies and research

Three main societies provide for scientific exchange among Chilean psychiatrists:

- The Society of Neurology, Psychiatry and Neurosurgery of Chile, founded in 1932, has a membership of 200 psychiatrists, in eight thematic working groups. It holds regular seminars, courses and a congress, and publishes two periodicals, the quarterly *Revista Chilena de Neuropsiquiatría*, and *Folia Psiquiátrica*, which appears three times a year
- The Chilean Society of Mental Health, founded in 1983, is a multiprofessional body; it has almost 300 members, more than 100 of whom are psychiatrists. Besides regular congresses and courses, it publishes one periodical, *Revista Psiquiatría y Salud Mental*.
- The Chilean Society of Psychiatry and Neurology of Childhood and Adolescence, which was founded in 1970.
- Research by psychiatrists is largely into the epidemiology of mental disorders, quality of life associated with mental disorders and handicaps, evaluation of programmes and facilities, and, in the clinical arena, depression, suicide, personality disorders, post-traumatic stress disorder, drug and alcohol problems and adolescent mental health problems.

## Mental health services

The public health sector, which provides medical services to 70% of the population, employed 168 general psychiatrists and 39 child psychiatrists in 2001. The numbers have been steadily increasing over the past 12 years.

The 28 territory general health services comprise a widely distributed primary healthcare network. This includes dispensaries and small, undifferentiated general hospitals, second-level specialty out-patient care, and large general hospitals with medical specialty wards, including psychiatry, in the main cities.

A new National Mental Health Plan issued in 2000 resumed developments made in the previous 10 years, and marked the beginning of a new period which will see a transition from the traditional model of centralised care meeting the spontaneous demand of the population, to a network of facilities and programmes in which multiprofessional teams develop appropriate responses to mental health problems and preventive practice.

Some examples are given below:

- A national programme for the treatment of depression through primary healthcare, with the necessary second-level support, met the goal of treating 18 000 women in 2001 and 24 000 in 2002. For 2003, the goal is to offer protocol-guided treatment to 66 000 women and men all over the country. One public health aim for 2010 is to reduce the prevalence of depression by 10% from the 7.5% rate measured in the 1990s.
- A national case register of patients with schizophrenia is supporting the prescription of clozapine and risperidone (in addition to the usual neuroleptics), through protocol-based distribution, to more than 3000

affected persons (83% of the estimated number of patients being treated within the public sector).

- Thirty-one day hospitals were opened in the year 2001, all over the country. This is a new type of psychiatric facility in Chile. Its goals are to diminish in-patient bed needs and the duration of hospitalisation; they provide more cost-effective care, nearer to patients' families. After a few months of operation, early evaluation has been promising.
- A growing number of treatment centres for drug and alcohol problems have been established since 2001. There are six treatment protocols in place: detoxification, dual pathology, ambulatory (first response, basic and intensive) and residential.
- A special form of consultation–liaison psychiatry service has been developed, called mental health consultation. Teams comprising at least one psychiatrist and one psychologist visit a particular primary care facility, once or twice a month, for a technical and planning meeting with the local team. The review of clinical problems of patients in the charge of both primary- and secondary-level teams is at the core of the visit.
- Some major changes are also occurring within the in-patient wards, such as the differentiation of short- and medium-term hospitalisation, with a maximum of 60 and 189 days respectively. This has introduced a new dynamism in in-patient care.
- Finally, a gradual reduction in hospitalisation for chronic patients, together with the development of supervised community residence facilities, is in progress. Initial results have been good. Half-way and more permanent homes for chronic patients, many of whom drop out of care from the existing four psychiatric hospitals, now have 700 residential places.

## Conclusion

Chilean psychiatrists are coping with changes in the mental healthcare model. The process of reform in the health sector represents an opportunity and new challenges.

# Ecuador

## Marcelo E. Cruz, Rachel Jenkins, Clare Townsend and Donald Silberberg

We assessed the mental and neurological health (MNH) situation of Ecuador in 2006–8, using the Mental and Neurological Health Country Profile (MNHCP) (Gulbinat *et al*, 2004; Jenkins, 2004; Jenkins *et al*, 2004), an instrument which helps to develop evidence-based MNH policy and services (Townsend *et al*, 2004). An extensive review of the literature was undertaken and consultations and consensus meetings (Schilder *et al*, 2004) were conducted with key mental and neurological health stakeholders, including consumers, carers and clinicians from the government and non-government sectors.

## Context

Ecuador, in the north-west of South America, has an area of 256 370 km² and a population of around 13 400 000. The population distribution has become younger in recent decades, with 61.9% aged 15–64 years. Nearly two-thirds (63.4%) of the population live in urban areas. The national fertility rate is 22.9 births per 1000. Life expectancy is 78 years for women and 72 years for men. The major ethnic groups are Mestizo (65%), Native Indigenous (25%), White (7%) and Black (3%). Official languages are Spanish and Quechua. Most of the population (95%) is Roman Catholic.

Other significant data are presented in Table 1.

Internal and external migration is significant. Over one million Ecuadorians emigrated to the USA and Europe following economic problems in 2000. The Colombian guerilla movement has forced the displacement of half a million Colombians into Ecuador and rural migration continues to increase the size of the slum areas in major cities.

Positive mental health and well-being is understood as emotional health; mental disorder and mental illness as loss of reason; neurological illness is described in terms of the associated disability; and personality disorder is understood as antisocial or delinquent behaviour. Discrimination against people with mental or neurological illnesses exists owing to cultural influences and ignorance. Mental and neurological disorders are considered physical and cultural ailments, and approximately 30% of the population (particularly those in the rural sector) regard mental and neurological conditions as punishments of nature.

Women primarily bear the burden of caring for people with mental and neurological disorders. There are significant levels of stigma and discrimination shown to people with MNH problems and to other vulnerable groups, including those who experience physical or intellectual disability, poverty, disease, the young and the aged. There is no recognition of the rights of people with disabilities, resulting in government failure to address the physical and MNH needs of these groups, until a start was made by the 2006 Organic Health Law.

Violence against women, associated with male jealousy and macho attitudes, is common. Alcohol misuse is high and commonly associated with unemployment, lack of close family, marital problems and debt. Drug misuse among children and young people is rising. This is frequently associated with parental migration, as it often causes young people to come under the care of grandparents. Homicide rates have tripled in the last 19 years, going from 6.5 per 100 000 people in 1985 to 19 per 100 000 in 2004. Drug- and alcohol-related criminal violence resulted in 2315 deaths in 2004.

**Table 1** Select national data, 2006

| **Measures** | |
|---|---|
| Gross national product | US$44 billion |
| National debt | US$11 billion |
| Economic aid | US$22 billion |
| Proportion of budget spent on health | 6% |
| Proportion of budget spent on mental health | 0.00006% |
| Annual income per capita | US$3216 |
| Proportion of population living below poverty line | 30% |
| Proportion of homeless people | 31% |
| Proportion of population with access to safe drinking water | 15% |
| Proportion of population with access to adequate sanitation | 43% |
| Unemployment rate | 8.8% |
| Inflation rate | 3.1% |
| Child immunisation coverage | 93% |
| Prison population | 14 400 male, 1600 female |

Source: Inec, *Indicadores Basicos de Salud* (2006).

# Social policy, health policy, legislation and human rights

Ecuador experienced social spending restrictions, economic reforms and economic restructuring in the 1980s, followed by the introduction of welfare legislation in 1992 and compulsory education in 2000. However, school non-attendance remains high. Alcohol is available only to those above 18 years of age; public tobacco advertising is restricted; and tobacco and alcohol are taxed. There is regulation of drink-driving and firearms.

Free maternity services are provided and there are childhood immunisation programmes. There are, however, no programmes aimed at: reducing substance misuse, tobacco or alcohol consumption; detecting and preventing high blood pressure; or promoting life skills in schools.

There is no national MNH policy in Ecuador. The Ministry of Public Health is the main body responsible for the regulation of MNH care. The 2006 Organic Health Law legislates for human rights in the field of MNH, and regulates the way in which involuntary admission is decided by family members, physicians, police officers and the justice system. The law guarantees patients access to their case-notes, but there is no tradition of enforcing constitutional rights.

## Estimates of need

Small-scale neuroepidemiological surveys were carried out in Ecuador in the 1980s, using a World Health Organization protocol (Cruz *et al*, 1985). Epilepsy prevalence figures (10–17/1000) are generally higher than those found in industrialised countries. Migraine headache has been found to affect 68 people per 1000 (Cruz *et al*, 1995). The prevalence of established cerebrovascular disease was 3.5 per 1000 and of peripheral neuropathies 15 per 1000. There are no community-level epidemiological data on mental disorders.

## Financial and human resources

The main obstacle to the purchasing and delivery of specialist care in Ecuador is lack of financial resources. Central government spending accounts for only a small proportion of national expenditure for mental and neurological illnesses. In 2008, 6% of the national budget (US$700 million) was allocated to general health. Of this, US$3 200 000 was allocated to MNH. MNH services are also financed through social security insurance, private insurance, fee for service, community financing, charity and donor funds (loans and grants). The cost of medicines is high, public health services are limited and private sector services are expensive. The approximate financial burden experienced by a family when a member is mentally or neurologically ill is approximately US$500 per month.

Ecuador has 4658 primary care doctors, 338 psychiatrists (or 2.3 per 100 000), 333 neurologists, 22 community psychiatric nurses and 1 psychiatric social worker.

Medical students receive 36 hours of training in psychiatry and 36 hours in neurology, spread over the 18 weeks of the internal medicine module. Psychiatric postgraduate training has been in place for the past 25 years, sponsored by the Central University of Ecuador, in Quito. It is a 3-year course, with eight students per year. A similar programme has been established recently by the University of Cuenca. There are no training programmes in psychiatric nursing.

## Services

Initial treatment is generally in the form of home-made medicines, products from local pharmacies or friends' advice. There are 721 primary care centres (169 in the state sector, 12 in the non-government sector and 540 private facilities). Specialist care is also available.

There are 1635 psychiatric beds in state-funded general and teaching hospitals. No information is available on the non-governmental and private provision of psychiatric beds.

It is a legal provision that psychotropic substances are available only through prescription. In Ecuador the financial expenditure on antidepressants and anticonvulsants alone is about US$120 million per year.

The 2006 Organic Health Law integrates traditional medicine within the national health system. Traditional healers include 'cleansers' (who clean the body of bad spirits), midwives, healers, shamans and witches. Other alternative/complementary medicine includes homeopathy, acupuncture and bioenergetics.

There are no programmes for MNH promotion or plans for training workers in this field. There are no policies for reducing mortality from physical illnesses in people with a mental or neurological illness, or initiatives to address suicide reduction or epilepsy and stroke prevention. There are no programmes for addressing the needs of children, older people or disadvantaged minorities, and initiatives are limited in areas such as incest, child abuse, domestic violence, trauma and rape.

The prison population totals 16 000, of whom 80% fulfil ICD–10 criteria for mental disorders and 10% deserve specialist attention. Medical services and therapeutic communities exist within prisons. Prisoners have access to primary care and psychiatric and psychological evaluation and in an emergency may be referred to specialist psychiatric services. There are protocols within the prisons for prevention of violence and crisis intervention. Two psychiatrists and 60 psychologists work in the prisons.

## Discussion

Key problems for MNH in Ecuador include limited resources and services. The main challenge is to establish a national MNH policy with widespread ownership by the key stakeholders. MNH policy needs to address stigma and discrimination, health promotion and illness prevention, and improved supply of and access to clinical and non-clinical services. MNH needs to be integrated into primary care, with supervision and support from specialist services which are decentralised to all districts, more specialised multidisciplinary personnel, and better access to low-cost medicines. Funding strategies are needed to address resource generation, allocation and audit. Access to care is restricted owing to scarce financial resources, cultural and religious beliefs, a weak primary care system, long distances from the main hospitals, concentration of specialist services in the main cities, discrimination and a lack of inter-sectoral liaison at local and national levels, including within public policy. Of particular concern is the total lack of research in this area or plans for training separate cadres of specialist care staff.

## Conclusion

Ecuador has significant MNH needs, aggravated by rising levels of emigration, and high levels of alcohol misuse and violence. Mental health services are mainly delivered by specialists, concentrated in the cities. There is a pressing need for decentralisation of services, for systematic support to primary care, and for inter-sectoral liaison in order to enhance access to mental health promotion, prevention and treatment.

## References

Cruz, M. E., Schoenberg, B. S., Ruales, J., *et al* (1985) Pilot study to detect neurologic disease among a population with high prevalence of endemic goiter. *Neuroepidemiology,* 4, 108–116.

Cruz, M. E., Cruz, I., Preux, P-M., *et al* (1995) Headache and neurocysticercosis in Ecuador, South America. *Headache,* 35, 93–97.

Gulbinat, W., Manderscheid, R., Baingana, F., *et al* (2004) The International Consortium on Mental Health Policy and Services: objectives, design and project implementation. *International Review of Psychiatry,* 16, 5–17.

Jenkins, R. (ed.) (2004) International project on mental health policy and services. *Phase 1: Instruments and country profiles. International Review of Psychiatry,* 16(1–2).

Jenkins, R., Gulbinat, W., Manderscheid, R., *et al* (2004) The Mental Health Country Profile: background, design and use of a systematic method of appraisal. The International Consortium on Mental Health Policy and Services: objectives, design and project implementation. *International Review of Psychiatry,* 16, 31–47.

Schilder, K., Tomov, T., Mladenova, M., *et al* (2004) The appropriate and use of focus group methodology across international mental health communities. The International Consortium on Mental Health Policy and Services: objectives, design and project implementation. *International Review of Psychiatry,* 16, 24–30.

Townsend, C., Whiteford, H., Baingana, F., *et al* (2004) The Mental Health Policy Template: domains and elements for mental health policy formulation. The International Consortium on Mental Health Policy and Services: objectives, design and project implementation. *International Review of Psychiatry,* 16, 18–23.

# Peru

Marta B. Rondon

---

Peru is a land of mixed cultures, multiple ethnic heritages and severe economic inequities. Its history goes back thousands of years, from accounts of the first inhabitants of the continent to the impressive Inca Empire, the rich Viceroyalty of Peru and the modern republic, which boasts one of the highest economic growth rates in South America. Yet, in spite of such complex cultural development, or perhaps because of it, 21st-century Peruvians have substantial difficulties establishing a national identity and recognising each other as members of the same community.

Persons with mental illness represent with poignant clarity 'the other' which we seem to have so much trouble accepting as equals in terms of dignity and rights. When we look at mental health in terms of legislation, services and human rights, therefore, we are faced with exclusion and discrimination, unequal and inefficient use of resources, and lack of public interest.

## Mental health as a component of public health

Peruvian psychiatrists have traditionally had a biopsychosocial approach to mental health and illness. Social psychiatry studies, under the leadership of Rotondo and Mariategui in the 1950s and early '60s, were fundamental in the conceptualisation of mental health as a cultural construct (Perales, 1989). Another interesting development is that of psychosomatic medicine, under the leadership of Seguin, which originated in the establishment of a psychiatric ward in a general hospital, long before the Declaration of Caracas so suggested, and which also is the precursor of the current interest in women's mental health and in the consequences of violence in the country.

As far back as the 1960s, pioneers such as Baltazar Caravedo and Javier Mariátegui saw mental illness as a major obstacle to the development of the country, and they pointed to the need to devote public effort and money to the promotion of mental health and the prevention and treatment of mental illness. Others have followed this path, especially after the results of a large epidemiological study by the National Institute of Mental Health were made public (Rondon, 2006).

## Mental health and disorders

Anxiety, depression and schizophrenia are considered to be the most relevant psychiatric disorders in Peru. The use of alcohol, the prevalence of interpersonal violence and the high tolerance of psychopathic attitudes have also been identified as important (Instituto Especializado de Salud Mental, 2002).

Perhaps more striking than the prevalence of disorders is the large number of people (14.5–41.0% of those surveyed), mostly women, who report feelings of unhappiness, preoccupation and pessimism (Instituto Especializado de Salud Mental, 2004).

Interpersonal violence, in all its modalities, plays a significant role in the production of psychiatric morbidity. Gender-based violence is widely tolerated, with roots in the complex culture of the country (Rondon, 2003). According to a World Health Organization multi-country study on violence against women, adult women in the Andean region of Cusco are the most physically abused females in the world, with those in Lima faring just slightly better (García-Moreno *et al*, 2005).

In the 1980s, the country suffered much political violence, largely targeted against the civilian population. This led eventually to the establishment of the Truth and Reconciliation Commission at the turn of the century. It has recognised that exposure to political violence during the internal armed conflict in the 1980s has inflicted severe psychological damage to the population involved, and has left sequelae of 'fear, as an everyday experience, both at the individual and the collective levels, the disintegration of familial and communal bonds, loss of the ability to protect and nurture children, a negative impact on social cohesion, and damage to the personal identity'. The plight of the victims is, therefore, a major mental health concern (Peruvain Truth and Reconciliation Commission, 2003).

## Policy and legislation

After a long story of failure to implement mental health plans and due to the intervention of the Pan American Health Organization (PAHO) and reiterated demands of non-governmental organisations and relatives of users of services, the Guidelines for Action in Mental Health were promulgated by the Ministry of Health in 2004. The guidelines adhere to certain principles: respect for the rights of 'persons' (not 'human rights', careful wording in keeping with restrictive abortion laws), equity, integrality, universality, solidarity, shared responsibility and dignity and autonomy. According to this document, the Peruvian policy on mental health includes:

- direction from the Ministry of Health's specialised office (the Direccion Ejecutiva, although it has no budget of its own for service delivery)

- integrated services for mental and physical health
- prevention and treatment integrated in a new efficient way of delivering services
- promotion of mental health, human development and citizenship
- multi-sectoral coordination for mental health
- creation of an information system
- human resources development
- planning, monitoring, evaluation and systematisation of all mental health actions
- participation of users and their relatives in mental health services.

Two years later, the National Committee of Health, a part of the National Health Council, produced and obtained approval for the *National Plan for Mental Health*, which set objectives and goals for the policy guidelines. The objectives of the plan were stated as positioning mental health as a fundamental right of all persons, strengthening the normative role of the Ministry of Health, ensuring universal access to mental health services via the re-engineering of existing services and promoting equity in mental healthcare, with special attention given to vulnerable populations. The plan set forth three general objectives, 12 specific objectives and 31 actions. It is not being implemented, however, because of constant changes within the Ministry of Health.

There is no mental health law and several issues such as involuntary hospitalisation and treatment and informed consent are not sufficiently covered by appropriate legislation, with consequent risks for both patients and providers.

# Service delivery

Mental health services are mostly provided in psychiatric hospitals: 75% of psychiatric beds are in the three large psychiatric hospitals in Lima, with other beds in psychiatric centres in Piura, Arequipa and Iquitos. General hospitals belonging to the Ministry of Health in Lima have psychiatric out-patient services but do not have any beds, whereas general hospitals in five regions do have in-patient facilities, although there is concern over the quality of services provided. Several regions lack psychiatric services of any kind, and so patients have to travel long distances. Mental health episodes represent 1.15% of the annual total of all episodes of patient care.

In the social security sector (which is based on health insurance for people in formal employment and their dependants only) all national referral hospitals and several national hospitals have beds, and there are psychiatric out-patient services in all tertiary establishments.

There is no mental healthcare at the primary level. The Ministry of Health has organised itinerant teams to attend to the needs of those affected by political violence with the purpose of supporting people in the affected communities; this includes promotion, prevention, attention and rehabilitation in mental health, as well as education in mental health with members of the community, especially primary health workers (Kendall *et al*, 2006).

The provision of psychiatric medications is very unequal: atypical antipsychotics and novel antidepressants are available in Lima and other large cities for insured patients, but outside the big urban centres not even the substances listed in the World Health Organization's list of essential medications can be obtained.

## Staffing and training

There are 602 psychiatrists registered with the Peruvian College of Physicians, eight of whom are child and adolescent psychiatrists. Seventy per cent of them live in Lima. Psychologists and specialised nurses are also located mostly in Lima, as are the few psychiatric social workers.

Of the 31 medical schools in Peru, five offer specialisation in psychiatry: three in Lima, one in Arequipa and one in Trujillo. Nonetheless, all undergraduate medical students receive a course on psychological medicine (centred on the doctor–patient relationship) and one course in clinical psychiatry.

Specialisation in psychiatry takes 3 years. Junior doctors have a chance to spend some time abroad to complete their training. The curriculum does not follow the World Psychiatric Association's core curriculum. The only recognised subspecialty is child and adolescent psychiatry, training for which lasts 2 years.

## Research

Between 2005 and 2008, there was a project funded by the Japanese International Cooperation Agency that involved physicians, other health personnel in secondary and primary care and members of the community in five Andean regions in the integral care of people affected by political violence.

After 2000 there was a strong impulse for epidemiological research in psychiatry and the Lima Metropolitana, Sierra, Selva and Fronteras studies were completed. There is some ongoing work using the data from these important studies, such as the cross-country comparison of gender-sensitive mental health indicators. There is also some interest in participating in multicentre drug studies, and some psychiatrists participate as patient recruiters in fourth-stage studies.

## Human rights issues

The unavailability and inaccessibility of mental healthcare is the most important human rights issue. For those who do receive services, the poor quality of care, the high cost of medication, the generally miserable condition of the hospitals and the lack of attention to safety conditions are prominent concerns. Mental Disability Rights International published in 2004 a very critical report on the conditions of mental hospitals, after which both the ombudsman and the Ministry of Health, with the participation of the Peruvian Psychiatric Association, looked into providers' awareness of human rights and the conditions of the service (Ministry of Health, 2005). The Peruvian Psychiatric Association provided workshops on human rights for psychiatrists and other mental health providers and drafted the Declaration of Cusco, which calls for special concern for patients' rights. However, only the establishment of a national health system and universal health insurance with clear, state-of-the-art and consensual practice guidelines will improve current conditions.

# References

García-Moreno, C., James, H. A. F. M., Ellsber, M., *et al* (2005) *Multi-country Study on Women's Health and Domestic Violence: Initial Results on Prevalences, Health Outcomes and Women's Responses*. WHO.

Instituto Especializado de Salud Mental (2002) Estudio epidemiologico metropolitano de salud mental. *Informe general. Anales de Salud Mental*, **18**, 1–2.

Instituto Especializado de Salud Mental (2004) Estudio epidemiológico en salud mental en ayacucho 2003. *Anales de Salud Mental*, **20**, 1–2.

Kendall, R., Matos, L. & Cabra, M. (2006) Salud mental en el Peru luego de la violencia politica: intervenciones itinerantes. *Anales de la Facultad de Medicina*, **67**, 184–190.

Ministry of Health (2005) *Comisión Especial para la supervisión del cumplimiento de los derechos humanos de las personas con enfermedad mental. Informe Final*. Ministry of Health.

Perales, A. (1989) Concepto de salud mental: la experiencia peruana. *Anales de Salud Mental*, **5**, 103–110.

Peruvian Truth and Reconciliation Commission (2003) *Final Report, Vol.* 6. Available at http://www.cverdad.org.pe (last accessed November 2008).

Rondon, M. B. (2003) From Marianism to terrorism: the many faces of violence against women in Latin America. *Archives of Women's Mental Health*, **6**, 157–163.

Rondon M. B. (2006) Salud mental: un problema de salud pública en el Perú. *Revista Peruana de Medicina Experimental y Salud Publica*, **23**, 237–238.

# Trinidad and Tobago

Hari D. Maharajh and Akleema Ali

The Republic of Trinidad and Tobago is the most southerly of the Caribbean island states. Trinidad is just 14 km from the coast of Venezuela. Trinidad covers an area of 4828 km² while Tobago, the sister isle, has an area of 300 km². The total population is approximately 1.3 million; 40.3% of the population is of East Indian descent, 39.6% of African descent, 18.4% mixed and 1.7% belong to other ethnic groups (Central Statistical Office, 2001). St Ann's Hospital in Port of Spain, the capital, was established in 1900 and is the country's only psychiatric hospital. There are two general hospitals, one in the north, at Port of Spain, and the other in the south, at San Fernando.

The per capita gross domestic product (GDP) is US$8948 and total health expenditure represents 5.2% of GDP. Life expectancy at birth is 67.3 years for males and 72.6 years for females; a healthy life expectancy at birth is projected at 58.9 years for males and 62.0 years for females. Adult mortality is 235 per 1000 population for males and 150 per 1000 population for females; the male child mortality rate per 1000 population is 24 and the female rate is 18 per 1000 population (World Health Organization, 2004). The literacy rate for males is 95.3% and that for females is 91.5% (World Health Organization, 2002).

## Early mental health policies (1848–1975)

Under British rule, the early treatment policies of the mentally ill in Trinidad paralleled the treatment of the insane in Britain. In 1848, an ordinance was passed to detain the criminally insane at the Royal Gaol. The Belmont Lunatic Asylum was established in 1858. The facility later transferred to the St Ann's Asylum, now renamed the St Ann's Hospital. For the following five decades, policies of treatment were custodial, with the use of malaria therapy for syphilis, insulin coma therapy, bromide mixtures, veronal and sulphonal, transorbital leucotomy, electroconvulsive therapy and immersion therapy in cold water.

The advent of chlorpromazine and the open-door policy of the 1950s heralded a period of aggressive treatment outside the hospital, with an emphasis on decentralisation and deinstitutionalisation as models of care. In that decade, two plans were also submitted: the Julien report of 1957 and the Lewis plan of 1959. In the latter, commissioned by the Ministry of Health, a recommendation was adopted for the creation of psychiatric units at the two general hospitals. In 1962, the Chan report recommended the subdivision of St Ann's Hospital into four autonomous units. However, this proposition received little attention.

# The Sectorisation Plan (1975)

The Sectorisation Plan, adopted from the French model, was introduced in Trinidad and Tobago in 1975. The goals of this programme related to both community and institutional care. Its objectives were:
- to provide psychiatric care as near as possible to the patient's own home
- to upgrade the facilities of St Ann's Hospital, to reduce its size and to rehabilitate and return to the community the majority of its patients
- to introduce additional subspecialist services (e.g. child guidance and geriatric services)
- to develop a system of consultation with the community, to ascertain their needs and their views
- to consult with community leaders of all sorts in the development of health attitudes and education programmes, aimed at prevention
- to integrate mental healthcare with general and public healthcare as far as possible
- to devise an effective system to evaluate this programme
- to provide in-patient psychiatric services for patients (a proportion of beds in each sector would be general hospital beds)
- to set up out-patient services, wherever possible at district health offices
- to establish day and night hospitals
- to develop geriatric services
- to establish rehabilitation services – halfway houses, sheltered workshops, industrial therapy units
- to organise preventive services (e.g. early identification and work with special risk groups).

The plan divided the country into five sectors, each serving a population of approximately 200 000. Multidisciplinary teams were assigned to each sector and the regional hospitals were used for admissions. It was reported that a wave of excitement and enthusiasm engulfed all those involved, as it was felt to be the dawn of a new era in psychiatry in Trinidad and Tobago (James, 1984).

In June 1975, St Ann's Hospital was divided into four autonomous units and, together with the psychiatric unit at Port of Spain General Hospital, admitted patients from the five well-defined geographical areas (sectors). Patients from the city of Port of Spain and from Tobago were admitted to the General Hospital unit. The psychiatric unit at the San Fernando General Hospital formed an extension of one of the St Ann's Hospital units. Out-patient clinics were set up in each sector. This was supported by Mental Health Act No. 30 of 1975, which empowered mental health officers to treat patients. There are at present 75 out-patient clinics held monthly.

Towards the end of 1976, the initial enthusiasm of the Sectorisation Plan waned, as it became evident that the major objective of the programme, which was the decongestion of St Ann's Hospital and the treatment of patients in the community, was not being achieved. Adequate clinic facilities were lacking and no provision was made for hostels, halfway houses or sheltered workshops (James, 1984). Since 1975, there have been no major changes in community mental health in the Republic.

## The regional health authorities

The Regional Health Authorities (RHA) Act No. 5 of 1994 led to the establishment of five health regions. This new policy proposed the realignment of the sectors to the RHA boundaries and a shift towards primary care. The RHA Act legislated for the decentralisation of all health services and the five regions were empowered to develop their own psychiatric services. This generated some concern, since the only mental hospital in the country was situated in the North West Region and there was some ambiguity surrounding the allocation of human resources and infrastructure.

In 2000, the RHA Act was amended. The five regions were reduced to four, the Central Region being incorporated into the North West Regional Health Authority (NWRHA). The system is still in transition, as there are now two parallel administrative bodies, the Ministry of Health and the RHAs. In 2000, the psychiatric unit at the Port of Spain General Hospital was closed by the NWRHA and in 2003 the Ministry of Health aligned part of the Central Region to the South West Region.

## A new mental health plan (2000)

Against the background of persisting problems with the mental health programme, the Trinidad and Tobago National Mental Health Policy and Plan was formulated by the Ministry of Health and the Pan American Health Organization (PAHO) in 1995 and approved by Cabinet in 2000. The two main goals of this programme were to encourage the development of the highest level of mental health and to promote an adequate level of individualised care for those who have a mental disorder (Ministry of Health, 2000). The objectives of this new plan closely followed those of the Sectorisation Plan of 1975 and are as follows:

- to educate the population regarding mental health and to promote healthy lifestyles
- to reverse negative perceptions about mental disorders
- to reduce the incidence of certain kinds of illnesses and disabilities

- to reduce mortality associated with certain kinds of mental disorder
- to provide adequate primary, secondary and tertiary care for persons with mental health problems, although with an emphasis on primary care
- to integrate mental health with general health services as far as possible
- to develop linkages with other governmental, non-governmental and consumer organisations
- to undertake evaluation, research and training for improvement of the mental health services.

The delivery of the mental health services will now be the responsibility of the RHAs, while the Ministry of Health will be involved in the formulation and evaluation of policies. The RHAs have also established a National Mental Health Commission (NMHC) and a Regional Mental Health Committee (RMHC) in every sector for the implementation of the National Mental Health Policy and Plan. These coordinating committees are expected to formulate and implement specific plans of action in mental health. The most important function of the NMHC includes the evaluation of the effectiveness and quality of services.

The following changes in the present system are proposed:

- St Ann's Hospital is to see a phased reduction in bed numbers, from 1026 to 600
- the Eric Williams Medical Complex will provide in-patient child psychiatry care
- four extended care centres will provide 30 beds – 10 for psychogeriatrics and 20 for rehabilitation
- San Fernando General Hospital will provide 30 beds for acute psychiatric care
- residential units of 125 beds will provide care for patients with low levels of dependency
- non-residential day care units and sheltered workshops will be established
- a 25-bed psychiatric unit will be reopened at the Port of Spain General Hospital.

Human resources are said to be the single most important component of the National Mental Health Policy and Plan. Multiprofessional teams will provide services at primary, secondary and tertiary levels. The Plan proposes to have, in each region, at least one health facility that provides child guidance services, psychology services and occupational therapy. In addition, drug dependency services are provided at Caura and St Ann's Hospital.

# Training

In 1987 a 4-year programme of the DM Psychiatry was introduced at the University of the West Indies. To date, approximately 20 psychiatrists have graduated. Continuing medical education (CME) is ongoing and there is a proposal to make it mandatory.

## Personnel

In 2001, there were 187 nursing aides and 1383 nursing assistants (Central Statistical Office, 2001). There are at present 7.92 psychiatric beds per 10000 population in the only mental hospital and 0.24 psychiatric beds per 10000 population in general hospitals. There are 22 trained psychiatrists, 6 psychiatrists in training and 23 psychiatric social workers.

## Conclusion

Psychiatry in Trinidad and Tobago remains a unique blend of current scientific knowledge purporting a neurobiological basis of diseases and traditional practices based on superstition, religion and folk medicine (Maharajh & Parasram, 1999). Over the years, changes have been minimal. Mental health planning for culturally diverse and secular communities are difficult to construct and even more difficult to implement. Policies must be tailored to suit the needs of the population, with solutions for people with mental disorders in developing countries (Jacob, 2001). The planning and delivery of services must have a clear focus and vision, supported by both efficient legal machinery and a willingness on the part of government to invest in a rolling programme of service improvement. Patients' rights and regard for the individual's autonomy are imperative. This is indeed a tall order for a developing country.

## References

Central Statistical Office (2001) *Statistics at a Glance*. Port of Spain: Central Statistical Office.

Jacob, K. S. (2001) Community care for people with mental disorders in developing countries. *Problems and possible solutions. British Journal of Psychiatry*, **178**, 296–298.

James, V. (1984) *A Review of Psychiatry in Trinidad and Tobago Over the Decade 1970–1980*. Port of Spain: St Ann's Hospital.

Maharajh, H. D. & Parasram, R. (1999) The practice of psychiatry in Trinidad and Tobago. *International Review of Psychiatry*, **11**, 173–183.

Ministry of Health (2000) *Mental Health Plan*. Port of Spain: Ministry of Health.

World Health Organization (2002) *Project Atlas: Country Profile – Trinidad and Tobago*. Geneva: WHO. Available at www.cvdinfobase.ca/mh-atlas/. Last accessed 29 April 2004.

World Health Organization (2004) *Countries – Trinidad and Tobago*. Geneva: WHO. See www.who.int/country/tto/en/. Last accessed 29 April 2004.

# Venezuela

## Edgard Belfort and Javier González

The Bolivarian Republic of Venezuela covers 916445 km²; to the north is the Caribbean Sea, to the south-east the Amazonian region and the plains of Brazil and Colombia, and to the west the Andes and the Colombian Guajira peninsula. Its estimated population (2004) is 25226 million, which is concentrated along the north coastal area, where the population density exceeds 200 inhabitants per km²; most of the territory remains almost uninhabited (fewer than 6 inhabitants per km²), in particular the border areas. The population is mainly urban: 70% live in cities with more than 50000 inhabitants.

The annual mean rate of population growth is 2%, approximately, but this is reducing in line with a progressive reduction in the birth rate (from 27.4 per 1000 inhabitants in 1994 to 22.3 per 1000 in 1998), fertility (3.17 children per 1000 women in 1994 to 2.93 in 1998) and an increase in emigration. The population is predominantly young: 54.4% are under 25 years of age, while the 25- to 64-year age group represents 41.3% of the population. Life expectancy is presently estimated at 72.8 years.

The budget assigned to health amounts to 3.9% of gross domestic product, or US$6402 per capita.

Constitutionally, Venezuela is a free and independent republic. It is also a federal state, consisting of 25 states and a capital district; Caracas is the capital city. According to the constitution, the states are autonomous and have political integrity. They are called on, however, to maintain the integrity of the nation and to obey and abide by national law.

## Health system

Civil rights and the state's duties to its citizens set out in the constitution provide the framework for the health system. The state must guarantee opportunities for education and development in an environment of freedom, and must preserve the dignity of its inhabitants, for example. The constitution requires that a technical committee organises the administration of healthcare in Venezuela. This committee has the following duties:

- to study and recommend programmes for the control of important epidemiological diseases
- to study and develop strategies aimed at eradicating some recurrent (high-prevalence) diseases of social importance
- to suggest action programmes to be developed in the National Commission for the Zoonoses
- to evaluate, from the epidemiological and malarial point of view, the status of the border states in order to suggest action programmes, considering in particular the health status of indigenous ethnic groups
- to coordinate the organisation of symposia in environmental hygiene, together with government, municipal authorities, schools and universities, and other civil bodies
- to promote community health
- to take on any other function defined by the Ministry of Health and Social Development (in Spanish MSDS) or its representatives.

There is, however, a need to democratise the health structure, to widen social participation, in order to consolidate the role of the MSDS.

# Mental health policies and programmes

There is a mental health policy, which covers promotion, prevention, treatment and rehabilitation. This policy, based on the 1990 Caracas Declaration, seeks to integrate psychiatric care within primary care; this involves the decentralisation of services through the provision of day-care hospitals, health centres, prevention programmes and community participation.

There is a national programme of mental health, contained in the Nation's Ninth Plan (which is a 5-year plan for economic and social development, from which the priorities of the executive power are derived). The public health sector in Venezuela accounts for 214 hospitals (181 general and 33 specialised hospitals) and a network of 4605 ambulatory clinics for medical care (in 890 urban and 3715 rural centres).

Psychiatric services are provided in both the public and the private sectors. The public system looks after a large portion of the population, but access to psychiatric care is restricted in rural areas. There are few specific services for children and elderly people, even in urban areas.

Psychiatric care tends to be centred on psychiatric hospitals. Patients are referred from general hospitals or other institutions. From the 1960s, 11 rural sanatoriums, which house around 1800 chronic mental patients, were established. The main objective of this project was to create a psychiatric community but unfortunately this was never accomplished. Currently these institutes serve the private sector.

There is an overall lack of practical psychiatric care, reflected in an under-provision of institutional structures and poor access to the health system.

# Mental health legislation

Venezuela does not rely on a specific law to regulate all aspects of mental health from a holistic perspective. Issues related to mental health are usually addressed in health codes or general health laws, which set out universal principles. Commissions and technical committees govern the administration of some services and regulate the organisations devoted to mental healthcare.

Resolution number 1223 (15 October 1992), however, does emphasise the responsibility of the MSDS to provide comprehensive medical care for people with a mental illness, oriented towards the patient's full recovery and his/her reintegration in society. The resolution also refers to the principles contained in the Caracas Declaration and asks general hospitals appointed by the MSDS to study and adopt procedures related to the admission of acute psychiatric patients; more specifically, it seeks to guarantee that at least 10% of beds are available for those with a mental disorder.

There was also a decree in 1992 to regulate the sanatoriums. It refers to the humanitarian treatment of patients, in particular their individual freedom and security; it also relates to the admission of patients, technical and professional assistance, specialised medical care, health records and the assumption of responsibilities in the event of injury to patients.

# Mental health financing

There are budget allocations for mental health. The primary sources of mental health financing, in descending order, are: tax revenue, social insurance, out-of-pocket expenditure by the patient and family, and private health insurance.

# Mental health training and facilities

Disability benefits for persons with mental disorders require a certificate provided by the Venezuelan Institute of Social Security.

Treatment for severe and acute mental disorders is available at primary level in some regions of the country, for example the states of Merida, Tachira and Zulia.

Regular training of primary-care professionals is not carried out in the field of mental health. However, there are eight regular training programmes (for a university degree) in general psychiatry and one training programme in child and adolescent psychiatry. These account for 2.82% of the total resources invested in postgraduate health education programmes.

The establishment and maintenance of mental health services are governed by the MSDS. The resources it provides are set out in Tables 1 and 2.

**Table 1** Central and regional mental health resources

| | Caracas metropolitan area | 22 states |
|---|---|---|
| Psychiatric hospitals | 2 | 4 |
| Ambulatory clinics | 7 | 30 |
| Day-care hospitals | 1 | 1 |
| Psychiatric units in general hospitals | 3 | 31 |
| Ambulatory clinics for children and adolescents | 1 | 1 |
| Psychiatric units for children and adolescents | 2 | 1 |

**Table 2** Numbers of psychiatric beds and professionals

| | Number per 10 000 population |
|---|---|
| Psychiatric beds | 1.15 |
| Psychiatric beds in mental hospitals | 0.29 |
| Psychiatric beds in general hospitals | 0.15 |
| Psychiatric beds in other settings | 0.76 |
| Psychiatrists | 0.4 |

# Scientific societies

The most important of the several psychiatric societies is the Venezuelan Society of Psychiatry, which has approximately 900 members. It is affiliated to the Latin American Psychiatric Association and the World Psychiatric Association. It organises scientific activities, workshops, symposia, meetings, and a national congress every 3 years.

# Mental health research

The areas of mental health being investigated, in descending order of amount of research activity, are as follows:
- affective disorders (including post-partum depression)
- schizophrenia and other psychotic disorders
- childhood mental and behavioural disorders
- anxiety disorders
- drug misuse and dependence
- suicide
- dementia
- learning disabilities
- stress disorders (including post-traumatic stress disorder)
- mental comorbidity of AIDS

- neuropsychiatric disorders
- eating disorders
- epilepsy.

## Violence and mental health

Venezuela has an internationally high rate of homicide (principally involving young men). Statistics from the Institute of Legal Medicine show a present average of about 100 violent deaths every week. The number of injuries is much higher. Between 1990 and 1999, the annual homicide rate increased in Venezuela from 13 to 25 per 100000 inhabitants. In Caracas, this rate increased from 44 to 81 homicides for every 100000 inhabitants in the same period. Most of these violent events take place during the weekends in the area called 'Great Caracas' and other urban areas in the country. This represents an enormous drain on health resources, and has a serious psychological impact, notably anxiety disorders and post-traumatic stress disorders. Such psychological effects have not been properly quantified. Violent events have important physical and psychological consequences for both the victim and others, and this represents a considerable burden for the health and rehabilitation services.

The overall mortality rate is 4.6 per 1000 inhabitants. Accidents are the third most common cause of death, whereas suicides and homicides rank seventh. These two categories account for the highest number of years of life potential lost (in Spanish AVPP), mostly among males. The useful years of life lost as a consequence of accidents and violent events are higher or equal to those caused by cancer or cardiovascular diseases, because they mainly affect the infant, juvenile and young adult population.

## Non-governmental organisations

Some non-governmental organisations run ambulatory clinics and there are associations that care for vulnerable groups. These organisations provide their own resources or obtain direct help from the government to carry out their projects, which often involve prevention, treatment and rehabilitation in the area of mental health.

## Information systems

Currently there is a lack of an information system or epidemiological study in mental health. The mental health system narrows its scope by reporting exclusively on mental disorders.

## Programmes for particular populations

The country has specific programmes for the mental health of children and for people affected by natural disasters. There is a National Institute of Child Psychiatry (Instituto Nacional de Psiquiatría del Niño) and also a 2-year programme for university-level child and adolescent psychiatry (see above). This is the only specialised programme in the field of mental health in Venezuela.

In Venezuela in 1999 there were massive land slides in Vargas state. A plan for psychological care and rehabilitation was created to care for any victims of future similar tragedies.

# Conclusion

Venezuela has long had adequate health plans and programmes, which have provided immediate responses, sometimes improvised ones, in the area of mental health. The problem has been in their implementation, since priorities have not been properly ascertained, experiences are not taken into account and on-going training and research are not promoted. Venezuela therefore needs to strengthen the implementation of health plans and policies, to meet needs in the area of health, to protect patients' rights, to preserve mental and physical integrity and, consequently, to guarantee the population a good quality of life.

# Further reading

Desjarlais, R., Eisenberg, L., Good, B., *et al* (eds) *(1996) World Mental Health: Problems and Priorities in Low-Income Countries.* New York: Oxford University Press.

Levav, I., Restrepo, H. & Guerra de Macedo, C. (1994) The restructuring of psychiatric care in Latin America: a new policy for mental health services. *Journal of Public Health and Policy,* **15**, 71.

San Juan, A. (2003) *Political Violence in Venezuela. Some Preliminary Approaches.* Caracas: Centro de Estudios para la Paz, Fundación Centro Gumilla.

World Health Organization (2001) *Atlas. Mental Health Resources in the World 2001.* Mental Health Determinants and Populations. Geneva: WHO Department of Mental Health and Substance Dependence.

# Index

Compiled by Linda English

**487**

**491**